Communicable Disease Control Handbook

Gary Porter-Jones,

JACKIE IRWIN
(via Sian ap Devi)

About the authors

Dr Jeremy Hawker is Regional Epidemiologist for the West Midlands region of England with the PHLS Communicable Disease Surveillance Centre. He is also Honorary Senior Lecturer and Head of the Academic Communicable Disease Epidemiology and Control Unit at the University of Birmingham. He was previously Consultant in Communicable Disease Control at Birmingham, UK.

Dr Norman Begg is the former Head of the Immunization Division of the Public Health Laboratory Service and has served as Deputy Director of the Communicable Disease Surveillance Centre. He is co-editor of 'Immunization against Infectious Disease', the book that describes immunization policy in the UK, and is former chair of the WHO European Advisory Group on Immunization. He is now Head of Medical Affairs at GlaxoSmithKline.

Dr Iain Blair is Consultant in Communicable Disease Control (CCDC) for Sandwell Health Authority (UK). He has also served as CCDC in two other districts and as a Regional Infectious Disease Epidemiologist. He is Honorary Senior Lecturer at the University of Birmingham, UK. He originally trained as a General Practitioner and has worked in Canada and the Middle East.

Dr Ralf Reintjes heads the Department of Hygiene, Infectious Disease Epidemiology, and Vaccinations in the Institute of Public Health in North Rhine-Westphalia, Germany. He is visiting Lecturer at the Universities of Bielefeld, Nijmegen, and Tampere. Previously he was a Fellow of the 'European Programme of Intervention Epidemiology Training (EPIET)' at the National Institute of Public Health and the Environment in the Netherlands and worked on several projects in various European countries.

Professor Julius Weinberg is Pro-Vice Chancellor (Research) at City University, London and is currently developing the National Electronic Library for Communicable Disease. He was previously Consultant Epidemiologist at the Communicable Disease Surveillance Centre and Head of Epidemiological Programmes at the Public Health Laboratory Service. He is accredited both in Clinical Infectious Disease and Public Health and previously worked in Zimbabwe and for WHO in the former Yugoslavia.

Contents

Section 4: Services and organizations

Section 5: Communicable disease control in Europe

Appendices: Resources for the CCDC

Foreword

When in 1983 I took up the post of Chief Medical Officer for England, if past experience was to be a reliable guide to the future, it seemed a reasonable bet that my main preoccupation would be with the increasing burden of cancer, coronary heart disease and stroke rather than with infections. But events turned out otherwise. A series of high-profile outbreaks due to well understood microbial agents, and another – AIDS – the epidemiology of which was at that time little understood, and which therefore cast a particularly sinister shadow, ensured that communicable disease was always in the front of my mind.

It should be recalled that this was the era when, at local level, communicable disease control had been much weakened by the abolition of the post of Medical Officer of Health in the 1974 reorganization of health services. Public health as a medical specialty had all but disappeared and specialists trained in communicable disease were few and far between. It was therefore crucial, if as Chief Medical Officer I was to do my job, that I should seek a partnership with the Communicable Disease Surveillance Centre (CDSC) at Colindale and its Director.

It therefore was Dr Spence Galbraith and his colleagues and successors who steered me through some spectacular outbreaks, most of which included fatalities. To quote a few examples, these included salmonellosis due to a popular brand of baby food, and a major outbreak of a similar illness from a different source at the Stanley Royd mental hospital in Wakefield; legionellosis due to an aerosol from the cooling tank of a new hospital in Stafford; listeriosis due to paté imported from Belgium, and botulism associated with yoghurt containing hazelnuts.

And in those early days what slender resources were available to CDSC! The Director with two consultant colleagues and a handful of helpers worked in a small prefabricated building situated in the car park of the Central Laboratory for Public Health. However, in part due to the intense media interest in the outbreaks, it was not difficult for me to persuade ministers to steer funds in that direction. Today I am glad to know CDSC employs 35 consultants and some 250 staff, and in addition to the fine office at Colindale there are 10 regional epidemiology offices in England, Wales and Northern Ireland. I am equally pleased to have seen the creation and development of greatly improved local provision of communicable disease control services, led by district Consultants in Communicable Disease Control. The pivotal role of such local services in the prevention, surveillance and control of communicable disease is the constant theme throughout this book.

The crucial influence on public health of Norman Fowler, the Cabinet Minister accountable for health in England from 1983–87 should be acknowledged. It was he who, following the critical findings of the public inquiries into the Stanley Royd and Stafford outbreaks, commissioned me to review the arrangements for communicable disease control in England[1]. He directed that the Inquiry should not simply consist of a catalogue of defects and shortcomings. It should in addition, in a constructive and if necessary radical way, address *'the future development of the public health function'*. It was this emphasis on 'development' when the political catchwords of the day were 'value for money', and 'efficiency and effectiveness', and 'general management' that set public health on the upward path to renaissance. It set the scene for the creation of the new specialty dedicated to the control of communicable diseases mentioned above.

While the *Communicable Disease Control Handbook* is not an official publication of the CDSC, it seems to me to incorporate all that is best in the tradition of that organization – sound science, attention to detail and an essentially practical approach. This will foster rapid corrective action when, as often occurs, an urgent response to a case or cluster is needed in the face of incomplete information. To pick out but a few points, I like particularly the list of thirteen universal precautions to prevent spread of infection, with its emphasis on handwashing properly carried out as the most important of all; how to respond to such everyday topics as rash and fever in children and illness in returning travellers; and what is the appropriate immediate action if one is asked to advise outside office hours, 'on-call', about such varied conditions as campylobacter, chickenpox, giardiasis or gonorrhoea, and a host of others.

This outstanding and I suspect unique handbook is packed with useful information. I believe it will prove to be an essential resource for those, not only within the United Kingdom but throughout Europe, who have responsibility for the identification and control of infectious disease. It will also be an indispensable text for students aspiring to a career in this important field.

Sir Donald Acheson KBE, DM, FRCP, FFPHM, FFOM.

---

1 *Public Health in England. The Report of the Committee of Inquiry into the Future Development of the Public Health Function.* London. HMSO Cm.289. Jan 1988.

Abbreviations

AIDS   Acquired immune deficiency syndrome

BCG   Bacille Calmette-Guérin (vaccine against TB)

CCDC   Consultant in Communicable Disease Control (local public health doctor with executive responsibilities for CDC)

CDC   Communicable Disease Control

CDR   Communicable Disease Report

CDSC   PHLS Communicable Disease Surveillance Centre

CICN   Community Infection Control Nurse

CJD   Creutzfeldt-Jakob disease

CNS   Central nervous system

CSF   Cerebrospinal fluid

DNA   Deoxyribonucleic acid

DTP   Diphtheria, tetanus and pertussis (whole-cell)

EHO   Environmental Health Officer

ELISA   Enzyme-linked immunosorbent assay

EM   Electron microscopy

EU   European Union

GP   General Practitioner (primary care physician)

GUM   Genitourinary medicine

HA   Health Authority

HAI   Hospital acquired infection

HBV   Hepatitis B virus

HCV   Hepatitis C virus

HCW   Healthcare worker

Hib   *Haemophilus influenzae* type b

HIV   Human immunodeficiency virus

HNIG   Human normal immunoglobulin

HUS   Haemolytic uraemic syndrome

ICD   Infection control doctor

ICN   Infection control nurse

ICT   Infection control team

IDU   Intravenous drug user

IFA   Indirect immunofluorescent antibody test

IgG   Immunoglobulin class G

IgM   Immunoglobulin class M

IPV   Inactivated poliovirus vaccine

LA   Local authority

MMR   Measles, mumps and rubella

MRSA   Methicillin resistant *Staphylococcus aureus*

OPV   Oral poliovirus vaccine

Pa   Pertussis vaccine (acellular)

PCR   Polymerase chain reaction

PHLS   Public Health Laboratory Service

RCGP   Royal College of General Practitioners

RNA   Ribonucleic acid

RSV   Respiratory syncytial virus

SCIEH   Scottish Centre for Infection and Environmental Health

sp   Species

SRSV   Small round structured virus

STI   Sexually transmitted infection

TB   Tuberculosis

UK   United Kingdom of Great Britain and Northern Ireland

VHF   Viral haemorrhagic fever

VRE   Vancomycin resistant *Enterococcus*

VTEC   Verocytotoxin producing *Escherichia coli*

VZIG   Varicella zoster immunoglobulin

WHO   World Health Organization (OMS)

Section 1
Introduction

1.1 How to use this book

This book has been written with the needs of those working in the field of communicable disease control in mind. It aims to provide an easy reference book providing practical advice for specific situations and also to provide a short textbook of the important background knowledge that underlies communicable disease control (CDC) activities. As such it should be of interest to public health physicians, epidemiologists, public health nurses, infection control nurses, Environmental Health Officers, microbiologists and those training to work in these and related fields.

Chapter 1.2 runs through the basic principles of transmission and control which underlie later chapters.

Section 2 addresses topics in the way they often present to CDC staff in the field, i.e. as syndrome-related topics rather than organism-based. Examples of problems that fit this classification are an outbreak of gastroenteritis of an (as yet) undetermined cause, or a needlestick injury. In these chapters, we discuss the differential diagnosis (infectious and non-infectious), including how to decide the most likely cause based on relative incidence, clinical and epidemiological differences and laboratory tests. We also give general advice on prevention and control, including how to respond to a case or cluster when the organism responsible is not yet known. When the organism becomes known, Section 3 should be consulted.

Section 3 is the more traditional approach to this type of book, although we have attempted to identify for each organism the elements that are most relevant to the developed countries of north and west Europe. We have used England and Wales (or the UK if appropriate) as an example in each instance, although where important differences in the epidemiology exist in other western European countries

we have drawn attention to this. For differences relating to surveillance and control in other countries, the relevant country-specific chapter in Section 5 should be consulted (e.g. those working in Germany should consult Chapter 5.7). British readers will mainly be spared this exercise.

The chapters in Section 3 conform to a standard pattern, which we hope will make instant reference easier. Most chapters are ordered as follows.

1 A short introduction mentioning the syndrome(s), common synonyms and the main public health implications of the organism.

2 A box of *suggested on-call action*. This relates only to what needs to be done if cases are reported outside of normal office hours. Further action may be needed during the next working day, which will be identified in 'response to a case'.

3 *Epidemiology* will give the relevant points on burden of disease and any important differences by age/sex/season/year/risk group in the UK. Any important international differences are noted.

4 Two sections deal with diagnosis of the infection: *clinical features* and *laboratory confirmation*. Both sections highlight the important points to practising CDC professionals. They are not meant as a substitute for clinical and microbiological textbooks.

5 *Transmission* details the main sources, reservoirs, vehicles and routes of spread of the organism. The main aim of this section is to give the investigator clues as to how a case or outbreak may have arisen, so as to aid identification and control.

6 *Pathogenesis* deals with the incubation period, infectious period (if communicable), infective dose (if known) and any important factors affecting immunity or susceptibility.

7 The final five sections relate to control of infection. These are mainly based on current practice in the UK (supplemented by our own views), although the principles will be equally relevant to other European readers.

These sections are:

• actions likely to be effective in the *prevention* of infection;

- *surveillance* activities relevant to the organism;
- suggested public health actions to be taken in *response to a case*;
- suggested approach to an *investigation of a cluster* of cases of that organism, and suggested actions to help *control of an outbreak*, including a *suggested case-definition* for use in an analytical study, where appropriate.

Diseases that occur rarely in Europe are summarized in the **tables** that follow Section 3.

Section 4 refers to the organization of CDC services and could be titled 'how to run a CDC service'. For the three authors who have worked as Consultants in CDC, this is the textbook that we wished we'd had on appointment! It deals with the services that a CDC department is expected to provide, including the non-communicable disease functions that have been attached to the CCDC/CPHM post in the UK. Some of those chapters are, of necessity, UK focused, although many (e.g. surveillance, outbreaks, hospital infection, clinical governance) will be of equal use to other European colleagues.

Section 5 gives a brief overview of structures for infectious disease notification and Public Health action in the 15 EU Member States, Norway and Switzerland. The objective of this section is to provide an orientation on public health structures relevant for infectious disease control in various European countries and to offer a starting point for further information on individual countries. Lengthy descriptions have been avoided, but Internet addresses for contact points in the countries and for further information, reports and data are given. Those readers interested in more detailed or extended information on infectious disease control structures in Europe could consult the report and dataset of the 'EU-Inventory on Communicable Disease Control' which was compiled by the Italian, English and Swedish national surveillance centres and financed by the European Commission.

Finally the three **appendices** detail further sources of information and advice for those undertaking communicable disease control functions routinely or on-call.

We are indebted to a number of individuals who have helped us in commenting on parts of the book, including Pat Saunders, Gervase Hamilton, Kathy Nye, Sarah O'Brien, John Watson, Carol Joseph, Jenny Millward, Jammi Rao, Mary Ramsay, Angus Nicoll, Liz Miller, Natasha Crowcroft, Douglas Harding, Sue Skidmore and numerous advisors for the country-specific chapters, including A. Bosman, J.J.H.M. Oostendorp, J. Tselendis, P. Ruutu, M. Sousa, G. Hernández Pezzi, F. Van Loock, S. Wallyn, R. Strauss, H. Götz, K. Ekdahl, B. Iversen, D. Coulombier, A. Tozzi, S. Samuelson, P. Huberty-Krau, D. Stürchler, A. Raeber, B. Smyth and M. Fitzgerald. Linda Parr's administrative skills were essential as was the help of Marcela Holmes, Audrey Cadogan and Elizabeth Callaghan at Blackwell Science. Finally, we are grateful to our families and work colleagues for their patience and support whilst we were preoccupied with this project.

1.2 Basic concepts in the epidemiology and control of infectious disease

The epidemiological framework

Identification

Infections can be identified by their clinical features and the use of appropriate laboratory procedures.

Infectious agent

A variety of models of disease causation have been proposed. The traditional model of infectious disease causation is the epidemiological triangle. It has three components: an external agent, a susceptible host and environmental factors that bring the host and the agent together.

The agent is the organism (virus, rickettsia, bacterium, fungus, protozoon or helminth) that produces the infection. Generally, these agents must be present for the disease to occur.

Host factors are characteristics or attributes that influence an individual's exposure, susceptibility or response to a causative agent. Age, sex, socio-economic status, ethnicity and lifestyle factors such as smoking, sexual behaviour and diet are among the host factors that affect a person's likelihood of exposure. Age, genetic makeup, nutritional and immunological status, other disease states and psychological makeup are among the host factors that affect a person's susceptibility and response to an agent.

Environmental factors are extrinsic factors that affect the agent and the opportunity for exposure. These include geology, climate, physical surroundings, biological factors, socio-economic factors such as crowding and sanitation and the availability of health services.

Occurrence

The pattern of occurrence of infectious disease varies with place and time. The same diseases in different communities show different patterns of occurrence.

A persistent level of occurrence with low to moderate levels of disease is referred to as *endemic*. A persistently high level of occurrence is called *hyper-endemic*.

An irregular pattern of occurrence with occasional cases occurring at irregular intervals is called *sporadic*.

Occasionally the level of disease rises above the expected level. When the occurrence of a disease within an area is clearly in excess of the expected level for a given time period, it is called *epidemic*. The degree and duration of the excess will vary with the disease, the place and the season. The terms outbreak or cluster are also used. When an epidemic spreads over several countries or continents it is called *pandemic*.

Epidemics can be classified according to the pattern of their spread through a population. An *epidemic curve* should be plotted, which is a frequency histogram of number of cases against date of onset (see Figs 4.3.1, 4.3.2 and 4.3.3).

A *common source* outbreak is one in which a group of persons is exposed to a common source of infectious agent or toxin. If the exposure takes place over a relatively brief period, a *point source* outbreak occurs. If the exposure is intermittent or continuous, the range of exposures and range of incubation periods broadens the peaks of the epidemic curve, so that an irregular pattern is observed.

An outbreak that is spreading gradually from person to person is called a *propagated* outbreak. In theory the epidemic curve of a propagated outbreak would have a successive series of peaks, reflecting increasing numbers of cases at intervals approximating the incubation period. Usually the epidemic wanes after a few generations because the number of susceptible people falls below a critical level. Some epidemic curves have both common source epidemic and propagated epidemic features because of secondary person-to-person spread. These are called *mixed epidemics*. Two rates are commonly used to describe the occurrence of infectious diseases:

Incidence = New cases over a given time period/persons at risk

Prevalence = Existing cases at a given point in time/persons at risk

The chain of infection

Transmission occurs when the agent leaves its *reservoir* or host through *a portal of exit* and is conveyed by some mode of *transmission* and enters through an appropriate *portal of entry* to infect a susceptible host. This is the *chain of infection*.

Reservoir

The reservoir of an infectious agent is any person, animal, arthropod, plant, soil or substance (or combination of these) in which the infectious agent normally lives and multiplies. It is dependent on the reservoir for survival and it reproduces itself there in such a way that it can be transmitted to a susceptible host.

The reservoir may be different from the *source* or *vehicle* of infection. This is the person, animal, object or substance from which an infectious agent actually passes to a host. Many of the common infectious diseases have human reservoirs which include clinical cases, those who are incubating the disease and convalescent carriers. *Colonization* is the presence of a micro-organism in or on a host, with growth and multiplication, but without any overt clinical expression or detected immune reaction in the host at the time the micro-organism is isolated. Shedding of an organism from a colonized host may be intermittent.

Infectious diseases that are transmissible from animals to humans are called *zoonoses*.

The *portal of exit* is the path by which an agent leaves the source host, which usually corresponds with the site at which the agent is localized—for example, respiratory tract, genito-urinary system, gastrointestinal system, skin or blood.

The *portal of entry* is the route by which an agent enters a susceptible host. This provides access to tissues in which the agent can multiply or a toxin can act.

For any given infection, understanding the chain of infection allows appropriate control measures to be recommended.

Mode of transmission

This is the mechanism by which an infectious agent is spread from a source or reservoir to a susceptible person. The mechanisms are detailed in Table 1.2.1.

Natural history of disease

This refers to the progress of a disease process in an individual over time without intervention. It starts with exposure to an infectious agent or the accumulation of factors sufficient to begin the disease process in a susceptible host. Usually a period of subclinical or inapparent pathological changes follows exposure, ending with the onset of symptoms. For infectious diseases this period is usually called the *incubation period*. For a given infectious disease, the characteristic incubation period has a range. For example, for hepatitis A the range is about 2–6 weeks, with a mean of three weeks. Although disease is inapparent during the incubation period, some pathological changes may be detectable with laboratory or other screening methods. Most screening programmes attempt to identify the disease process during this early phase of its natural history, because early intervention may be more effective than treatment at a later stage. The onset of symptoms marks the transition from the subclinical to the clinical disease. Most diagnoses are made during this stage. In some people the disease may never progress to a clinically apparent illness. In others the disease process may result in a wide spectrum of clinical illness, ranging from mild to severe or fatal.

Infectious period

This is the time during which an infectious agent may be transferred directly or indirectly

Table 1.2.1 Modes of transmission of infectious agents

Types of transmission	Examples
Direct transmission This may be by direct contact such as touching, biting, kissing, sexual intercourse or by droplet spread on to the mucous membranes of the eye, nose or mouth during sneezing, coughing, spitting or talking. Droplet spread is usually limited to a distance of one metre or less	*Direct route* Infections of the skin, mouth and eye may be spread by direct contact simply by touching an infected area on another person's body or indirectly through a contaminated object such as a shared towel or hat. Examples are scabies, head lice, ringworm and impetigo. Sexually transmitted infections are also spread by the direct route

Continued

Table 1.2.1 *Continued*

Types of transmission	Examples
	Respiratory route Sneezing, coughing, singing or even just talking may spread respiratory droplets from an infected person to someone else close by. Examples are the common cold, influenza, whooping cough and meningococcal infection
	Faecal–oral route Gastrointestinal infections can also spread directly by the faecal–oral route when faeces are transferred to a susceptible host by direct contact
Indirect transmission This may be *vehicle*-borne involving inanimate materials or objects (*fomites*) such as toys, soiled clothes, bedding, cooking or eating utensils, surgical instruments or dressings; or water, food, milk or biological products such as blood. The agent may or may not multiply or develop in or on the vehicle before transmission	*Faecal–oral route* Faeces contaminate food or objects like toys or toilet flush handles. Animal vectors such as cockroaches, flies and other pests may transfer faeces. Environmental surfaces may be contaminated. This is particularly important in viral gastro-enteritis when vomiting occurs, since the vomit contains large numbers of infectious viral particles. Examples of infections spread in this way are food poisoning and hepatitis A
It may be *vector-borne*. This in turn may be *mechanical* and includes simple carriage by a crawling or flying insect as a result of soiling of its feet or proboscis or by passage of organisms through its gastro-intestinal tract. This does not require multiplication or development of the organism. It may be *biological* when some form of multiplication or development of the organism is required before the arthropod can transmit the infected form of the agent to man when biting	*The blood-borne route* There is transfer of blood or body fluids from an infected person to another person through a break in the skin such as a bite wound or open cut or through inoculation or injection. Blood-borne infections include infection with HIV, and hepatitis B and C infections. Spread can also occur during sexual intercourse
	Respiratory route Droplets from the mouth and nose may also contaminate hands, cups, toys or other items and spread infection to others who may use or touch those items
Airborne spread Airborne spread is the dissemination of a microbial aerosol to a suitable port of entry, usually the respiratory tract. Microbial aerosols are suspensions of particles that may remain suspended in the air for long periods of time. Particles in the range 1–5 microns are easily drawn into the alveoli and may be retained there. Droplets and other larger particles that tend to settle out of the air are not considered airborne. Microbial aerosols are either droplet nuclei or dust	Examples are infection with *Legionella*, *Coxiella* and in some circumstances TB

from an infected person to another person, from an infected animal to man or from an infected person to an animal or arthropod. In diseases such as diphtheria and streptococcal infection in which the mucous membranes are involved from the time of first exposure, the communicable period is from that time until the infecting agent is no longer shed from the involved mucous membranes. Some diseases are more communicable during the incubation period than during the actual illness. In other diseases such as tuberculosis, syphilis and *Salmonella* infection, the communicable period may be lengthy and intermittent. The communicable period may be shortened by antibiotic treatment.

Susceptibility and resistance

This describes the various biological mechanisms that present barriers to the invasion and multiplication of infectious agents and to damage by their toxic products. There may be inherent resistance in addition to immunity as a result of previous infection or immunization. The following terms are used to describe an infectious disease according to the various outcomes that may occur after exposure to its causative agent:

> • *Infectivity*: the proportion of exposed persons who become infected—also known as the attack rate.
> • *Pathogenicity*: the proportion of infected persons who develop clinical disease.
> • *Virulence*: the proportion of persons with clinical disease who become severely ill or die.

Hepatitis A in children has low pathogenicity and low virulence. Measles has high pathogenicity but low virulence, whereas rabies is both highly pathogenic and highly virulent. The *infectious dose* is the number of organisms that are necessary to produce infection in the host. The infectious dose varies with the route of transmission and host susceptibility factors.

Because of the clinical spectrum of disease, cases actually diagnosed by clinicians or in the laboratory often represent only the tip of the iceberg. Many additional cases may remain asymptomatic. People with subclinical disease may nevertheless be infectious and are called carriers.

Preventing spread of infection: universal precautions

It is not always possible to identify people who may spread infection to others, therefore precautions to prevent the spread of infection must be followed at all times. These routine procedures are usually called universal precautions (see below). All blood and body fluids are potentially infectious, and universal precautions are necessary to prevent exposure to them, including avoiding injury by sharp objects.

Universal precautions to prevent the spread of infection

1 Practice good basic hygiene with regular handwashing.
2 Cover wounds or skin lesions with waterproof dressings.
3 Avoid contamination of person and clothing with blood and body fluids.
4 Disposable gloves and aprons should be worn when attending to dressings, performing aseptic techniques or dealing with blood and body fluids.
5 Handle and dispose of sharps safely.
6 Avoid puncture wounds, cuts and abrasions in the presence of blood.
7 Avoid using sharps if possible.
8 Protect eyes, mouth and nose from blood splashes.
9 Know what to do if there is a sharps injury or blood splash incident.
10 Clear up blood spillages promptly and disinfect surfaces.
11 Dispose of contaminated waste safely.
12 Know how to deal with soiled linen.
13 Clean, disinfect and sterilize equipment as appropriate.

Handwashing

Handwashing is the single most important part of infection control.

An effective hand wash technique (see Fig. 1.2.1) using liquid soap and water is sufficient for routine handwashing and will remove 90–95% of micro-organisms acquired during normal patient contact. Each handwashing step consists of five strokes backwards and forwards. All parts of the hand should be washed. Particular attention should be paid to thumbs, fingertips, interdigital spaces and the centre of the palm. These are the parts that are most often missed. Jewellery should be removed before handwashing. Fingernails should be kept short and free from varnish.

Liquid soap is preferable to bar soap. Paper towels should be used to dry the hands thoroughly. Nailbrushes if used should be single-use. Alcohol hand-rub following handwashing will remove a further 4% of micro-organisms and has an effect on the normal skin flora. Alcohol hand-rub can be used for aseptic procedures or when caring for susceptible patients; it can also be used as an alternative to soap and water on clean hands. It is not recommended as the only method. If an alcohol hand-rub is used, hands should be washed periodically with soap and water. In treatment rooms where aseptic techniques are carried out there should be a separate hand basin with elbow- or wrist-operated taps. Hands should be washed:

1 when arriving at and leaving the workplace;
2 before and after direct contact with patients;
3 after contact with patient's blood or body secretions;
4 after removing protective clothing and gloves;
5 after using the toilet;
6 after handling soiled items;
7 before handling food;
8 before any clean or aseptic technique;
9 before and after eating;
10 before and after smoking.

Managing diarrhoea and vomiting: enteric precautions

• Affected persons should stay away from others until the diarrhoea has stopped.
• Affected persons should not prepare or handle food for other people until they have been symptom-free for 48 h.
• Care should be taken when changing nappies or clearing up after someone who has been sick or had diarrhoea. If cleaning up diarrhoea or vomit, the surface should be washed with detergent and water, disinfected, rinsed and allowed to dry. Paper towels or disposable cloths should be used for cleaning.
• If possible the patient should use the toilet as usual. If a commode or bedpan is used it should be carefully emptied in the toilet bowl after use, washed with disinfectant, rinsed and allowed to dry. Hands should be washed after attending to the patient.
• Toilet bowls, seats, flush handles, door handles and taps should be cleaned frequently with a suitable household cleaner and wiped with a disinfectant. Rubber household gloves should be worn.
• Baths should be rinsed thoroughly and disinfected after use. Set aside a towel for the personal use of affected people.
• Soiled clothing and bedding should be washed on a hot washing machine cycle. Articles that are heavily soiled can be soaked beforehand in a disinfectant or a sanitizer. Sluicing should be avoided but a prewash cycle may be used. Rubber household gloves should be worn. After loading clothing into the washing machine the outer surfaces should be wiped down with disinfectant. This is particularly important if the machine is in the kitchen.
• Different brands and types of disinfectants can be used. Bleach or disinfectant conforming to British Standard 5197 or 6424 is recommended. The disinfectant should be diluted according to the manufacturer's instructions. Keep disinfectants away from children. If using bleach remember that it can remove the colour from fabrics and carpets and can irritate the skin.

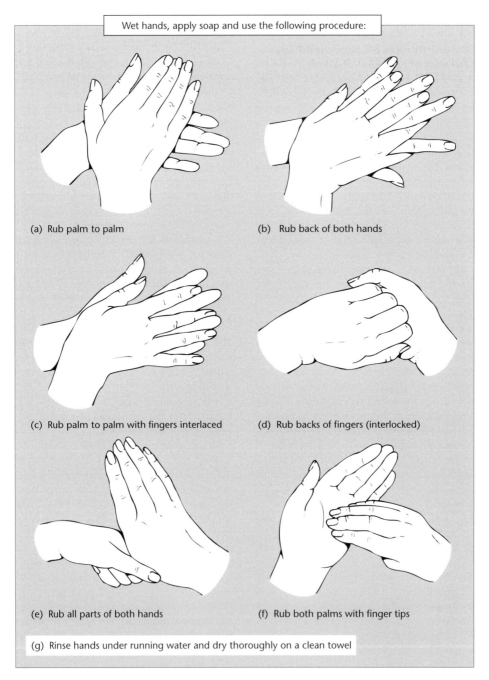

Wet hands, apply soap and use the following procedure:

(a) Rub palm to palm

(b) Rub back of both hands

(c) Rub palm to palm with fingers interlaced

(d) Rub backs of fingers (interlocked)

(e) Rub all parts of both hands

(f) Rub both palms with finger tips

(g) Rinse hands under running water and dry thoroughly on a clean towel

Figure 1.2.1 How to wash hands correctly and reduce infection. Reproduced with permission from J.C. Lawrence (1985) The bacteriology of burns. *Journal of Hospital Infection*, **6** (Suppl. B): 3–17.

• Children should stay away from school until they are well again and two full days have passed since the diarrhoea has stopped.

• People with certain jobs are more likely to spread infection. These are: people working in food businesses and catering jobs that involve handling food, and nurses and other carers, particularly those looking after infants or the elderly. Affected persons in these jobs should stay away from work for at least two full days after the diarrhoea has stopped.

Section 2
Common topics

2.1 Meningitis and meningism

Meningitis is inflammation of the meninges. Meningism is the group of signs and symptoms that accompanies the inflammation. The symptoms of meningism are headache, neck stiffness, nausea or vomiting and photophobia. The classical physical sign of meningism is a positive Kernig's test, however, this may be negative in mild cases. Typical features of meningism are uncommon in infants and young children, who are usually simply floppy and pale with fever and vomiting. A bulging fontanelle may be present in a young infant.

Meningitis is, a notifiable disease in many countries. This is, however, a rather unhelpful term for communicable disease control purposes, as the most important causal agent of meningitis, *Neisseria meningitidis*, can present as septicaemia without any features of meningitis. Meningococcal septicaemia presents with a typical haemorrhagic rash (see Plate 1, facing p. 22), which may be accompanied by shock, circulatory collapse, and confusion or coma. Many patients with meningococcal disease will have features of both meningitis and septicaemia (see Chapter 3.48).

Infectious and other causes

Meningitis is the most common cause of meningism, however, meningism can occur in the absence of meningitis (Table 2.1.1). It may accompany upper lobe pneumonia, urinary tract infection and other febrile conditions. Cerebrospinal fluid (CSF) examination is normal in these conditions. Meningism without fever can also occur in non-infectious conditions, the most important of which is subarachnoid haemorrhage; malignancy affecting the meninges can also present as meningism.

Clinical and epidemiological differences

Many infectious agents can cause meningitis.

Acute meningitis is nearly always either viral or bacterial; fungal and protozoal infections occasionally occur, mainly in the immunosuppressed patient.

In 1999, 2094 cases of acute meningitis (all causes) were notified in England and Wales (Table 2.1.2). The overall number of notified cases has remained relatively constant in recent years.

Viral meningitis

Viral meningitis is common. However, most cases are mild or inapparent. In 1999 there were 211 notified cases in England and Wales (Table 2.1.2). This represents only a small fraction (approximately 1%) of the true incidence, as only the more severe cases are investigated.

The most common cause is an enterovirus infection (either an echovirus or coxsackie virus) (Table 2.1.3). In enterovirus meningitis there is sometimes a history of a sore throat or diarrhoea for a few days before the onset of headache, fever and nausea or vomiting. The headache is severe, however, there is no alteration of neurological function. Meningism is usually present to a greater or lesser degree. Recovery is usually complete and rapid (within a week). The CSF is clear, with 40–250 cells, all lymphocytes, elevated protein and normal glucose. An enterovirus infection can be confirmed by detection of virus in a faecal sample or by serology. Enterovirus meningitis occurs mainly in later summer. It affects all age groups, although it is commonest in preschool children.

Mumps can cause meningitis, although it is now rare in countries where MMR vaccine is used. It is easily recognized by the accompanying parotitis. The diagnosis can be confirmed by detection of specific IgM in blood or saliva, or by serology.

In herpes simplex meningitis the illness is more severe and may persist for weeks. It is associated with primary genital herpes.

Non-paralytic poliomyelitis can present as meningitis, indistinguishable clinically from other causes of enteroviral meningitis. Poliovirus is detectable in faeces or CSF.

Table 2.1.1 Differential diagnosis of meningism

Cause	Distinguishing features
Viral meningitis	Fever, clear CSF with a lymphocytosis and raised protein
Bacterial meningitis	Fever, purulent CSF with a neutrophil pleiocytosis, raised protein and lowered glucose
Other febrile conditions	Fever. Normal CSF
Subarachnoid haemorrhage	No fever. Abrupt onset, rapid deterioration Bloodstained CSF
Meningeal malignancies	No fever. Insidious onset Variable CSF features

Table 2.1.2 Notifications of meningitis by cause in England and Wales in 1999

Meningococcal	1145
Pneumococcal	237
Haemophilus influenzae	29
Viral	211
Other specified	194
Unspecified	278
All causes	2094

Table 2.1.3 Causes of viral meningitis

Common
Echovirus
Coxsackievirus

Rare
Poliovirus
Mumps virus
Herpes simplex type 2
Herpes zoster
Influenza types A or B
Arbovirus
Rubella
Epstein–Barr virus

Bacterial meningitis (Table 2.1.4)

Bacterial meningitis is a medical emergency. The clinical presentation depends on the age of the patient, and the infecting organism. In the neonate, the presentation is non-specific, with features of bacteraemia. The infant is febrile, listless, floppy and does not feed. There may also be vomiting, drowsiness, convulsions or an abnormal high-pitched cry. In this age group, the commonest causes are *E. coli* and group B streptococci.

Signs and symptoms in older infants and young children are also non-specific. Meningococcal infection is the commonest cause at this age and is often accompanied by a haemorrhagic rash (see Chapter 3.48).

In older children and adults the symptoms are more specific. Fever, malaise and increasing headache are accompanied by nausea and often vomiting. Photophobia may be extreme. Meningism is usually present. Meningococcal infection is also the commonest cause in this group and the typical rash of meningococcal septicaemia may be present. Patients with rapidly advancing meningococcal disease may, over the course of a few hours, develop hypertension, circulatory collapse, pulmonary oedema, confusion and coma.

Other causes of acute bacterial meningitis in older children and adults are uncommon. *Haemophilus influenzae* meningitis occasionally occurs in unvaccinated children or adults; it has a slower onset than meningococcal meningitis and a rash is rare. Pneumococcal meningitis also has a more insidious onset and the symptoms are less specific than meningococcal meningitis. It usually occurs in adults with an underlying risk factor such as dura mater defect due to trauma or surgery, chronic intracranial infection, asplenia, terminal complement deficiency or alcoholism. *Listeria* meningitis presents either as a neonatal infection following intrapartum exposure or as a food-borne illness in older children and young adults, often in the immunosuppressed.

Tuberculous meningitis is a manifestation of primary tuberculosis, which occurs mainly in children and young adults. It has an insidious onset; meningism is usually mild and other features (except fever) are often absent.

Laboratory diagnosis

With the exception of tuberculosis, bacterial meningitis causes neutrophil pleiocytosis in the CSF, with raised protein and lowered glu-

Table 2.1.4 Causes of bacterial meningitis

Neonate	Infant/preschool child	Older child/adult
Common		
E. coli	N. meningitidis	N. meningitidis
Group B streptococci		S. pneumoniae
Uncommon		
L. monocytogenes	H. influenzae	L. monocytogenes
N. meningitidis	S. pneumoniae	Staphylococci
Staphylococci		H. influenzae
		M. tuberculosis

cose. A Gram stain will often demonstrate the typical appearance of the infecting organism, allowing a definitive diagnosis to be made.

Conventional culture of CSF and blood should always be carried out, however, these may be negative, particularly if the patient has been given antibiotics before hospital admission. In addition a CSF specimen may not be available, as clinicians are often reluctant to undertake a lumbar puncture.

A number of non-culture diagnostic techniques are now available. These include polymerase chain reaction (PCR) diagnosis for meningococcal disease (see Box 3.48.1 for suggested investigations) and serology. Other useful investigations include throat swab and microscopic examination of a rash aspirate if present.

General prevention and control measures

Hygiene. Enteroviral meningitis usually spreads as result of environmental contamination, particularly under conditions of crowding and poor hygiene. General hygiene measures such as handwashing will help prevent spread. This is particularly important in hospitals.

Immunization. The routine childhood immunization schedule ensures protection against meningitis caused by mumps, polio, *Haemophilus influenzae* type b (Hib), *Neisseria meningitidis* group C and tuberculosis. Polysaccharide vaccines are also available for *N. meningitidis* (serogroups A, C, Y and W135)

and *S. pneumoniae* (23 serogroups) although neither of these vaccines is currently suitable for routine use in infants.

Chemoprophylaxis is indicated for close contacts of meningococcal and Hib disease (see Chapters 3.48 and 3.35) and investigation for close contacts of TB (Chapter 3.78). It is not necessary for contacts of pneumococcal or viral meningitis.

Food safety. *Listeria* meningitis is preventable by avoiding high-risk foods such as soft cheese, pate and cook-chill foods, particularly for the immunosuppressed and in pregnancy.

Optimizing case management. In cases of suspected meningococcal disease, general practitioners and casualty officers should be urged to administer preadmission benzylpenicillin (see Chapter 3.48).

Response to a case or cluster

A case or cluster of meningitis is a highly emotive and newsworthy event. The first priority when a case is notified is to establish the diagnosis. This requires close liaison with clinicians and microbiologists to ensure that appropriate investigations are carried out. If the initial diagnosis is viral meningitis, then no further action is needed at this stage, although it may be necessary to provide information to GPs and parents if the case appears to be linked with others.

If bacterial meningitis is suspected, then further measures will depend on the cause. Again, optimum investigation is essential as the nature of the public health response differs for each organism. Chemoprophylaxis, and sometimes also vaccination, is indicated for cases due to *N. meningitidis* or *H. influenzae* (see Chapters 3.48 and 3.35). With the introduction of Hib vaccine, meningococcal infection is by far the most likely diagnosis in a patient with acute bacterial meningitis and it may sometimes be appropriate to initiate control measures before laboratory confirmation.

In the UK, useful information leaflets on meningitis are available from the National Meningitis Trust and the Meningitis Research Foundation (see Appendix 1).

2.2 Gastrointestinal infection

Every year in the UK, approximately 1 in 30 people attend their general practitioner with an acute gastroenteritis (usually diarrhoea and/or vomiting) and many more suffer such an illness without contacting the health service. Although an infectious cause is not always demonstrated, there is strong epidemiological evidence to suggest that most of these illnesses are caused by infections. A wide variety of bacteria, viruses and parasites may cause gastrointestinal infection; the most commonly identified ones in the UK are listed in Table 2.2.1. Less common but highly pathogenic infections may be imported from abroad, including amoebic or bacillary dysentery, cholera, typhoid and paratyphoid fevers. Other infectious causes of gastroenteritis include other *E. coli*, *Bacillus subtilis*, *Clostridium difficile*, *Giardia lamblia*, *Vibrio parahaemolyticus*, *Yersinia enterocolitica* and viruses such as adenovirus, coronavirus and astrovirus. Non-infectious causes of acute gastroenteritis include toxins from shellfish, vegetables (e.g. red kidney beans) and fungi, and chemical contamination of food and water (see Section 3.88.6).

Laboratory investigation

Identification of the causative organism is dependent upon laboratory investigation, usually of faecal samples. It is important that such samples are taken as soon after the onset of illness as possible, as the likelihood of isolating some pathogens (e.g. viruses) decreases substantially within a few days of onset. Collecting more than 2 mL of faeces and including the liquid part of the stool will increase the chances of a positive result. Delay in transport to the laboratory, particularly in warm weather should be minimized; if delay is likely, samples should be refrigerated or stored in a suitable transport medium. A local policy on sampling and transport should be agreed with the local microbiology laboratory. Samples of vomit may sometimes be helpful. In both cases, the patient should receive instructions on the collection and storage or transport of the specimen. Serology may be helpful if some cases become jaundiced. It is often difficult to distinguish between bacterial and chemical food-borne gastroenteritis on clinical grounds, although some toxins cause an unpleasant taste and/or burning in the mouth or throat. If a chemical cause is suspected, advice on sampling should be obtained from a toxicologist (e.g. public analyst).

Prevention and control

Vaccines are not yet available against the major causes of gastrointestinal infection and so public health efforts concentrate on reducing exposure to the organisms responsible. Much gastrointestinal infection is either food-borne or spread from person to person. The role of the consumer in demanding safe food via pressure on government and food retailers is under-developed in the UK; indeed public opinion is against food irradiation which many experts feel could make an important contribution to reducing food-borne illness.

At the local level, prevention of such spread is achieved by:
• Working with food businesses and staff to reduce the likelihood of contamination of

Table 2.2.1 Differential diagnosis of gastrointestinal infection

Organism	Laboratory confirmed (annual average, England and Wales**) Cases (no.)	Outbreaks (no.)	Incubation period (approx.) Usual	Range	Clinical clues in outbreaks Symptoms*	Severity	Other features
Campylobacter	44000	9	2–5 days	1–10 days	D often with blood Abdominal pain ± fever	Usually lasts 2–7 days	Peaks in early summer
Salmonella	28200	120	12–36 h	6–72 h	D often with fever. Maybe myalgia, abdominal pain, headache	Can be severe Lasts several days to 3 weeks	Peaks in late summer
Rotavirus	15100	15	24–72 h	24–72 h	Watery D, fever, vomiting ± respiratory symptoms	Usually lasts a few days, but occasionally severe	Usually children, common in winter
Shigella sonnei	4830	7	24–72 h	12–96 h	Often watery D Maybe mucus	Self-limiting in 3–5 days	Often children or institutions: secondary spread common
Cryptosporidium	4650	8	6–13 days	1–28 days	D, bloating and abdominal pain common	Self-limiting but lasts up to 4 weeks	Severe in immunocompromised. Increase in spring and autumn
Hepatitis A	3450	n/a	Mean = 28 days	15–45 days	Fever, nausea, malaise. Jaundice fairly specific but not sensitive	Worse in adults Lasts up to 4 weeks	Children may be asymptomatic
SRSV	1600	200	15–50 h	4–77 h	Nausea/vomiting common. Cramps, mild D may occur	Usually mild, lasts 1–2 days	Secondary spread common. More common in winter
E. coli O157	680	11	3–4 days	1–9 days	D, blood not uncommon	Variable, may be very severe, e.g. HUS, TTP	Consider in all cases of bloody diarrhoea
Other shigellae	650	1	24–72 h	12–96 h	D, mucus, blood, fever and colic common	Lasts average of 7 days. Often severe	Often imported, secondary spread common
Clostridium perfringens	330	25	8–18 h	5–24 h	D, abdominal pain common (vomiting and fever are rare)	Usually mild and short-lived. Lasts approx. 1 day	Usually failure of temperature control post cooking
Bacillus cereus	40	4	1–6 h for syndrome of nausea, vomiting + abdominal pain 6–24 h for syndrome of diarrhoea and abdominal pain			Usually mild and short-lived. Lasts approx. 1 day	Often from rice or pasta. High attack rate
Staphylococcus aureus	30	3	2–4 h	0.5–8 h	Vomiting, abdominal pain (diarrhoea rare). Often abrupt onset	May be very acute	Food handler may have skin infection

* D = Diarrhoea, which can be defined as three or more loose stools in 24 hours.
** Average number of reports p.a. to PHLS/CDSC, 1990–99 (cases) or 1992–99 (outbreaks).

food (from the environment, food handlers or cross-contamination), inadequate cooking and storage at inadequate temperatures. The Hazard Analysis Critical Control Point (HACCP) system has proven to be a powerful tool for use by the food industry in identifying and assessing hazards in food, and establishing control measures needed to maintain a cost-effective food safety programme. Important features are that HACCP is predictive, cheap, on-site and involves local staff in the control of risk. In the UK, this approach is reinforced by inspection of premises by the Environmental Health Department of the Local Authority and other enforcement agencies.

• Use of statutory powers: UK Local Authorities can exclude cases or carriers of infection from work or school and compensate them for any loss of earnings. Other powers include seizure of food and closure of premises that present an 'imminent risk to Public Health'. Officers of the Environmental Health Department usually exercise these powers. The Meat Hygiene Service (part of the Food Standards Agency) is the enforcing authority for licensed fresh meat/poultry premises in Great Britain.

• Advising the general population on safe food handling and the reduction of faeco–oral spread. This includes the importance of hand-washing immediately after going to the toilet and before handling or eating food. This is of vital importance, as approximately 80% of people with gastrointestinal infection do not consult the health service when ill.

• Adequate infection control policies in all institutions including hospitals, nursing and residential homes, schools and nurseries, including use of enteric precautions (see Chapter 1.2) for cases of diarrhoea or vomiting.

• Regular surveillance to detect outbreaks and respond to individual cases. Food poisoning (proven or suspected and including water-borne infection), dysentery and viral hepatitis are all statutorily notifiable to the proper officer of the relevant UK Local Authority (usually the CCDC), as are cholera, paratyphoid and typhoid fever (as is the case in most European countries). There are, however, no generally accepted clinical case-definitions for these notifiable infections and there may often be no laboratory confirmation of the organism

responsible. It is therefore often necessary to initiate action before the causative organism is known. Arrangements should also be in place for reporting of isolates of gastrointestinal pathogens from local microbiology laboratories to the CCDC (see Table 4.2.2). However, around 90% of cases seen by general practitioners are not identified by either of these systems.

Response to individual case

It is not usually possible to identify the organism causing gastroenteritis on clinical grounds in individual cases. The public health priorities in such cases are as follows.

• To limit secondary spread from identified cases by provision of general hygiene advice to all and by specific exclusion from work/school/nursery of those at increased risk of transmitting the infection (see Box 2.2.1).

• To collect a minimum dataset to compare to other cases to detect common exposures or potential outbreaks. It is best to collect such data on standardized forms, and a subset should be entered on a computerized database (e.g. CoSurv in UK) for both weekly and annual analysis. A possible dataset is given in Box 2.2.2.

• Ideally, a stool sample would be collected from all clinical notifications of food poisoning or dysentery to look for clusters by organism/type, to detect potentially serious pathogens requiring increased intervention, and to monitor trends.

A local policy to address these priorities should be agreed with local EHOs, microbiologists and clinicians. The role of the primary care practitioners in public health surveillance and in preventing secondary spread is of particular importance and needs to be emphasized regularly (e.g. via a GP newsletter).

Response to cluster

The most common setting for a cluster of clinical cases of gastroenteritis is in an already defined cohort, e.g. in a nursing home or amongst attendees at a wedding. Such a situation is slightly different to investigating a laboratory-identified cluster.

> **Box 2.2.1 Groups that pose an increased risk of spreading gastrointestinal infection**
>
> **1** Food handlers whose work involves touching unwrapped foods to be consumed raw or without further cooking.
> **2** Staff of healthcare facilities who have direct contact, or contact through serving food, with susceptible patients or persons in whom an intestinal infection would have particularly serious consequences.
> **3** Children aged less than five years who attend nurseries, nursery schools, playgroups, or other similar groups.
> **4** Older children and adults who may find it difficult to implement good standards of personal hygiene – for example, those with learning disabilities or special needs; and in circumstances where hygienic arrangements may be unreliable – for example, temporary camps housing displaced persons. Under exceptional circumstances (e.g. *E. coli* O157 infection) children in infant schools may be considered to fall into this group.
>
> Guidelines for the exclusion of cases in risk groups 3 and 4 assume that, once cases have recovered and passed normal stools, they can subsequently practice good hygiene under supervision. If that is not the case, individual circumstances must be assessed.
>
> Source: PHLS Salmonella Committee, 1995.

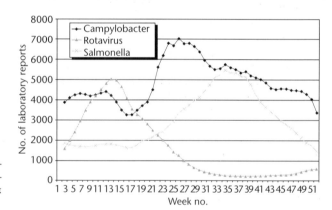

Figure 2.2.1 Seasonal distribution of gastrointestinal pathogens, 1994–1998, England & Wales (3 week rolling averages).

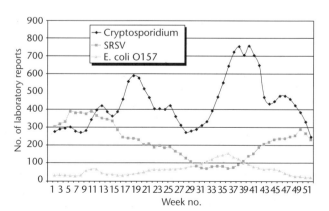

Figure 2.2.2 Seasonal distribution of gastrointestinal pathogens, 1994–1998, England & Wales (3 week rolling averages).

Box 2.2.2 Possible district data set for investigation of cases of gastrointestinal infection

---

Administrative details (name, address, telephone, date of birth, GP, unique number*)

Formally notified?   Yes/No

Descriptive variables (age*, sex*, postcode*)

Date * and time of onset

Symptoms

Diarrhoea	Yes/No
Nausea	Yes/No
Vomiting	Yes/No
Fever	Yes/No
Abdominal pain	Yes/No
Blood in stool	Yes/No
Malaise	Yes/No
Headache	Yes/No
Jaundice	Yes/No

Others (specify):_____

Duration of illness

Stool sample taken? (source, date, laboratory)

Microbiological result (organism details*, laboratory, specimen date)

Food history: functions, restaurants, takeaways

Food consumed in last five days (for unknown microbial cause)

Raw water consumed outside the home in previous 14 days

Other cases in household?

Travel abroad?

Animal contact?

Occupation, place of work/school/nursery

Advised not to work?

Formally excluded?

Part of outbreak?*

   Organism-specific questions may be added if microbiological investigation reveals an organism of particular public health importance (e.g. *E. coli* O157, *Cryptosporidium*, *S. typhi*, *S. paratyphi*).

* *Minimum dataset to be recorded in computerized database*

• It is important to discover the microbiological agent. Following discussion with the relevant microbiologist (e.g. the local Public Health Laboratory in most of England and Wales) stool specimens should be obtained without delay from 6 to 10 of the patients with the most recent onset of illness and submitted to the laboratory for testing for all relevant organisms, including *E. coli* O157, viruses and enterotoxin-producing bacteria (the laboratory may not test for all these routinely). The identity of the agent will affect the urgency of the investigation (e.g. to prevent further exposure to a source of *E. coli* O157), the control measures to be introduced (e.g. to limit person-to-person spread of SRSV in institutions) and provide valuable clues as to how the outbreak may have happened (e.g. inadequate temperature control in a *Bacillus cereus* outbreak).

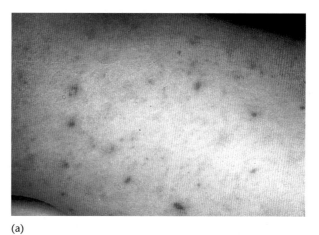

(a)

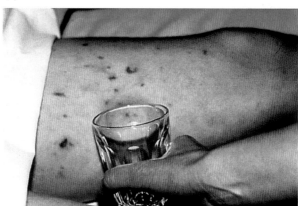

Plate 1 Testing for the non-blanching rash of meningococcal septicaemia with a glass. (a) Early-stage rash; (b) tumbler test.

(b)

• As microbiological results will not be available for a number of days, clinical details should be collected from all reported cases so that the incubation period, symptom profile, severity and duration of illness can be used to predict which organism(s) are most likely to be the cause (Table 2.2.1). The likelihood of different microbiological causes also varies by season (Figs 2.2.1 and 2.2.2). There may also be clues as to whether the illness is likely to be food-borne or spread person-to-person (Box 2.2.3). In many such outbreaks a formal hypothesis-generating study is not necessary, and it is often possible to progress to an analytical study to investigate possible food vehicles early in the investigation (see Chapter 4.3).

• The environmental component of the investigation is often illuminating as to why the outbreak happened, i.e. how did an infectious dose of the organism occur in the identified food vehicle. This investigation will look at:

(i) food sources, storage, food preparation, cooking procedures, temperature control after cooking and reheating;

(ii) symptoms of gastrointestinal or skin disease, or testing for faecal carriage in food handlers;

(iii) general state of knowledge of the staff and condition of the premises;

(iv) examination of records of key controls, such as temperature and pest controls;

(v) whether samples of food are available for examination/analysis and whether environmental swabbing or water sampling is appropriate.

Box 2.2.3　Clues as to whether an outbreak of gastro-enteritis could be food-borne or spread from person to person

May suggest food-borne	**May suggest person-to-person**
Dates of onset (epidemic curve) clustered indicating a point source outbreak. incubation	Dates and times of onset do not cluster, but occur in waves coinciding with the period of the responsible pathogen.
All wards, classes, buildings or units supplied by the kitchens or food supplier are affected.	Patients and staff in a single ward, class, building or unit are affected.
Food handlers and catering staff are affected.	People in the households of staff members or pupils are also affected.
Clinical features and laboratory tests indicate an organism predominantly spread via food and water rather than person-to-person, e.g. *C. perfringens*, *B. cereus*.	Clinical features and laboratory tests suggest organism predominantly spread from person to person, e.g. Rotavirus, *Shigella*.
Environmental investigation reveals poor food handling practices or premises.	Environmental investigation reveals poor infection control practice or hygiene facilities.

Warnings
• Some food-borne outbreaks may be prolonged by person-to-person spread.
• Food-borne outbreaks may be due to a continuing source.
• Some outbreaks may be augmented by environmental contamination.

• General control measures to prevent spread from those affected can be instituted early, as can addressing important problems identified in the environmental investigation. This includes the exclusion from work of infected food handlers and measures to avoid secondary spread from cases. More specific measures can be instituted when the organism and vehicle are identified (see appropriate Chapter in Section 3).

2.3 Community-acquired pneumonia

Respiratory tract infections are the most common infectious disease in developed countries, and pneumonia remains one of the most common causes of death. Community (as opposed to hospital) acquired pneumonia (CAP) affects all ages, although its incidence increases dramatically beyond 50 years of age. Other risk factors include chronic respiratory disease, smoking, immunosuppression (including HIV/AIDS) and residence in an institution. Approximately 20% of cases require hospitalization, of which 5–10% die.

In general, the symptoms of CAP are fever, cough, sputum production, chest pain and shortness of breath, with accompanying chest X-ray changes. The most common causes of CAP are listed in Table 2.3.1. Although the clinical picture cannot be used to diagnose individual cases, clues may be obtained to help identify the causes of outbreaks.

Rare causes of pneumonia for which there may be an environmental cause (most likely abroad) include anthrax, brucellosis, hantavirus, histoplasmosis, leptospirosis and plague. Similar symptoms may also be seen in exacerbations of chronic respiratory disease and non-infective respiratory conditions, e.g. pulmonary oedema, pulmonary infarction, alveolitis (may follow exposure to inorganic particles) and eosinophilic pneumonias (may be associated with drugs or parasites).

Laboratory investigation

Microscopy and culture of sputum remains the mainstay of diagnosis, although about a third of pneumonia cases do not produce sputum, culture is only moderately sensitive and contamination with oropharyngeal flora is not an uncommon event. Blood culture is highly specific but relatively insensitive.

Serology has been the mainstay of diagnosis for viral and 'atypical' causes, but this is often not diagnostic until 2–6 weeks into the illness. *Mycoplasma*-specific IgM may be apparent rather earlier.

Influenza and RSV may be cultured from nasopharyngeal swabs or aspirates, and viral antigen or DNA may also be detected from these specimens. *Legionella* antigen may be detected in urine and pneumococcal antigen in sputum, serum or urine, even if antibiotics have already been given.

A proportion of cases may be infected with more than one pathogen.

Prevention and control

• Immunization of elderly and those with chronic disease and immunocompromised with influenza and pneumococcal vaccines.
• Immunization of children against *Haemophilus influenzae* type b.
• Reduction of smoking.
• Promotion of breastfeeding.
• Avoiding overcrowding, especially in institutions.
• Good infection control in institutions.
• Environmental measures to reduce *Legionella* exposure.
• Surveillance of community-acquired pneumonia, especially for influenza, *Mycoplasma*, *Legionella*, *Coxiella* and *Chlamydia psittaci*. Surveillance of antibiotic-resistant pneumococci.
• Reporting of outbreaks in institutions to public health authorities.

Table 2.3.1 Differential diagnosis of community-acquired pneumonia

Organism	Percent of cases*	Clinical clues**	Epidemiological clues
Streptococcus pneumoniae	29	Acute. Rusty sputum, fever, chest pain. Prominent physical signs	More common in infants, elderly, unvaccinated and in winter
Mycoplasma pneumoniae	9	Gradual onset, scanty sputum, headache, malaise, sore throat	Epidemics every 4 years. Often affects younger patients
Influenza A	8	Headache, myalgia, coryza, fever, sore throat	May be seasonal community epidemic. Affects the unvaccinated
Chlamydia pneumoniae	6	Hoarseness, sore throat, scanty sputum, sinus tenderness. Insidious onset	Often affects young adults. No obvious seasonality
Gram-negative bacteria	6	Severe. Acute onset. Redcurrant jelly sputum	Particularly common in nursing homes. More likely if chronic respiratory disease, diabetes, alcohol
Haemophilus influenzae	5	Purulent sputum. Onset may be insidious	Often associated with chronic lung disease and elderly
Legionella pneumophila	4	Anorexia, malaise, myalgia, headache, fever. Some with diarrhoea, confusion and high fever. Upper respiratory symptoms rare	May be associated with aerosol source. More common in summer and autumn. Male excess
Staphylococcus aureus	4	Often serious. May be ring shadows on X-ray	May complicate influenza infection. More common in nursing homes
Parainfluenza	2	Croup or wheezing. Ear or upper respiratory infection	Mostly affects children. Also affects immunocompromised
Chlamydia psittaci	2	Fever, headache, unproductive cough, myalgia. May be rash	Possible link to birds. May be severe
Influenza B	1	Headache, myalgia, coryza, fever, sore throat	May be seasonal community epidemic. Affects the unvaccinated
Coxiella burnetii	1	Fever, fatigue, chills, headache, myalgia, sweats. May be weight loss or neurological symptoms	Possible link to sheep, other animals or animal products. May be increase in April–June. Male excess, rare in children
RSV	1	Wheezing, rhinitis, fever	Peaks every December and January. Causes outbreaks in nursing homes
Adenovirus	0.7	Fever, sore throat, runny nose	Usually children or young adults (e.g. military recruits). Highest in January–April

* Average from a number of prospective studies of patients admitted to hospital (Farr and Mandell, 1988). Will vary according to epidemic cycles.

** Clinical picture is not a reliable indicator of organism in individual cases.

Response to a case

• If resident or attender at institution, or if severely ill, investigate to obtain microbiological cause.
• Follow up individual cases of legionellosis, psittacosis and Q fever for source of organism.
• Advise personal hygiene, particularly handwashing, coughing and disposal of secretions.
• Limit contact with infants, frail elderly and immunocompromised.

Response to a cluster

• Discuss investigation with microbiological colleagues. A suitable set of investigations could be the following.
   (i) Take nasopharyngeal aspirates or nose and throat swabs from most recently infected cases for virus culture, PCR and antigen testing.
   (ii) Take serum samples from recovered cases or those with date of onset 10 days or more ago.
   (iii) Send sputum samples for microbiological culture.
   (iv) Send blood cultures from febrile cases.
   (v) Send urine for *Legionella* and pneumococcal antigen.
• If an institutional cluster, isolate or cohort cases until cause known. Stop new admissions. Avoid discharges to institutions containing elderly, frail or immunocompromised individuals.
• Collect data on immunization history (influenza, pneumococcus), exposure to water and aerosols, animals, birds and other potential sources of *Legionella*, *Coxiella* and *Chlamydia psittaci*.
• Advise community cases on hygiene measures (handwashing, coughing, discharges, etc.) and to avoid individuals susceptible to severe disease (e.g. elderly, chronically ill).
• Specific interventions as appropriate to identified cause.

2.4 Rash in pregnancy

Infectious and other causes

There are many possible causes of a rash in a pregnant woman. Most causes are noninfectious and include drug reactions and allergies. The important differentiating feature from an infectious cause is the absence of fever. Infectious causes are relatively uncommon, but important because of the potential harm to the developing fetus. Rubella, parvovirus B19, varicella and syphilis can all cause severe congenital disease or intrauterine death.

Clinical and epidemiological differences

Viral infections in pregnancy are often mild or inapparent with variable or absent fever. The exceptions are varicella, which presents with a characteristic rash, and measles. Bacterial infections are more severe and usually accompanied by a high fever (with the exception of syphilis). The clinical presentation of each of the infections in Table 2.4.1 is described in more detail in the relevant chapters.

The most common infections in pregnancy are parvovirus B19 (1 in 400 pregnancies), varicella (1 in 500 pregnancies) and the enteroviruses. Rubella and measles are now both rare, due to successful immunization programmes. Bacterial causes of rash in pregnancy are very uncommon.

Table 2.4.1 Infections that may present with a rash in pregnancy

Viral
Rubella
Parvovirus B19
Varicella-zoster
Measles
Enterovirus
Infectious mononucleosis
Bacterial
Streptococcal
Meningococcal
Syphilis

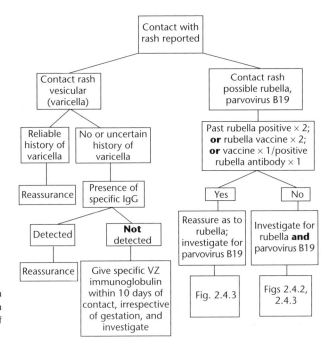

Fig. 2.4.1 Investigation of a pregnant patient in contact with a rash illness. With permission of PHLS Working Group.

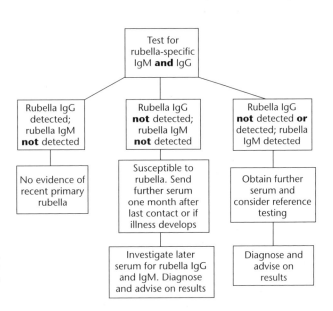

Fig. 2.4.2 Investigation for rubella of a pregnant woman exposed to a rash illness. With permission of PHLS Working Group.

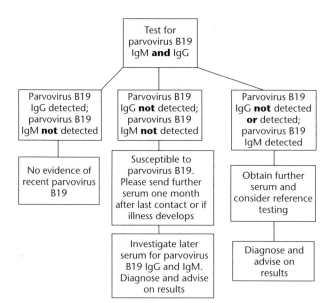

Fig. 2.4.3 Investigation for parvovirus B19 of a pregnant woman exposed to a rash illness. With permission of PHLS Working Group.

Laboratory investigation

The laboratory investigation of suspected meningococcal and streptococcal disease and syphilis is described in Chapters 3.48, 3.72 and 3.25, respectively.

Where a viral infection is suspected, it is important to exclude varicella, parvovirus B19 and rubella. Varicella can usually be diagnosed on the basis of the typical vesicular rash, but where there is doubt, serology should be performed. Rubella and parvovirus B19 can both be diagnosed by detection of IgM in saliva or serum.

The investigation of a pregnant woman who has been in contact with someone with a rash illness is more complex. The aim of investigation is to determine whether the contact case has varicella, rubella or parvovirus B19, and whether the pregnant patient is susceptible to these three infections. The three algorithms in Figures 2.4.1–3 describe the laboratory investigation recommended in the UK.

Prevention and control

Rubella infection in pregnancy can be prevented both directly, by vaccination of susceptible women of childbearing age, and indirectly, by universal childhood immunization (which reduces circulation of wild virus and thus prevents exposure). All pregnant women should be screened for rubella in each pregnancy and vaccinated postpartum. Rubella vaccine is a live vaccine and should not be given during pregnancy, although the risk to the fetus is theoretical and immunization in pregnancy is no longer an indication for termination of pregnancy.

Varicella vaccine is licensed in some countries (not the UK) and can be used, like rubella vaccine, for both direct prevention of varicella in pregnancy (by vaccination of susceptible women) and indirect prevention (universal childhood immunization). A specific varicella zoster immunoglobulin (VZIG) is available for postexposure prophylaxis of susceptible women exposed in the first 20 weeks of pregnancy or within 21 days of the estimated date of delivery (see Chapter 3.7).

No specific measures are available for prevention of parvovirus B19 in pregnancy, although pregnant women may wish to avoid outbreak situations, and healthcare workers who have been in contact with B19 infection should avoid contact with pregnant women for 15 days from the last contact or until a rash appears (see Chapter 3.55).

Response to a case

Laboratory investigations should be undertaken as described above. Pregnant women with varicella, rubella or parvovirus B19 should be counselled regarding the risks to the fetus and managed accordingly by the obstetrician. The public health management of the close contacts is the same as for non-pregnant cases (see Chapters 3.55, 3.65 and 3.7).

Response to a cluster

As for response to a case, but consider community-wide vaccination programme for clusters of rubella or measles.

2.5 Rash and fever in children

Rashes in children are common (Table 2.5.1). Where fever is present, this usually means the cause is infectious. In the absence of a fever, a non-infectious cause (e.g. allergy or drug reaction) is the most likely cause, although in some infections, e.g. enterovirus infections, the fever may be mild or absent.

Table 2.5.1 Causes of rash in children

Common
Infection
Drug reaction
Allergy
Rare
Inherited bleeding disorder
Leukaemia
Purpura

Clinical and epidemiological differences

In addition to fever, other features that suggest an infectious cause are the presence of swollen lymph nodes, general malaise, and a history of recent contact with another case. A full vaccination history should always be obtained from a child with a rash.

There are four main types of rash: vesicular, maculopapular, punctate and haemorrhagic. Vesicular rashes have a blister-like appearance and sometimes contain fluid. Maculopapular rashes are flat or slightly raised and there is sometimes joining together of areas of the rash. Punctate rashes have small, discrete pin-point lesions. Haemorrhagic rashes look like bruising. The main causes of each type are shown in Table 2.5.2.

Laboratory investigations

General investigations which are useful in differentiating infectious from non-infectious causes are a full blood count, erythrocyte sedimentation rate, blood culture, specimens for viral culture and an acute serum sample for serology. Other investigations will depend on the possible differential diagnoses. A saliva test should be obtained if measles or rubella is suspected.

Prevention and control

General hygiene measures such as hand-washing may help limit the spread of some infectious causes of rashes. Transmission of measles, rubella, meningococcal disease (serogroup C) and chickenpox are all preventable by vaccination (see Chapters 3.47, 3.65, 3.48 and 3.7, respectively).

Response to a case

• Obtain clinical details, especially whether fever present.
• Check vaccination status.
• Obtain history of contact with other case(s).
• Most childhood rashes are mild and do not warrant any specific public health action.

Table 2.5.2 Types of rash. From E. G. Davies *et al. Manual of Childhood Infections.* British Paediatric Association, 1996, with permission

	Prodrome	Fever	General malaise	Distribution of rash	Pruritus	Special features
Vesicular rashes						
Chickenpox	None or short Coryzal	Mild to moderate	Mild	Mostly truncal	Yes	Contact with sufferers is common; crops
Dermatitis herpetiformis	Nil	Nil	Nil	Trunk	Yes	Sporadic cases eventually leave depigmentation
Eczema herpeticum	Nil	Moderate to high	Moderate	In areas of eczema	Yes	May be seriously ill
Hand, foot and mouth disease	Nil	Minimal	Minimal	Palms, soles and inside mouth	No	Often occurs as minor epidemics
Herpes simplex gingivostomatitis	Nil	Moderate to high	Moderate (may be dehydrated)	Mouth and lips	Yes (at onset)	Frequent history of contact with cold sores
Impetigo	Nil	Nil	Nil	Face and hands	Yes	Vesicles often replaced by yellow crusting
Insect bites	Nil	Nil	Rare	Variable	Yes	Usually isolated lesions
Molluscum contagiosum	Nil	Nil	Nil	Variable	Yes	Characteristic pearly vesicles with central dimples

Maculopapular and punctate rashes

Enteroviral infections	Short	Mild	Mild	General	No	Rash often pleomorphic
Fifth disease	Uncommon; mild fever and respiratory symptoms	Mild, if any	Minimal	Face ('slapped cheeks') trunk and limbs	No	Rash may come and go. Heat brings it out. Can have a reticular pattern
Glandular fever	Malaise, mild fever and sore throat	Moderate	Common	General	No	Exudate in throat especially marked swollen glands and spleen
Kawasaki disease	Mild fever, malaise and sore throat	Moderate to high and persistent	Mild to moderate	General	No	Palms and soles, lips and conjunctivae affected
Measles	Rising fever, cough and conjunctivitis	Moderate to high	Substantial	Around ears, then face, then trunk. Confluent	No	Koplik's spots in mouth before rash on 4th day of illness
Meningococcal disease	None or short with coryza or fever	Variable	Profound	Variable	No	Petechial rash may be preceded by maculopapular rash
Pityriasis rosea	Nil	Nil	Nil	Trunk	Initially	Usually in older children; herald patch at onset
Roseola infantum	High fever and irritability	Moderate	Moderate	Trunk then face	No	Dramatic improvement in child when rash appears on 4th or 5th day

Continued on p. 32

Table 2.5.2 Continued

	Prodrome	Fever	General malaise	Distribution of rash	Pruritus	Special features
Rubella	Short, mild fever and malaise	Mild	Mild or absent	Face then trunk and limbs	No	Posterior occipital lymphadenopathy
Scarlet fever	Fever and sore throat	Moderate to high	Moderate	Face, then rapidly generalized	No	Rash blanches on pressure; strawberry tongue and perioral pallor
Haemorrhagic rashes						
Acute lymphoblastic leukaemia	Mild, non-specific	Absent or mild/moderate	Moderate	Anywhere, including mucous membranes	Nil	Pallor, lymphadenopathy and hepatosplenomegaly may be present
Henoch–Schönlein purpura	Mild, sometimes symptoms of upper respiratory tract infection	Mild or moderate	Moderate	Mainly limbs, especially legs and buttocks	No	Rash is urticarial initially. Arthralgia, joint swelling and abdominal pain often present
Idiopathic thrombocytopenic purpura	Nil to mild	Nil	Nil	Anywhere, including mucous membranes	Nil	Child is usually well, apart from effects of bleeding
Inherited bleeding disorder	Nil	Nil	Nil	Anywhere, including mucous membranes	Nil	Spontaneous bruises. Family history may be present
Meningococcal disease	None or short with coryza or fever	Variable	Severe	Variable	No	Petechial rash may be preceded by maculopapular rash

• Exclusion from school is indicated for the vaccine-preventable diseases (see above) and for scarlet fever (see Chapter 3.72).

• Chemoprophylaxis (and sometimes vaccination) should be given where meningococcal infection is suspected (see Chapter 3.48).

Response to a cluster

As per a case, although it will often be important to give out information to parents and GPs to allay anxiety and to increase disease awareness.

2.6 Illness in returning travellers

The increasing numbers of international travellers and destinations have increased the opportunity for people to come into contact with organisms that they would not routinely meet and the likelihood of such infections presenting in countries in which they are unfamiliar. Over 600 million people spend a night in a foreign country each year. Infectious disease complications of travel depend on the destination, but in some places more than 50% of travellers will fall ill.

The possibility of an imported infection should be considered early in all investigations of infectious disease.

Infectious causes

Imported causes of fever include malaria, enteric fevers, pneumonias (including Legionnaires' disease), hepatitis, tuberculosis and schistosomiasis. Falciparum malaria is a medical emergency. Malaria has a variety of clinical presentations (see Section 3.46) and usually presents within 3 months of return, but may occasionally take one year.

Travellers' diarrhoea usually occurs during travel or soon after return. The most frequently identified pathogen causing travel-ler's diarrhoea is toxigenic *Escherichia coli*. In some parts of the world (North Africa and South-east Asia), *Campylobacter* predominates. Other common causative organisms include *Salmonella*, *Shigella*, rotavirus, and the Norwalk agent. The longer the history, the more likely the cause is to be parasitic, e.g. *Giardia*, *Entamoeba histolytica* or *Cyclospora*, rather than bacterial or viral.

In addition to causes of pharyngitis that are common in the UK, potentially serious causes are diphtheria and, in a febrile patient who has visited rural West Africa, Lassa fever. Diphtheria and leishmaniasis may both present with cutaneous lesions. Hepatitis A, B, C and E viruses may all be contracted abroad.

Epidemiological differences

The organisms that should be considered depend upon the location(s) that have been visited. Careful travel histories are important; it may be necessary to consult an expert who knows the local epidemiology of disease.

• Where has the person been (country)?
• Which districts (urban, rural)?
• Staying where (luxury hotels, camping)?
• Doing what (healthcare, animals)?
• Exactly when (incubation periods)?
• Precautions taken (vaccines, prophylaxis, lifestyle)?

The possibility of a highly infectious exotic infection, such as a viral haemorrhagic fever (VHF) should be considered and advice sought from specialists as necessary. VHF is more likely if an individual has been staying in rural areas, or has been in contact with other possible cases. As the geographical range of these diseases is not known they should be considered whenever the clinical picture warrants, although confirmed cases are rare (Table 2.6.1).

Prevention and control

See Chapter 4.10.

Response to a case

For febrile illnesses:

Table 2.6.1 Approximate number of imported infections into England and Wales each year

Malaria	1000
Enteric fever	250
Hepatitis A	200
Viral haemorrhagic fever	<1

- determine likely exposure;
- malaria should be excluded if there is any possible exposure in a patient who is unwell;
- enteric precautions for cases with diarrhoea;
- exclusion and contact tracing as appropriate for cholera, diphtheria, hepatitis A or B, paratyphoid and typhoid fevers (see specific chapters in Section 3);
- if haemorrhagic fever is seriously considered, the nearest unit with special expertise should be contacted urgently;
- inform national surveillance unit of incidents of potential significance, e.g. VHF, Legionnaires' disease, outbreak of food poisoning and imported infections that should be reported to WHO under the International Health Regulations (yellow fever, cholera, plague).

Acute travellers' diarrhoea is usually self-limiting and does not require antibiotic therapy. Chronic bowel problems which persist after return home may be postinfectious sequelae, such as lactose intolerance or irritable bowel syndrome or an initial presentation of inflammatory bowel disease. Rare infectious causes of chronic bowel symptoms include *Giardia intestinalis*, *Cyclospora cayetanensis*, *Cryptosporidium* species, and *Entamoeba histolytica*.

Investigation of a cluster

The absence in Western Europe of essential vectors in the life cycle of an organism and better sanitary conditions mean that the conditions for onward transmission do not exist for many imported infections. Secondary cases are unusual.

For those that can occur in UK, determine if cluster is a result of primary exposure abroad (tell national centre), or secondary transmission in UK (investigate mechanism).

2.7 Sexually transmitted infections

Sexually transmitted infections (STIs) are infections that are spread by direct sexual contact. Table 2.7.1 lists the common infectious agents that cause STIs, their clinical features and common sequelae.

Other organisms that are less commonly sexually spread include cytomegalovirus, *Campylobacter*, *Entamoeba histolytica*, *Giardia lamblia*, hepatitis A virus, shigellae and group B streptococci.

Diagnosis depends on clinical features and the results of appropriate laboratory investigations including culture, serology, ELISA and PCR (see Table 2.7.1).

Why are STIs important?

Sexually transmitted infections are an increasingly important cause of ill health. In addition to the initial episode of infection with its accompanying discomfort and distress they may result in long-term complications such as infertility, ectopic pregnancy and genital cancers. Many of these complications specifically affect young women. The costs of maintaining NHS services for diagnosing and treating STIs and their complications are considerable. STIs may have other hidden costs. STIs such as gonorrhoea in men can be an indicator of sexual behaviour that may carry a risk of transmission of HIV infection. STIs that result in genital ulceration may enhance HIV transmission. Programmes and interventions that reduce STI incidence have enormous potential for health gain.

Table 2.7.1 Clinical features and laboratory confirmation of acute STIs

Infection and infectious agent	Clinical features and sequelae	Diagnosis
Genital chlamydial infection *Chlamydia trachomatis*	Many cases asymptomatic In women may be cervicitis and urethritis May be complicated by pelvic inflammatory disease, tubal damage, infertility and ectopic pregnancy In men, urethritis and possibly epididymitis	Infection may be confirmed by enzyme immunoassay, direct fluorescent antibody test, ligase chain reaction (may be used on urine), polymerase chain reaction or culture of cervical or urethral samples
Bacterial vaginosis *Gardnerella vaginalis*, anaerobic coccobacillus, other anaerobes including *Bacteroides*	Vaginal discharge and itching There is debate about the importance of sexual transmission	Wet mount of the discharge reveals vaginal epithelial cells studded with so-called clue cells
Chancroid *Haemophilus ducreyi*	A painful ulcerating genital papule appears 4–10 days after exposure. If untreated, suppurating lymphadenopathy follows	Diagnosis is confirmed by a Gram-stained smear or culture on special media
Genital candidiasis *Candida albicans*	Vaginitis with irritation and discharge *C. albicans* is a vaginal commensal and infection is often endogenous although sexual spread may occur In males infection is often asymptomatic but irritation and a rash on the glans penis may occur	The organism can be identified in a Gram stain or wet mount or by culture
Genital herpes Herpes simplex virus (HSV). Usually HSV-2 but HSV-1 causes 20% of cases	Primary infection produces painful vesicles or ulcers on the penis, labia, cervix and adjacent genital areas. There may be fever and malaise. Healing occurs within 17 days. In the majority of cases, recurrent secondary episodes, usually less severe, occur as often as once a month due to HSV latency in local nerve ganglia. Precipitating factors include menstruation, sexual intercourse and stress. Subclinical attacks are common and are important in transmission Serious HSV infection of the neonate may be acquired during delivery	Genital herpes has a typical appearance and can be confirmed by viral isolation
Genital warts Human papillomaviruses (HPV)	Sessile warts are 1–2 mm in diameter and affect dry areas of skin. Condylomata acuminata are large fleshy soft growths and occur particularly when cellular immunity is depressed. Genital warts are often multiple and may occur anywhere on the external	HPV cannot be cultured Diagnosis may be made histologically on examining cervical cytology specimens Polymerase chain

Continued on p. 36

Table 2.7.1 *Continued*

Infection and infectious agent	Clinical features and sequelae	Diagnosis
	genitalia and within the vagina. Subclinical HPV infections of the genitalia are common. Certain HPV types are associated with genital tract neoplasia Possible sequelae are carcinoma of anus, cervix, penis and vulva	reaction-based assays are now available that are capable of distinguishing more than 25 different HPV types
Gonorrhoea *Neisseria gonorrhoeae*	Cervicitis in females and urethritis in males, with purulent discharge. Anorectal and oropharyngeal infection can occur. Incubation period is 2–5 days Sub-clinical infection is common and an important source of transmission. Salpingitis is a complication in 10–15% of females but local complications in males are uncommon Possible sequelae are neonatal infection, pelvic inflammatory disease, ectopic pregnancy, infertility, epididymitis, urethral stricture, septic arthritis	Urethral or cervical swabs should be requested. Gram-negative diplococci may be seen on microscopy. *N. gonorrhoea* may be cultured
Non-chlamydial non-gonococcal urethritis	*Ureaplasma urealyticum* and *Mycoplasma hominis* are causes of urethritis and pelvic inflammatory disease. Possible sequelae are infertility and ectopic pregnancy	Specific diagnostic tests for these organisms are not usually clinically indicated
Granuloma inguinale *Calymmatobacterium granulomatis*, a Gram-negative coccobacillus	Destructive ulcerating genital papules appear 1–12 weeks after exposure Possible sequelae are genital lymphoedema, urethral stricture	Biopsy of the edge of the ulcer shows Donovan bodies on appropriate staining
Human T-cell lymphotropic virus	Leukaemia, lymphoma, tropical spastic paraparesis	Tests for HTLV specific antibodies are available
Lymphogranuloma venereum Types L-1, L-2, and L-3 of *Chlamydia trachomatis* distinct from those that cause trachoma and oculogenital infection	Starts with a painless penile vesicle 1–4 weeks after exposure. This heals but is followed 1–2 weeks later by fever and regional lymphadenopathy, which leads to suppuration and fibrosis that become chronic	Diagnosis is made by serology, culture of aspirates or direct fluorescence of smears
Syphilis *Treponema pallidum*, a spirochaete	The clinical manifestations of syphilis are varied The primary and secondary stages are characterized by mucocutaneous lesions. The primary chancre occurs on average 21 days after exposure. A variable secondary rash follows after 6–8 weeks, often with fever and malaise. Gummata (tertiary lesions)	The diagnosis of syphilis is based upon clinical examination and demonstration of *T. pallidum* in early infectious lesions by dark ground microscopy.

Continued

Table 2.7.1 *Continued*

Infection and infectious agent	Clinical features and sequelae	Diagnosis
	appear after several years. Almost any organ of the body can be affected Transplacental spread of *T. pallidum* may result in fetal death, prematurity or congenital syphilis Possible sequelae are fetal and neonatal infection, neurological and cardiovascular disease	Serological tests aid the diagnosis of secondary, latent and tertiary syphilis
Trichomoniasis *Trichomonas vaginalis,* a flagellated protozoan	Vaginitis with offensive discharge Asymptomatic urethral infection or colonization common in males	Motile organisms may be seen on unstained wet preparation

Surveillance in England and Wales

The effective management of infectious disease depends on good surveillance. This is as true for STIs as for any other infections.

Data on sexually transmitted infections are available from the KC60 returns. These record the number of initial contacts by diagnosis and sex, and are sent quarterly by all genito-urinary medicine (GUM) clinics to the CDSC on behalf of the Department of Health. Male patients who are thought to have acquired their infections through homosexual contact and age group are recorded for selected infections.

In their current form, since clinics do not service defined catchment populations, this aggregated data is of limited use below regional or national level. However the individual patient data that is aggregated to produce the KC60 returns is collected by each clinic on the clinic computer system and is available for surveillance purposes. This includes area of residence and ethnic group.

A second data source is laboratory reports to the CDSC of positive laboratory isolations of genital *Chlamydia*, herpes simplex and gonorrhoea.

Surveillance data are reported by CDSC in the sexually transmitted disease quarterly reports and there is an annual supplement of KC60 data (*CDR Weekly*: http://www.phls.co.uk). *Communicable Disease and Public Health* publishes regular articles on the epidemiology of STIs.

STI surveillance data can also be found at the Internet: Public Health Laboratory Service (http://www.phls.co.uk), Eurosurveillance Weekly (http://www.eurosrv.org), Morbidity and Mortality Weekly Report (http://www.cdc.gov) and the World Health Organization's Weekly Epidemiological Record (http://www.who.ch/wer/wer_home.htm).

The most recent data from GUM clinics in England demonstrate large and significant increases in cases of acute STIs in most regions. Between 1996 and 1997 total GUM clinic STI diagnoses in England rose by 9% and between 1997 and 1998 they rose by a further 5%. These rises follow similar substantial rises between 1995 and 1996 and were most pronounced amongst teenagers and homosexual and bisexual men (Table 3.25.1). London and the rest of the Thames regions have the greatest burden of STIs and the epidemiology of most STIs in those regions is influenced more by sex between men than in other areas. The continued growth in the numbers of acute STIs is occurring despite sexual health education and intervention programmes and reinforces the need to redouble efforts to improve sexual health and collect good quality STI surveil-lance data.

Prevention and control of STIs

The source of STIs is controlled by early diag-nosis of cases of infection and prompt effective treatment. Contacts are actively followed up and offered diagnostic testing and prophylac-tic antibiotics if appropriate.

All pregnant women are screened for syphilis by serology and increasingly there is opportunistic screening for genital chlamydia infection in women at increased risk.

Genito-urinary medicine (GUM) clinics are open access clinics that offer free, confidential services and treatment for all sexually trans-mitted infections (STI) including HIV infec-tion. A national network of GUM clinics was created as a result of the Venereal Disease Reg-ulations 1916.

Transmission of STIs is controlled by promoting safer sexual behaviour, includ-ing condom use, through education and information.

Vaccines are not available for the major STIs but susceptible individuals and populations may be offered hepatitis A and hepatitis B im-munization.

Table 2.8.1 Non-infectious causes of jaundice

Drug reaction (paracetamol, phenothiazines, alcohol)
Recent anaesthetic
Haemolysis (e.g. due to G6PD deficiency, sickle cell disease)
Physiological (in the neonate)
Toxin causing liver damage
Primary biliary cirrhosis
Gallstones
Biliary or pancreatic cancer
Genetic disorders

Table 2.8.2 Infectious causes of jaundice

Common
Viral hepatitis
Malaria

Uncommon
Acute infections of the biliary system (cholecystitis, cholangitis, pancreatitis)
Leptospirosis
Epstein–Barr virus infection
Cytomegalovirus
Yellow fever

2.8 Jaundice

Differential diagnosis

The differential diagnosis of jaundice includes many infectious and non-infectious causes. In a previously well patient with acute onset of jaundice, the most likely cause is viral hepatitis.

Viral hepatitis can be clinically distin-guished from other causes of jaundice by the presence of a prodrome of fever, anorexia, nau-sea and abdominal discomfort. The liver is often enlarged and tender. There may be a his-tory of travel to endemic areas, contact with a case or high-risk behaviour. Bilirubin is pre-sent in the urine, and serum transaminase levels (ALT, AST) are markedly elevated.

In viral hepatitis, the fever usually subsides once jaundice has developed. If the fever persists, other liver infections should be considered, such as Epstein–Barr virus or leptospirosis.

Laboratory investigations to distinguish be-tween the different types of viral hepatitis and other liver infections are covered in the rel-evant chapters.

Prevention and control

General measures for the prevention of gastrointestinal infection (Chapter 2.2) and blood-borne virus infection (Chapter 2.11) will help prevent jaundice due to viral hepati-tis. Malaria prophylaxis is covered in Chapter

3.46. Vaccines are available for hepatitis A (Chapter 3.29), hepatitis B (Chapter 3.30) and yellow fever (Chapter 3.86).

Response to a case

Determine whether infectious or non-infectious cause. No specific public health measures are needed for non-infectious causes. For infectious causes, specific measures will usually be indicated, depending upon the causal agent. Assume blood, body fluids and (until one week after start of jaundice) stools are infectious until cause known.

Investigation of a cluster and response to an outbreak

Investigate to determine whether infectious or non-infectious cases. For non-infectious cases, consider common toxic exposure. For infectious cases, the response will depend upon the causal agent.

2.9 Infection in the immunocompromised

Ageing, improved medical care, new treatments and new pathologies mean that it is increasingly common for patients to have impaired immunity. Infection should be considered in any immunocompromised person who becomes unwell; the risk of infection by both common and unusual pathogens is increased and infection may present in unusual ways in unusual sites.

Particular opportunistic infections may be associated with specific immune defects, such as invasive aspergillosis with neutropenia and intracellular organisms with T-cell defects. Therefore knowledge of the aetiology of the immune defect may guide preventative measures, investigation and therapy.

Treating infection in the immunocompromised is highly specialized; this chapter concentrates upon issues that might be of concern to a public health specialist.

Epidemiology

Organism and syndrome(s)

Infections with common organisms usually respond to routine treatment. Of major concern is infection with antibiotic-resistant or unusual organisms that may not be recognized. Immunocompromised patients are often exposed to healthcare facilities, and to courses of antimicrobials, and are therefore at increased risk of infection with resistant organisms.

The major public health role is in the identification of risk, and ensuring systems are in place to minimize the risk of infection in the immunocompromised. This entails close liaison with clinical colleagues.

Activities can be considered by cause of compromise, or by preventative action.

Causes of immunosuppression

- Physiological: extremes of age.
- Impaired anatomical barriers: burns, catheters, intubation.
- Impaired cellular or host defence: genetic or acquired, underlying malignancy, chronic infection, immunosuppressive drugs.

Specific causes of immunosuppression and public health issues

Underlying conditions

HIV

Associated infections: *Pneumocystis*, TB, *Cryptosporidium*, CMV.

HIV-positive patients are particularly at risk when they associate with other immunocompromised patients in healthcare surroundings. Services should be organized to minimize transmission of likely pathogens, in particular TB. Outbreaks of resistant TB associated with healthcare have occurred.

Post splenectomy

Associated infections: capsulate bacteria, malaria.

Post splenectomy or as a consequence of hyposplenism, patients are at risk of infection from capsulate bacteria, particularly *S. pneumoniae*, *N. meningitidis*, *H. influenzae*. Asplenic children under 5, especially those with sickle cell anaemia or splenectomized for trauma, have an infection rate of over 10%. Most infections occur in the first two years following splenectomy, however, the increased risk of dying of serious infection is almost certainly lifelong.

Splenectomized patients and those with functional hyposplenism should receive (asplenia is not a contraindication to routine immunization):
• pneumococcal immunization;
• *Haemophilus influenzae* type b vaccine (if not already immune);
• conjugate meningococcal group C immunization;
• influenza immunization;
• prophylactic antibiotics are recommended for all children aged up to 16 (oral phenoxymethylpenicillin or an alternative).

Asplenic patients are at risk of severe malaria, so the importance of preventive measures should be stressed for travellers.

Patients should carry a card to alert health professionals to their risk of overwhelming infection. Splenectomized patients developing infection despite measures must be given a systemic antibiotic and urgently admitted to hospital.

Prevention of infection in the immunocompromised

Prevention through immunization

• Pneumococcal infection;
• *H. influenzae;*
• influenza;
• meningcococcal C.

Prevention through prophylaxis

• Pneumocystis (oral trimethoprim/ sulphamethoxazole);
• malaria chemoprophylaxis;
• penicillin in hyposplenism.

Prevention through managing the environment

Boiling water: the Bouchier Report of 1998 on *Cryptosporidium* in water supplies clarifies which groups are at particular risk of *Cryptosporidium* infection. Patients with T-cell deficiency are advised to boil their drinking water. This group includes:
• HIV-positive patients with a low T-cell count.
• Children with severe combined immunodeficiency (SCID).
• Others with specific T-cell deficiencies.

Fungal infection and building work

Outbreaks of fungal infection have been associated with building work occurring close to healthcare areas which immunocompromised patients have frequented. Consideration to relocating services should be made if major building work is undertaken.

Reducing exposure

Treatment of TB and HIV-positive: examining the geographical layout of services so that infected and at-risk patients do not come into contact.

Avoid healthcare staff who are zoster susceptibles working with immunocompromised individuals, or vaccinate non-immune healthcare workers.

Travel advice

Immunocompromised patients are at increased risk of travel-related infection. Asplenic patients are at risk of severe malaria, patients with AIDS are at risk from GI parasites. Advising such patients requires detailed knowledge of the epidemiology of disease in the area they are planning to visit and the underlying cause of immunosuppression.

Laboratory diagnosis

A search for infection, including blood and urine cultures and a chest X-ray, will be necessary as soon as an immunocompromised patient spikes a fever. Opportunistic organisms that do not cause disease in the immunocompetent must be sought but it should be remembered that immunocompromised patients are most often infected by common pathogens, so these should be considered first.

Surveillance

All units treating significant numbers of immunocompromised patients should have ongoing surveillance of infection in place, and be aware of the risk of outbreaks in the patient population.

Investigation of a cluster

Clusters of infection in the immunocompromised should be investigated with urgency. A cluster suggests a group of vulnerable people exposed to a common source, for example, fungal spores following building work near a ward containing immunocompromised patients, or exposure on a unit for HIV-positive individuals to a case of open TB.

Control of an outbreak

Rapid removal of any source. If necessary closure of a ward if environmental contamination is feared.

2.10 Eye and skin infections

Eye infections

The conjunctivae and outer structures of the eye are prone to infection with a range of micro-organisms. Such infections are common and affect all age groups. It is estimated that trachoma affects 600 million people throughout the world, and 10–20 million are blinded by it. Overcrowding, lack of water for washing and an abundant fly population are risk factors. The wearing of contact lenses may predispose to infection with the *Acanthamoeba*. Pain, redness and purulent discharge are the main features of acute conjunctivitis.

Infection of the deeper layers of the eye may result from trauma or local or blood-borne spread. The fetal eye may be infected *in utero*. Clinical features include pain, swelling, blindness, cataract and retinitis.

Laboratory investigation

Microscopy and culture of samples of conjunctival fluid or pus are the main methods of laboratory diagnosis.

Prevention and control

- Promote personal hygiene, especially hand and face washing.
- Minimize hand–eye contact.
- Do not share personal items, especially eye make-up, eye-droppers, etc.
- Ensure infection control best practice in healthcare settings.
- Wear eye protection in industrial premises as appropriate.
- Report outbreaks in schools and institutions to public health authorities.

Response to a case

- Confirm diagnosis in the laboratory wherever possible.
- Treat promptly if a bacterial cause is suspected.
- Advise on measures to minimize spread to others.

Response to a cluster

- Strict application of measures to prevent further spread.
- Consider exclusion of affected persons from school or work.

Table 2.10.1 Causes of eye infections

Conjunctivitis	
Viral conjunctivitis	Adenoviruses serotypes 3 and 7
	Adenoviruses types 8, 11 or 17 (epidemic keratoconjunctivitis)
	Enterovirus type 70, Coxsackievirus type A24 (acute haemorrhagic conjunctivitis)
	Measles virus
Bacterial conjunctivitis	*S. pneumoniae, S. aureus, S. pyogenes, H. influenzae, N. gonorrhoea*
Chlamydia trachomatis conjunctivitis	Inclusion conjunctivitis (TRIC conjunctivitis): serovars D–K
	Trachoma: serovars A–C
Ophthalmia neonatorum	*C. trachomatis, S. aureus, N. gonorrhoea*
Loiasis	Caused by *Loa loa*, a filarial nematode. The adult worms migrate through the subcutaneous tissues including the conjunctiva producing itching, pain and oedema
Periocular infections	
Stye (external hordeolum)	*S. aureus*
Acute chalazion (internal hordeolum)	
Blepharitis	
Phthiris pubis (crab lice)	
Acute or chronic dacryocystitis, inflammation of the lacrimal sac	*S. aureus* and *S. pneumoniae*
Preseptal cellulitis	Staphylococci and streptococci, *H. influenzae*
Orbital infections	
Acute infection of the orbit	*S. aureus, S. pyogenes, S. pneumoniae, H. influenzae*
Keratitis (inflammation of the cornea)	Viruses: Herpes simplex, Herpes zoster
	Bacteria: *S. pneumoniae, S. aureus*, various Gram-negative bacilli, particularly *Pseudomonas aeruginosa*
	Fungi: in the immunocompromised individual or in association with topical steroid usage
	Protozoa: *Acanthamoeba*
	Nematode: *Onchocerca volvulus*
Endophthalmitis	
Infection of the intraocular tissues	*S. pneumoniae, S. aureus, N. meningitidis*
	Fungi: *Candida albicans*
	Toxocara
	Toxoplasma
	Cytomegalovirus
	Rubella

Skin infections

Healthy intact skin is the body's first line of defence against pathogenic micro-organisms. Part of this defence depends on the skin's normal flora, a mixture of Gram-positive and Gram-negative bacteria.

Infection may follow a breach of intact skin, there may be blood-borne spread to the skin from a distant focus of infection or there may be toxin-mediated damage.

Skin infections affect people of all ages; risk factors are trauma, surface or nasal colonization with bacteria, diabetes, immunosuppression, oedema, lack of skin care and poor personal hygiene.

The features of skin infection include rash, swelling, pain, fever and ulceration and discharge. A wide range of infectious agents can cause skin infections (Table 2.10.2).

Laboratory investigation

Pus, vesicle fluid, tissue fluid, skin scrapings or biopsies may be submitted for microscopy, culture or histology. Systemic infections may be diagnosed serologically.

Prevention and control

• Prompt identification and treatment of cases if appropriate.
• Promote personal hygiene, especially handwashing, and discourage the communal use of personal items.
• Ensure infection control best practice in health care settings, including adherence to antibiotic policies.
• Report outbreaks in schools and institutions to public health authorities.

Response to a case

• Confirm diagnosis in the laboratory wherever possible.
• Treat promptly where appropriate.
• Advise on measures to minimize spread to others.

Response to a cluster

• Strict application of measures to prevent further spread.
• Consider exclusion of affected persons from school or work.

Table 2.10.2 Causes of skin infection

Bacterial	*Staphylococcus aureus*
	Streptococcus pyogenes
	Neisseria meningitidis
Mycobacterial	Leprosy
	Tuberculosis
Viral	Papilloma (wart)
	Molluscum contagiosum
	Orf
	Herpes simplex
	Varicella-zoster
	Coxsackie
	Parvovirus
Fungal	Ringworm
Parasitic	Leishmaniasis
	Schistosomiasis
	Scabies
	Tumbu fly

2.11 Blood-borne viral infections

Human immunodeficiency virus (Chapter 3.36), hepatitis B (Chapter 3.30) and hepatitis C (Chapter 3.31) are the main viruses of public health importance that are spread indirectly by the blood-borne route. These are covered in detail in individual chapters.

Preventing exposure in the health and social care workplace

Health and social care workers should adhere to safe working practices and work in a safe environment to prevent occupational exposure to blood-borne viruses. The general precautions recommended to prevent the spread of infection, including blood-borne infection, are listed in Chapter 1.2.

Further precautions relevant to blood-borne viruses:

1 Use a container approved to BS7320 to dispose of sharps. Do not re-sheath needles.

2 Protect eyes, mouth and nose from blood splashes. Personal protective clothing and equipment should be used as follows:

• Gloves: use when there may be direct contact with body fluids, non-intact skin, or mucous membranes.

• Plastic aprons: use where contamination of clothing is possible.

• Impermeable gowns: use where there is likelihood of spillage of large volumes of blood or body fluids.

• Protective eyewear and masks: goggles or visor and mask should be worn where there is a risk of blood or body fluid splashing into the face.

3 Ensure that all at-risk staff are vaccinated against hepatitis B (see Chapter 3.30).

4 Take action when there is a sharps injury or blood splash incident (see below).

• Clean up spillages of blood or body fluids, **however small**, immediately.

• Open wounds must be covered with a waterproof dressing. Staff with fresh open cuts or active dermatitis of the hands and arms should if possible avoid clearing up blood spillages.

• Wear disposable non-seamed latex or vinyl gloves and an apron.

• If there is broken glass never pick it up with your fingers, even if wearing gloves. Use a paper or plastic scoop and dispose in the sharps box.

• For a small spillage, cover with chlorine-releasing granules to soak up the spillage. Do not use on urine since chlorine may be released.

• For large spillage, the spill should be soaked up first with paper towels. Sodium hypochlorite (10000 p.p.m. available chlorine) should then be poured on to the area and left for 10 minutes.

• As the application of sodium hypochlorite may discolour carpets, these spillages should be cleaned with warm soapy water or carpet cleaner and dried. Carpets are best avoided in areas where spillages are likely. Splashes of blood or body fluid on to the skin should be washed off immediately with soap and water. If a mop and bucket are used, these should be washed with detergent and water after use and stored dry.

• Place used paper towels in plastic sack for disposal as clinical waste.

• Rinse area with hot water and detergent.

• Dispose of gloves and apron as clinical waste.

• Wash hands.

5 Dispose of contaminated waste safely.

• Clinical waste is defined as waste of human or animal origin or waste arising from healthcare activities which may prove hazardous or cause infection in any person coming into contact with it.

• Healthcare workers who produce waste are bound by a duty of care imposed by Section 34 of the Environmental Protection Act 1990 and the Environmental Protection (Duty of Care) Regulations 1991 in the UK.

• The waste producer should conduct a local risk assessment to determine which wastes are clinical and whether they are potentially infectious. This determines the most appropriate storage, collection, transport and disposal arrangements for the waste. If the risk assessment identifies the need to treat the waste as clinical waste, the waste must be placed into the correct storage container and the appropriate waste disposal stream.

• Sharps must go into an approved container (UN 3291, BS 7320).

• Infectious waste should go into a UN-approved container (UN 3291) or yellow plastic bag.

• Yellow plastic bags and waste containers may be returned to base by the staff member. If a large quantity of waste is produced then arrangements should be made for the local authority or some other contractor to provide a clinical waste collection service.

• Waste collection authorities have a duty to collect household waste but they have to be requested to collect clinical waste and they can make a charge for this.

• In the domestic setting the healthcare worker should instruct the householder on the most appropriate disposal technique and provide an initial supply of storage containers, sharps boxes or yellow bags if appropriate.

• Some waste arising from a healthy individual may be treated as household waste including sanitary towels, tampons, condoms, nappies, stoma bags, incontinence pads, pregnancy kits, etc. This noninfectious waste may be disposed of with household waste but it should be wrapped before it is placed in a refuse sack or dustbin.

• Urine and faeces and other body fluids can be safely disposed of down the toilet into the sewage system. A bedpan washer, disinfector or macerator can be used.

6 Know how to deal with soiled linen.

• When handling soiled linen, a plastic apron should be worn and guidelines issued by the laundry contractor should be followed. Generally linen should be stored in a closed plastic bag before being machinewashed using a cold prewash followed by a hot wash at the highest temperature setting.

• Water-soluble bags should be used if they are available, inside a secondary colour-coded bag (usually red) for dispatch to the laundry.

• Heat-labile material may require a chemical disinfectant added to the rinse cycle.

7 Clean, disinfect and sterilize equipment as appropriate.

• Wherever practical, use disposable items. For other items, cleaning with soap and water will be adequate in most circumstances.

• Household bleach is usually supplied at a strength of 100000 parts per million (p.p.m.) free chlorine. Add one part bleach to nine parts cold water in order to make a solution for disinfecting blood and body fluids (10000 p.p.m.). For general use, such as disinfecting work surfaces, a 1000-p.p.m. solution of bleach is adequate (i.e. 1 in 100 dilution of household bleach).

• Undiluted Milton is equivalent to a strength of 10000 p.p.m. For general use, such as disinfecting work surfaces, a 1 in 10 (1000 p.p.m.) dilution is adequate.

• All dilutions become ineffective with time and should be freshly made up every day.

8 Know how to handle laboratory specimens safely.

• Aprons and gloves should be worn when taking specimens. Eyewear should also be used if splashes are possible.

• Only staff who have been trained should take and handle specimens. Phlebotomy staff should not take blood from patients with HCV or HIV infection; this should be done by the medical staff requesting the investigation. Phlebotomy staff can take blood from patients with HBV infection provided they are known to be immune.

• If available and appropriate, Vacutainer equipment should be used.

• The patient should be appropriately restrained.

• A biohazard label should be used.

• All infectious substances that are sent by mail have to comply with UN 602 packaging requirements.

• Known HIV/HBV/HCV patients should not have blood glucose monitoring carried out using bedside blood glucose monitoring equipment.

Sharps injuries and blood splash incidents

The risk of HCV transmission after percutaneous exposure to infectious blood is 3%. This is intermediate between the risk of transmission of HBV (30%) and HIV (0.3%).

The PHLS Communicable Disease Surveillance Centre operates a surveillance scheme in England and Wales for healthcare workers who have been exposed to HIV, HBV or HCV during their work.

Action following a sharps injury, a blood splash or other exposure incident

Advice is often requested when someone has a blood contamination incident—for example, a stab with a needle or contamination of an open wound with blood where the source of the blood may not be known.

There is a risk of HBV transmission following an exposure incident, which depends on the nature of the exposure, the HBV status of the source and the HBV status of the recipient (see Table 3.30.3). At the present time in the UK the risk of other blood-borne viral infections such as HIV and HCV infection is very small.

The action to be taken is summarized as follows:

1 Follow recognized first aid procedures. The injured area should be encouraged to bleed and washed with soap and water. Contamination of eyes, nose and mouth should be flushed with water. Attend occupational health department (OHD), general practitioner or accident department as appropriate.

2 Wounds should be cleaned, sutured and dressed as appropriate.

3 Tetanus toxoid should be administered according to standard protocols if indicated.

4 Report to Occupational Health Department, line manager and record in incident book. If source is known to have confirmed HBV, HIV or HCV report to CDSC. In the UK a report may be required to be made to the health and safety authorities according to the Reporting of Incidents, Diseases and Dangerous Occurrences Regulations (RIDDOR).

5 Record details and assess significance of exposure. Significant exposures are penetration of skin by a sharp object contaminated by blood or other body fluid or contamination of eyes, inside of mouth or nose or non-intact skin by blood or **bloodstained** body fluid.

6 Give person accelerated course of hepatitis B immunization or reinforcing dose as appropriate. Human normal immunoglobulin (HNIG) should only be needed if source is known to be HBsAg-positive or the exposed person is a known vaccine non-responder.

7 If source is identifiable, assess HCV and HIV risk. If either is a possibility, with consent, consider testing source for anti-HCV and anti-HIV. Counselling and testing should not be carried out by the staff member who has sustained the injury. With consent, obtain blood sample from exposed person (5–10 mL serum) for storage at −70 °C for two years. Arrange follow up for exposed person. As a minimum the person should be tested for anti-HCV and anti-HIV after six months. Person should report any hepatitic illness. Occupationally acquired HCV infection should be reported to CDSC (or appropriate institution in other countries). Immunization is not available for HCV, and HNIG is not effective. Consider postexposure prophylaxis (PEP) with antiviral drugs if source known to be HIV-infected.

8 If source is not identifiable or not available for testing, reassure exposed person that transmission of HCV and HIV is unlikely.

For an exposure in the community Step 7 may be omitted.

Employment policies

At present there is no vaccine, passive immunization, or effective routine post-exposure treatment available to protect against hepatitis C infection. All staff undertaking exposure-prone procedures should be immunized against HBV and have their immune status confirmed. All other staff at risk of blood-borne infections should ensure that they are fully immunized against HBV.

Any employee found to be infected with a blood-borne viral infection should be offered confidential counselling and guidance on the likely cause of the disease, the possibility of treatment and any effect upon their work.

In the UK, guidelines for healthcare workers with blood-borne viral infections who carry out *exposure-prone procedures* (see Chapter 4.6) have been published. Advice on individual cases is also available.

There should be a policy which outlines the action that would be taken in the event of a worker who carries out exposure-prone procedures being deemed unfit to continue undertaking such procedures. The policy should address sick leave, re-deployment, assessment for treatment, re-training, and any necessary compensation or ill-health retirement package.

Education and training

During induction training all staff should be made aware of the risks of blood-borne viruses and the ways in which they are controlled. There should be an annual infection control update for all staff at risk.

Advice for people living with blood-borne viral infections

All persons found to be infected with a blood-borne virus should be considered potentially infectious and should be counselled concerning infectivity. The following advice should be given:

1 Keep cuts or grazes covered with a waterproof plaster until the skin has healed.

2 Avoid sharing your razor or toothbrush (or anything which might cut the skin or damage the gums and cause bleeding). Use your own towel and face cloth.

3 If you cut yourself, wipe up any blood with paper tissues and flush these down the toilet. Wipe any surfaces where blood has been spilt with household bleach diluted in cold water (1 part bleach to 9 parts water). Do not use this on your skin or on any fabrics. In these circumstances wash thoroughly with soap and water.

4 Tell any helpers that you are a carrier of a blood-borne virus and that blood precautions should be taken. If available they should wear plastic gloves. Otherwise they can use a towel or cloth to prevent them from getting blood on to their skin.

5 If your clothing is soiled with blood or other body fluids, wash them using a prewash and hot washing machine cycle.

6 Dispose of used tampons straight away by flushing down the toilet by burning or by putting in your rubbish after first sealing inside a plastic bag.

7 If you go for medical or dental treatment,

Table 2.11.1 Advice on sexual intercourse, pregnancy and birth

	HCV	HBV	HIV
Sexual intercourse	If you are in a stable relationship with one partner you may not feel the need to start using condoms, however it is advisable to avoid sexual intercourse during a menstrual period. Otherwise condom use should be encouraged and safe sex should continue to be promoted for the prevention of HIV and other sexually transmitted infections.	Condom use recommended until sexual partners are immunized against HBV and have had immunity confirmed.	Condom use recommended.
Pregnancy and birth	The risk of transmission from mother to child appears to be very low. At the present time there is no need to advise against pregnancy based on HCV status alone. Mothers who are viraemic should not breastfeed.	Newborn infants of HBV carrier mothers must start immunization at birth.	The risk of transmission from mother to child can be reduced by anti-viral treatment in pregnancy, caesarean section and avoiding breastfeeding.

tell your doctor or dentist you have a blood-borne viral infection.

8 Do not donate blood or carry an organ donor card.

9 Do not have acupuncture, tattooing, earpiercing or electrolysis.

10 If you are an injecting drug user do not share your works and dispose of used needles and syringes safely by putting them in a rigid container with a lid. If possible use a local needle exchange scheme. Return used works to the scheme in the special plastic sharps bin.

11 Sexual intercourse, pregnancy and birth: see Table 2.11.1.

12 If you have HCV infection you should limit weekly alcohol consumption to less than 21 units for women and 28 units for men.

13 Blood-borne viral infections are not infectious under normal school or work conditions. There is no need to stay away from school or work.

Section 3
Diseases

3.1 Amoebic dysentery

Infection by the protozoan parasite *Entamoeba histolytica* usually presents as an intestinal infection, which may include dysentery.

Suggested on-call action

- Exclude cases in high-risk groups for transmission of gastrointestinal infections (Box 2.2.1).
- If other non-travel related cases known to you or reporting laboratory/clinician, consult local outbreak plan.

Epidemiology

Although much more common in tropical countries, amoebiasis does occur in Europe: approximately 720 cases per annum are reported in England and Wales. Infection is most common in young adults and is unusual in preschool children, especially infants. Increased risk is reported in mental handicap institutions, amongst gay men and in travellers abroad.

Clinical features

Intestinal infection may be asymptomatic; an intermittent diarrhoea with abdominal pain; amoebic colitis presenting as bloody diarrhoea; and a fulminant colitis with significant mortality in the malnourished, pregnant, immunosuppressed or very young. Extraintestinal disease includes liver, lung and brain abscesses.

Laboratory confirmation

The diagnosis is confirmed by demonstrating either the trophozoites or cysts of *E. histolytica* on microscopy of very fresh stool samples. Three specimens are required to exclude amoebiasis. Many cysts are non-pathogenic (often called *E. dispar*) but morphologically indistinguishable from *E. histolytica*: immunological and isoenzyme ('zymodeme') differences can be used by reference laboratories to identify these organisms. Invasive disease may be diagnosed by serology.

Transmission

E. histolytica is predominantly spread by environmentally resistant cysts excreted in human faeces. Transmission may occur via contaminated water or food, or direct faeco–oral contact. Cysts resist standard water chlorination. Acute cases pose only limited risk.

Pathogenesis

The incubation period is usually 2–4 weeks but a range of a few days to years has been reported.

The infectious period depends upon the excretion of cysts in the stool and may last several years. In acute dysentery only trophozoites are passed in the stool: these die within minutes in the environment.

Recovered patients appear to be immune to reinfection in almost all cases.

Prevention

- Avoid faecal contamination of water supplies, plus adequate water treatment (e.g. filtration).
- Good personal (e.g. handwashing) and food hygiene.
- Care with food and water for travellers in developing countries.

Surveillance

Cases should be reported to the local public health department: notify as 'dysentery' in UK. Laboratory isolates should also be reported to national surveillance systems.

Response to a case

- Exclude cases in groups at increased risk of spreading infection (Box 2.2.1) until 48 h after first normal stool.

• If no history of travel abroad, then obtain detailed food history for the period 2–4 weeks before onset, including drinking water.
• Enteric precautions. Hygiene advice to case and household.
• Screen household contacts. Discuss with microbiologist further investigation of positives. Consider treatment for those with prolonged excretion of pathogenic cysts, especially if in risk group for spreading infection.

Investigation of a cluster

• Check to ensure not due to travel abroad: inform relevant national centre if associated with particular country.
• Organize further testing to ensure that reported cases have infection with pathogenic *E. histolytica*.
• For symptomatic cases, obtain detailed food and water consumption history for period 2–4 weeks before onset of symptoms. Check home/work/travel against water supply areas.
• Look for links with institutions with potential for faeco–oral spread, e.g. young adults with learning difficulties or camps with poor hygiene facilities.
• Consider transmission between gay men.

Control of an outbreak

• Rarely a problem in developed countries. Response will depend upon source identified.
• Enteric precautions and treatment of cases and carriers. Exclusion of those in risk groups (Box 2.2.1).
• Sanitary disposal of faeces, handwashing, food hygiene and regular cleaning of toilet and kitchen areas.

Suggested case-definition for an outbreak

Demonstration of trophozoites **or** diarrhoea and demonstration of cysts.

3.2 Anthrax

Anthrax is a potentially serious infection caused by *Bacillus anthracis*, an organism which forms spores that may survive for many years. There are concerns that it is an agent which might be used in a biological attack.

Suggested on-call action

• Ensure case admitted and treated.
• Identify likely source of exposure and other individuals who may have been exposed.
• Ensure exposed individuals are clinically assessed.

Epidemiology

Anthrax is a zoonosis, acquired from contact with infected herbivores or their products, which has been eliminated from the UK and most of northern Europe. There are rare sporadic cases in the UK, usually resulting from occupational exposure, in particular to animal carcasses, hides, hair and wool. There is occasional concern about renovating old buildings where animal hair may have been used in the construction, although these have not been associated with cases.

Anthrax is endemic in many parts of the world, such as the Middle East, Africa and the former Soviet Union. In these areas it is usually a disease of rural herdsmen. Imported infection is rare.

Clinical features

The clinical manifestations are dependent upon the route of infection.

Cutaneous anthrax (over 90% of cases): infection is through the skin. Over a few days a sore which begins as a pimple grows, ulcerates and forms a black scab, around which are purplish vesicles. There may be associated oedema. Systemic symptoms include rigors, headache and vomiting. The sore is

been linked to the method of making fried rice employed in Chinese restaurants. The rice is boiled, allowed to drain at room temperature (to avoid clumping), stored and then flash-fried at insufficient temperature to destroy preformed heat-stable toxin. Attack rates of near 100% have been reported from such outbreaks.

Other reported food vehicles include pasta dishes, vanilla sauce, cream, meatballs, boiled beef, barbecue chicken and turkey loaf. Attack rates of 50–75% are reported for these outbreaks.

Nosocomial infection and cases in intravenous drug users have both been reported.

Pathogenesis

The incubation period is approximately 2–3h (range 1–6) for the vomiting illness and 8–12h (range 6–24) for the diarrhoeal syndrome.

B. cereus is not thought to be communicable between person and person.

The infectious dose is at least 10^3/g, with most outbreaks reporting contamination of 10^5/g.

People at increased risk of severe infection include those with sickle-cell disease, patients with intravascular catheters and those with immunosuppressive or debilitating medical conditions.

Prevention

Store cooked foods at above 60°C or below 10°C before re-heating or consumption. Limit storage time and reheat thoroughly.

Surveillance

• Infection by *Bacillus cereus* should be reported to local public health departments: in the UK, notify as 'Food Poisoning'.
• Report to regional and national surveillance systems.
• Ensure laboratories test for *B. cereus* when an increase in cases of vomiting or diarrhoea with abdominal pain is noted.

Response to a case

• Collect data on food consumption in 24h before onset of symptoms. Ask particularly about meals out of the house.
• Although secondary spread of *B. cereus* does not occur, it is sensible to exclude risk groups with diarrhoea or vomiting until 48h after these symptoms cease. Microbiological clearance is not necessary before return.
• No need to screen contacts unless as part of an outbreak investigation.

Response to a cluster

• Discuss further investigation, e.g. serotyping and toxin production, with microbiologist.
• Undertake hypothesis-generating study covering food histories, particularly restaurants, social functions and other mass catering arrangements.

Control of an outbreak

• Identify and rectify faults with temperature control in food preparation processes.

Suggested case-definition for an outbreak

Clinical. Either:
• vomiting occurring 1–6h *or*
• diarrhoea occurring 6–24h
after exposure to potential source.

Confirmed: as above, plus toxin-producing *B. cereus* cultured from stool or vomit.

Box 3.3.1 *Bacillus subtilis—licheniformis* **group**

Recently recognized food-borne pathogens transmitted via inadequate post-cooking temperature control of foods such as meat or vegetable pastry products, cooked meat or poultry products, bakery products, sandwiches and ethnic meat/seafood dishes.

B. subtilis causes a predominantly emetic illness with an incubation of 10 minutes to 14 hours (median = 2.5 hours) and *B. licheniformis* a predominantly diarrhoeal illness with incubation 2–14 hours (median 8 hours). *B. amyloliquifacians* and *B. pumilis* are rarely reported.

Investigation and control measures are similar to *B. cereus*.

3.4 Botulism

Botulism is caused by a neurotoxin produced by *Clostridium botulinum*. In north and west Europe its main significance is as a rare cause of food-borne infection with a potentially high mortality: one suspected case warrants immediate investigation.

Suggested on-call action

A suspected case of botulism should be viewed as an emergency for investigation.

- Ensure case admitted to hospital.
- Obtain food history as a matter of urgency.
- Obtain suspect foods.
- Identify others at risk.
- Inform appropriate authorities (e.g. CDSC and Food Standards Agency).

More details in 'response to a case' section.

Epidemiology

Only four cases were notified in England and Wales in the period 1990–99, although in 1989 an outbreak affecting 27 people occurred. Reported cases of botulism are more common in Italy (40 cases per annum) and Germany (15 cases per annum). The age, sex and ethnic distribution of cases will usually reflect the consumption patterns of the implicated foods.

Clinical features

The neurotoxin classically causes acute bilateral cranial neuropathies manifesting as a dry mouth, difficulty in swallowing, double vision, slurred speech and blurred vision. Symmetrical descending muscle weakness may follow, affecting upper and then lower limbs and causing shortness of breath with risk of respiratory failure. There may be initial vomiting or diarrhoea followed by constipation. There is usually no fever or sensory loss. Mortality of up to 10% is reported.

C. botulinum may also cause infant (intestinal) botulism and wound botulism, both of which also produce a flaccid paralysis.

Laboratory confirmation

The toxin may be detected in serum, faeces, vomit, gastric fluid or food. The organism may also be cultured from faeces, gastric fluid and food. The aid of the relevant reference laboratory should be enlisted and suspect foods and clinical specimens sent immediately by courier: in England and Wales this is the Food Safety Microbiology Laboratory at the Central Public Health Laboratory. As *C. botulinum* is ubiquitous in the environment, any isolate in food should be shown to be of the same 'cultural group' or produce the same toxin type as the cases. Toxin types A, B and F are mainly associated with human disease, with type B being the most common in Europe. It may take up to eight days for reliable negative results to be available.

Infant botulism may occasionally be caused by *C. baratii* or *C. butyricum*.

Transmission

Illness results from the ingestion of preformed toxin. Although boiling inactivates the toxin, spores may resist 100 °C for many hours. These may multiply (producing toxin) when conditions are favourable, i.e. anaerobic, above pH 4.6 and at room temperature (usually 10–50 °C, but in some cases as low as 3 °C). These conditions occur in underprocessed foods such as home-cured hams or sausages, and foods contaminated after canning and bottling, e.g. canned salmon in the UK and bottled vegetables in Italy. The contaminated food may be consumed directly or used as an ingredient for another product. *C. botulinum* spores are ubiquitous in the environment and can be found in dust, soil, untreated water and the digestive tracts of animals and fish. Toxin type E is particularly associated with fish products.

Pathogenesis

The incubation period is usually 12–36 h but extremes of 2 h to 10 days are reported. In general, the shorter the incubation period the higher the ingested dose and the more severe the disease.

Although demonstrable in the faeces of cases, botulism is not communicable from person to person.

The dose of toxin needed to cause symptoms is very low, with illness resulting from nanogram quantities of ingested toxin.

There appears to be no acquisition of immunity to botulinum toxin, even after severe disease. Repeated illness is well recognized.

Prevention

• Care with commercial or home canning processes.
• Avoid consumption from food containers that appear to bulge (possible gas from anaerobic organisms). Avoid tasting potentially spoilt food.
• Refrigeration of incompletely processed foods. Boiling for 10 minutes before consumption would inactivate toxin in home-canned foods.
• High index of clinical suspicion and urgent investigation and response to cases.

Surveillance

Botulism is statutorily notifiable in all EU countries: in the UK clinicians should notify clinical cases as 'suspected food poisoning' to the CCDC for urgent investigation.

Laboratories should report positive toxin or culture results from patients to the relevant national centre as a matter of urgency.

Response to a case

• Clinicians or laboratories should report suspected cases immediately to the relevant public health officer for urgent investigation: in England and Wales this is the CCDC.
• Take urgent food history from case or, if not possible, other reliable informant (e.g. spouse). Take details of all foods consumed in five days before illness. Ask specifically about any canned foods or preserved foods.
• Obtain any leftovers of any foods eaten in last five days, including remains from uncollected domestic waste and unopened containers from the same batch. This prevents further consumption and allows storage under refrigeration by the laboratory in case later testing appropriate.
• Organize testing of foods at highest suspicion (e.g. canned food eaten 12–36 h before onset) with reference laboratory.
• Inform appropriate national authority: in England and Wales, inform CDSC of all cases and inform Food Standards Agency if commercial food product suspected.
• Case-finding: any other suspected cases in local hospitals or laboratories or known to national centre? Compare food histories if so.
• Ensure case admitted to hospital for investigation and treatment, and that others exposed to suspect food informed and assessed. If indi-

cated, arrange for supply of botulinum anti-toxin to clinician in charge of case.
• No exclusions required for cases or contacts if well enough to work.

Investigation of a cluster

• Treat individual cases as indicative of a significant public health risk and investigate as above.
• Compare food histories if more than one case. Specifically ask *each* case about *each* food reported by all other cases.
• Organize laboratory testing of *any* food reported by more than one case.
• Check preparation details of any food reported by more than one case to see if anaerobic conditions could have been created for any component and/or it was stored at room temperature after cooking.
• Remember, as well as canned or bottled produce, unexpected food vehicles have been reported from recent incidents, including sautéed onions (kept under butter), hazelnut yogurt (canned purée used in preparation), baked potatoes (kept in foil) and honey.

Control of outbreak

• Identify and remove any implicated food.
• If commercially produced food, organize recall of product: in the UK contact the Food Standards Agency, to activate the Food Hazard Warning System.

Suggested case-definition for use in outbreak

Confirmed: clinically compatible case with demonstration of botulinum toxin in blood, faeces, vomit or gastric aspirate.
Clinical: acute bilateral cranial neuropathy with symmetrical descending weakness.
Provisional: any three from dysphagia, dry mouth, diplopia, dysarthria, limb weakness, blurred vision or dyspnoea, in an alert, non-febrile patient with no sensory deficit. Review when clinical investigations complete.

Severe systemic illness relating to soft tissue inflammation in injecting drug users

In early summer 2000, severe infection with a high case fatality rate due to toxin producing *Clostridium novyi* type A was reported in injecting drug users who had injected heroin in Glasgow and other parts of the UK and Ireland.

On-call action

Advise on appropriate laboratory investigation using advice notes available from PHLS (or other national agency).

Epidemiology

Those affected were injecting drug users who had injected heroin intramuscularly or subcutaneously. Thirty-eight cases and 17 deaths were reported from Scotland alone between April and June 2000. *C. novyi* is well known as a cause of severe infection in domestic animals.

Clinical features

The illness is characterized by local inflammation at an injection site, which is followed by hypotension and circulatory collapse. There is a very high white blood cell count. Cases usually have a temperature of less than 40°C and may look and feel quite well before deteriorating dramatically over a period of a few hours.

Laboratory confirmation

Blood and tissue cultures yield multiple organisms including group A streptococcus, *Staphylococcus aureus*, *Clostridium* species and *Bacillus* species. The definitive cause appears to be toxin-producing *Clostridium novyi* type A, an anaerobic spore-forming organism, although in a number of cases *Clostridium perfringens* was found.

Transmission

C. novyi type A is found in soil and animal faeces. Spores may contaminate batches of illicit heroin and can survive preparation for injection including mixing with citric acid and heating. When injected into tissues or muscle rather than intravenously, the anaerobic conditions allow multiplication and the production of a toxin that enters the circulation causing damage to vital organs.

Pathogenesis

The incubation period is unknown. The infection is not spread from person to person.

Prevention

Injecting drug users should be advised:
- smoke heroin instead of injecting;
- if injecting, inject into a vein do not inject into muscle or under skin;
- don't share needles, syringes with other drug users;
- use as little citric acid as possible to dissolve the heroin;
- if swelling, redness, or pain develops at an injection site seek prompt medical attention.

Surveillance

Public health departments may learn of cases from the local intensive care unit, consultant microbiologist, infectious disease consultant or staff of community drug services. Cases should be reported to national authorities (e.g. CDSC). An enhanced surveillance system was temporarily set up in the UK in 2000.

Response to a case

Drug injectors who develop swelling, pain and redness at an injection site should seek immediate medical attention. Surgical debridement and early treatment with antibiotics active against anaerobes (penicillin, metronidazole, clindamycin) may be life-saving.

Investigation of a cluster

Sudden death is not uncommon in drug users. All possible cases should be compared to the case definition (see below). Cases of infection should be investigated in the usual way. Staff of community drug services may be able to assist. Enquiries should be made about sources of heroin, method of injecting, use of citric acid and other users who may be affected.

Control of an outbreak

The CCDC with drug services staff should alert injectors that contaminated heroin is circulating and advise on steps that can be taken to prevent infection.

Case-definition

An IDU admitted to hospital or found dead with soft tissue inflammation (abscess, cellulitis, fasciitis, or myositis) at an injection site *and* either severe systemic toxicity (total peripheral white blood cell count $>30 \times 10^9$/L and sustained systolic pressure <90 mmHg despite fluid resuscitation) or evidence at necropsy of a diffuse toxic or infectious process, including pleural effusion and soft tissue oedema or necrosis at an injection site.

3.5 Brucellosis

Bacteria of the genus *Brucella* cause brucellosis (undulant fever, Malta fever, Mediterranean fever), which may present as an acute febrile disease or a chronic illness.

Suggested on-call action

None usually necessary.

Epidemiology

About 500 000 cases of human brucellosis are reported worldwide annually; up to a third of infections may be unrecognized. Fewer than 20 cases have been reported in England and Wales in each of the recent years. *Brucella melitensis* in sheep and goats remains the most important source of brucellosis. Farmers, veterinarians and abattoir workers are at particular risk of acquiring disease.

Brucellosis has been eradicated in much of northern Europe and most cases are acquired abroad. It remains common in the Mediterranean, Arabian Gulf, Latin America, Africa, and parts of Asia.

Clinical features

About half the recognized cases present with an acute, often severe, systemic febrile illness, sometimes associated with cough, arthralgia or testicular pain. Others present with localized suppuration, often involving bones or joints, particularly the spine. Splenomegaly and lymphadenopathy occur in about 15% of cases. Chronic disease may last for years, with non-specific features of fatigue, malaise and little or no fever. Neuro-psychiatric features may predominate.

Laboratory confirmation

Routine: Definitive diagnosis is provided by culture of *Brucella* from blood, bone marrow, or pus. However, the yield is often poor. The laboratory should be prepared to prolong culture, which may take 10 days or longer. Bone marrow culture produces the highest yield and may remain positive for some days after antimicrobial chemotherapy starts.

Reference: Serology using agglutination tests remains the mainstay of diagnosis. The 2-mercaptoethanol agglutination, Coombs test and ELISA are in use. Interpretation of results is difficult. Sensitivity in chronic infection is poor. Serologic tests have to be interpreted in the light of clinical data and the local prevalence.

Transmission

Brucellosis is a zoonotic disease. *B. melitensis* is associated with goats and sheep, *B. abortus* with cattle and *B. suis* with pigs (occasionally acquired from dogs, deer, elk). Transmission is either by direct contact with infected animals or tissues (blood, urine, aborted fetuses, placenta), or following consumption of contaminated milk or milk products. Airborne infection in stables, laboratories and abattoirs has also been described.

Pathogenesis

The incubation period is 5–60 days. Presentation of the chronic form, or as bone or joint disease, may take very much longer.

There is no person-to-person spread. The duration of acquired immunity is uncertain.

Prevention

The prevention of human disease is dependent on the control of brucellosis in the animal population. Mass testing, with slaughter of infected herds, has virtually eliminated endemic brucellosis in N. Europe, USA, Israel and Japan. A vaccine is available for cattle but is unsuitable for human use.

Pasteurization of milk will diminish the risk to populations in endemic areas.

Surveillance

Brucellosis is a notifiable disease in many countries. In England and Wales it is statutorily notifiable if occupationally acquired. Cases should be reported to public health authorities on suspicion, so that steps can be taken to identify the source.

Response to a case

Individual cases should be investigated to determine the source of infection. The authorities in the country in which the infection is believed to have been acquired should be informed. If the case has not been abroad, possible animal exposure should be sought.

Others who may have been exposed should be offered serological investigation.

Investigation of a cluster

As cases seen in N. Europe are imported, a cluster usually results from a common exposure at a single point. Occasionally the source may be difficult to identify if it is sold widely in an endemic area, through markets or small traders.

Control of an outbreak

The mainstay of control is the identification and eradication of infected livestock.

Suggested case-definition for an outbreak

Clinical: an acute illness characterized by fever, night sweats, undue fatigue, anorexia, weight loss, headache, and arthralgia.

Confirmed: clinical case with isolation of *Brucella* spp. from a clinical specimen, or demonstration by immunofluorescence of *Brucella* spp. in a clinical specimen, or fourfold or greater rise in *Brucella* agglutination titre between acute and convalescent serum specimens obtained at least 2 weeks apart.

3.6 *Campylobacter*

Campylobacter species cause diarrhoeal and systemic illnesses in humans and animals, and are the most commonly identified cause of infectious intestinal disease in developed countries. Although food-borne outbreaks are rarely identified, occasional large outbreaks due to contaminated milk or water may occur.

Suggested on-call action

- Exclude symptomatic cases in high risk groups (Box 2.2.1).
- If you or reporting clinician/microbiologist aware of potentially linked cases, consult outbreak control plan.

Epidemiology

Over 50000 laboratory-confirmed cases are reported annually in England and Wales (1997–99), although true community incidence is much higher, at an estimated 8.7 per 1000 population. The number of confirmed cases rose consistently between 1978 and 1998 (but not in 1999), partially due to improved ascertainment. Fortunately deaths are rare, with an estimated annual mortality of about 25 in the UK.

Infection occurs at all ages. Laboratory-reported cases are highest in children under five, show a secondary peak in young adults and decline slightly after 30 years of age. Amongst hospitalized patients, a third peak occurs in those aged 60–80. Positivity rates (number of confirmed *Campylobacter* infections per faecal specimen routinely submitted) are highest in 15 to 24-year-olds. There is a slight male excess in cases, particularly in young adults.

Campylobacter infections occur all year round, but there is a sharp peak in late spring and early summer, slightly earlier than that seen for *Salmonella* (Fig. 2.2.1), which then declines in late summer. This pattern is similar to that seen in most developed countries, although in Scandinavian countries, a second peak occurs after the winter holiday season, and outbreak-associated cases occur regularly in the spring and autumn in the United States.

Certain groups are at increased risk of *Campylobacter* infection due to increased exposure, including those with occupational contact with farm animals or meat, travellers to developing countries, gay men (including infection with other *Campylobacter* species) and family contacts of cases. *Campylobacter* infection is the most commonly identified cause of travellers' diarrhoea in Scandinavia and the second most common (after enteropathogenic *Escherichia coli*) in the UK. *Campylobacter* infection is hyperendemic in developing countries.

Clinical features

Campylobacter infection may vary from asymptomatic (about 25% of cases) to a severe disease mimicking ulcerative colitis or acute appendicitis. Most diagnosed cases present as acute enteritis with symptoms of diarrhoea, abdominal pain, fever, malaise and nausea. There may be a prodromal period of fever, headache, myalgia and malaise for approximately 12–24 h before onset of intestinal symptoms. Diarrhoea varies from loose stools to massive watery stools, with an average of 10 stools per day on the worst day. Nearly half of diarrhoeal cases also have blood in the stool, usually appearing on the second or third day. Abdominal pain may be prominent, is often described as constant or cramping rather than colicky, and may be relieved by defaecation.

Most cases settle after 2–3 days of diarrhoea and 80–90% within one week. Complications include reactive arthritis and Guillain–Barré syndrome.

Although difficult to distinguish from other causes of intestinal infection in individual cases, *Campylobacter* might be suspected as the cause of an outbreak due to the combination of abdominal pain and fever, and/or the presence of bloody diarrhoea or faecal leucocytes. However, *E. coli* O157 may cause a similar picture.

C. jejuni is responsible for most campylobacteriosis and *C. coli*, which may be less severe, for most of the rest. Other species such as *C. fetus* and *C. lari* are uncommon causes of diarrhoea in immunocompetent individuals, but can cause severe systemic illness in debilitated patients.

Laboratory confirmation

The mainstay of diagnosis is culture of the organism from faecal samples. Sensitivity is increased if samples are delivered to the laboratory on the day of collection; if this is not possible, samples should be either refrigerated or stored in a suitable transport medium. Culture of *Campylobacter* requires different conditions than for other enteric pathogens. Provisional results may be available after overnight incubation. Confirmation that the colonies are *Campylobacter* requires simple microscopy, but identification of the species depends upon latex agglutination (quick but costly) or biochemical tests (takes 1–2 days). Typing (e.g. serotype and/or genotype) of *C. jejuni* or *C. coli* may be available from reference laboratories if required for epidemiological purposes.

Microscopic examination of fresh diarrhoeal stool specimens may permit a rapid presumptive diagnosis, although sensitivity is only 60% compared to culture. *Campylobacter* is sometimes isolated from blood cultures in acute illness. Serological testing may be useful for retrospective diagnosis in countries like the UK with a low background rate of asymptomatic illness, although it does not differentiate between species, and cross-reactions occur. *Campylobacter* may be isolated from food or environmental specimens after enrichment culture.

Transmission

Campylobacteriosis is a zoonosis. It is found worldwide in the gastrointestinal tract of birds and mammals. Many animals develop a lifelong carrier state. Humans are not an important reservoir. Transmission from animals to man occurs predominantly via ingestion of faecally contaminated food or water. Campylobacters do not normally survive well in the environment as they are not tolerant of atmospheric oxygen levels, but their survival time increases as the temperature declines. They are also sensitive to drying, acid, high salt concentrations, chlorine and temperatures over 48 °C. The main routes of infection are:

Water-borne

Campylobacter excretion by wild birds causes contamination of open waters, and the organisms can survive for several months in water below 15°C. Large outbreaks have occurred from the use of untreated surface water in community water supplies. There may also be failures in 'treated' water supplies. Smaller outbreaks have occurred from the storage of water in open-topped tanks, which risk contamination by bird or rodent faeces. Deliberate or accidental ingestion of raw water can cause infection in those undertaking outdoor activities, e.g. trekkers, canoeists, etc.

Milk-borne

Campylobacters are commonly found in bulked raw milk samples. Infected animals may contaminate milk with faeces or excrete the organism via infected udders. *Campylobacter* can survive in refrigerated milk for three weeks and, when ingested, milk protects the organisms from the effect of gastric acid. Properly conducted pasteurization destroys the organism. Consumption of raw or inadequately pasteurized milk has caused large outbreaks of campylobacteriosis, and contributes to endemic infection.

Contamination of milk after pasteurization may also occur: in the UK, home delivery of milk in foil-topped bottles left on the doorstep is a temptation for birds such as magpies and jackdaws. The birds peck through these tops and contaminate the milk with *Campylobacter*. This may contribute to the early summer peak in infection in certain areas of the UK.

Poultry and other foods

In the majority of sporadic cases in developed countries, *Campylobacter* probably entered the kitchen on contaminated meat. Chicken carcasses are the most commonly contaminated, but pork, lamb and beef may also be affected. Contamination of these meats is usually with *C. jejuni*, with the exception of pork for which almost all are *C. coli*. The contamination can lead to illness in one of three ways: contamination of hands leading to accidental ingestion; inadequate cooking, especially of chicken, and a particular risk for barbecues; and cross-contamination of foods which will not be cooked, either via hands or via utensils such as knives and chopping boards. Fortunately *Campylobacter* does not multiply on food, which reduces the risk of large food-borne outbreaks. Normal cooking kills *Campylobacter*, and viable organisms are reduced tenfold by freezing, although freezing cannot be assumed to have made contaminated poultry safe.

Other food vehicles that have been reported include shellfish contaminated by sewage and mushrooms contaminated by soil.

Consumption of contaminated food and water is the likely cause of most cases of travel-associated campylobacteriosis.

Direct transmission from animals

Approximately 5% of cases in the UK are thought to occur through contact with infected pets. The most likely source is a puppy with diarrhoea or, less often, a sick kitten, and the most likely victim a young child. Transmission from asymptomatic pets has also been reported. Children may also be exposed to excreting animals on farm visits.

Occupational exposure to excreting animals or contaminated carcasses is also well recognized.

Person-to-person spread

Although the transmissibility of *Campylobacter* is low, person-to-person spread does occur. The index case is usually a small child who is not toilet-trained. The victim may be the person responsible for dealing with soiled nappies. Vertical transmission has also been documented.

Secondary spread has not been documented from asymptomatic food handlers or hospital staff.

Pathogenesis

The incubation period is inversely related to the dose ingested. Most cases occur within 2–5 days of exposure, with an average of three days, but a range of 1–10 days' incubation is possible.

The infectious period lasts throughout the period of infection, although once the acute illness is over the risk is very low. The average duration of excretion is 2–7 weeks, falling exponentially after the end of symptoms. Treatment with erythromycin usually terminates excretion, but it is rarely necessary to attempt to do this.

The infective dose is usually 10^4 organisms or above, but food vehicles which protect the organism against gastric acid (fatty foods, milk, water) can result in an infectious dose of as little as 500 organisms.

Immunity develops in response to infection, with antibodies that protect against symptomatic infection against the same strain and some cross-reacting strains. Patients with immune deficiencies or chronic illnesses may develop severe disease with *C. jejuni* or rarer pathogens such as *C. fetus*.

Prevention

- Chlorination of all drinking water supplies.
- Pasteurization of all milk for retail sale.
- Reducing infection in poultry and animal farms, particularly via water supplies, and other ways of introducing infection into poultry sheds.
- If unable to prevent contaminated meat leaving the slaughterhouse, gamma-irradiation of carcasses is effective, although not popular with the public.
- Adequate hygiene in commercial and domestic kitchens, particularly the avoidance of cross-contamination.
- Adequate cooking, especially of poultry.
- Protecting doorstep milk against birds.
- Handwashing after contact with faeces, nappies, meat or animals, including on farm visits.
- Conventional disinfectants are active against *Campylobacter*.
- Advice to travellers abroad.

Surveillance

Campylobacter infection is notifiable in the UK as suspected 'food poisoning', of which it is the most commonly reported cause. Laboratory isolates of *Campylobacter* species should be reported to local public health departments and the national surveillance system. However, most community infection caused by this organism is not reported to surveillance systems. A routinely available serotyping or genotyping scheme for all isolates is required.

Response to a case

- Enteric precautions for case (see Chapter 1.2).
- Exclude from work/nursery if in risk group (see Box 2.2.1) until 48h after first normal stool. No microbiological clearance necessary.
- Antibiotic treatment unnecessary unless severe or prolonged illness.
- Obtain history of food consumption (particularly chicken, unpasteurized milk or untreated water), travel and contact with animals.
- Investigate illness in family or other contacts.

Investigation of a cluster

- Discuss further microbiological investigations of epidemiological relevance with reference laboratory, e.g. serotyping or genotyping of strains to see if similar. Ensure that local laboratories retain isolates for further investigation.
- Obtain details from cases on:
  source of water supply (failure of treatment?);
  source of milk supply (failure of pasteurization?);
  functions attended (food-borne outbreak?);
  foods consumed, particularly consumption of undercooked chicken or, if *C. coli*, pork;
  bird-pecked milk;
  farm visits (age-distribution of cases may support this);
  occupation/school/nursery;
  travel abroad or in UK.

Control of an outbreak

- Exclude symptomatic cases if in risk groups, and ensure enteric precautions followed.
- Re-enforce food hygiene and handwashing. Look for ways in which food or water could have become contaminated.
- Prevent use of unpasteurized milk or untreated water.

Suggested case-definition for outbreak

Clinical: diarrhoea or any two symptoms from abdominal pain, fever, nausea, with onset 2–5 days after exposure in person with link to confirmed case.

Microbiological: isolate of outbreak strain from faeces or blood. As carriage of any type of *C. jejuni* in asymptomatic controls in the UK is only about 1%, but 25% of cases of *Campylobacter* infection are asymptomatic, clinical component of case-definition could be waived if appropriate typing results are available.

3.7 Chickenpox and shingles (varicella-zoster virus infections)

Chickenpox is a systemic viral infection with a characteristic rash caused by varicella-zoster virus (VZV), a herpes virus. Its public health importance lies in the risk of complications in immunosuppressed and pregnant patients, and the potential for prevention by vaccination. Herpes zoster (shingles) is caused by reactivation of latent VZV whose genomes live in sensory root ganglia of the brain stem and spinal cord.

Suggested on-call action

Assess clinical status of close contacts and arrange for VZIG if appropriate (see Box 3.7.1).

Epidemiology

Chickenpox occurs mainly in children, although the incidence in older children and adults is rising in the UK and some other Western countries. There are epidemics every 1–2 years, usually in winter/spring. More than 90% of adults have natural immunity. Herpes zoster occurs mainly in middle or older age.

Mortality is low, although it increases with age. There are an average of 26 deaths from chickenpox in England and Wales annually.

Clinical features

There is sometimes a prodromal illness of fever headache and myalgia. The diagnostic feature is the vesicular rash, which usually appears first on the trunk. They start as small papules, develop into clear vesicles which become pustules and then dry to crusts. There are successive crops of vesicles over several days. The hands and feet are relatively spared.

A more fulminant illness including pneumonia, hepatitis or disseminated intravascular coagulation may affect the immunocompromised, neonates and occasionally healthy adults, particularly smokers. Congenital varicella syndrome occurs following infections in the first five months of pregnancy, although most risk appears to be in weeks 13–20.

Herpes zoster begins with pain in the dermatome supplied by the affected sensory root ganglion. The trunk is a common site. The rash appears in the affected area and is vesicular and rapidly coalesces. It is very painful and persists for several days and even weeks in elderly people.

Laboratory confirmation

This is rarely required as the clinical features are so specific. If necessary, VZV is readily demonstrable from vesicular fluid in both chickenpox and shingles; serology is also available and can be used to demonstrate immunity.

Transmission

Man is the only reservoir. Carriage does not

occur. Chickenpox is highly infectious; herpes zoster very much less so. Transmission is by direct person-to-person contact, by airborne spread of vesicular fluid or respiratory secretions, and by contact with articles recently contaminated by discharges from vesicles and mucous membranes. The risk of transmission is high; the attack rate in susceptible exposed children is 87%.

Pathogenesis

The incubation period for chickenpox is two to three weeks, usually about 15–18 days.

Cases are infectious for up to 5 days before the onset of the rash (usually 1–2 days) until 5 days after the first crop of vesicles. Infectivity may be longer in immunosuppressed patients. Most transmission occurs early in the disease.

Patients with herpes zoster are usually only infectious if the lesions are exposed or disseminated. Infectivity is increased in immunosuppressed patients.

Prevention

Varicella vaccine is available in many European countries and the US, but is not yet licensed in the UK. It is, however, available on a named patient basis for immunocompromised individuals (especially children with leukaemia or solid organ transplants) and non-immune healthcare workers. The vaccine is a live attenuated preparation. The schedule is one dose in children and two doses a month apart in adults.

Surveillance

Chickenpox is notifiable in Scotland, but not in the rest of the UK. Laboratory diagnosis is rare, so local surveillance depends on informal sources such as schools. The CCDC may also be contacted with a request for specific immunoglobulin in an immunosupressed or pregnant contact. Trend data can be obtained from sentinel general practices.

Response to a case

Children with chickenpox should be excluded from school until five days from the onset of rash. Healthcare workers with chickenpox should stay off work for the same period. No exclusion criteria need to be applied to individuals with herpes zoster.

In most circumstances, no further action is required. There are, however, some situations in which postexposure prophylaxis with human varicella-zoster immunoglobulin (VZIG) is indicated. VZIG is indicated for non-immune individuals with a clinical condition which increases the risk of severe varicella and who have significant exposure to chickenpox or herpes zoster (Box 3.7.1).

VZIG is available from public health laboratories, CDSC and (in Scotland) regional transfusion centres. It should be given within 10 days of exposure.

The dose (i.m. injection) is:

0–5 years	250 mg (1 vial)
6–10 years	500 mg (2 vials)
11–14 years	750 mg (3 vials)
15 years and over	1000 mg (4 vials)

Response to a cluster/outbreak

In most outbreaks there will be no specific action in addition to the exclusion criteria and issue of VZIG described above.

Hospital outbreaks pose special problems because of the risk of transmission to immunosuppressed and pregnant patients. It may be worthwhile screening staff in contact with these high-risk groups for VZ antibody. Non-immune staff could then either be vaccinated, or where there is significant exposure to VZ virus (see above), excluded from contact with high-risk patients for 8–21 days after exposure.

Suggested case definition for an outbreak

Physician diagnosis of chickenpox or herpes zoster.

Box 3.7.1 How to determine whether VZIG is required postexposure

1 Is the contact at risk of severe disease? Include:
- immunosuppressed patients;
- infants whose mothers develop chickenpox (but not zoster) in the period 7 days before to 28 days after delivery;
- non-immune infants exposed to chickenpox or zoster in the first 28 days of life;
- pregnant women exposed during the first 20 weeks of pregnancy or within 21 days of the estimated day of delivery.

2 Is the exposure significant? Consider:
- type of infection in index case. VZIG is only indicated for exposure to chickenpox or to the following: disseminated herpes zoster, exposed herpes zoster lesions or immuno-suppressed patients with herpes zoster.
- timing of exposure. VZIG is only indicated for exposures between 2 days before, to five after, onset of rash.
- closeness and duration of contact. The following are significant: contact in the same room for 15 minutes or more; face to face contact; contact in the same hospital ward.

3 Is the contact already immune?

Individuals with a history of chickenpox are immune and do not require VZIG. Those without a history should be tested for VZ antibody, as many will be immune.

3.8 *Chlamydia pneumoniae*

Chlamydia pneumoniae, also known as TWAR, has recently been recognized as the third species of *Chlamydia* and is a relatively common cause of atypical pneumonia and other respiratory infections. The organism may also have a role in development of atherosclerosis.

Suggested on-call action

None required unless outbreak suspected.

Epidemiology

Data from the United States show annual incidence rates of 6–9% in 5 to 14-year-olds falling to 1.5% for adults, leading to an overall seroprevalence of 50% by about age 30. Incidence is low in the under 5s, but infection/reinfection may occur at any age. No seasonal pattern has been demonstrated but there is evidence of 2–3-year cycles of high and low endemicity. Infection probably occurs worldwide and has been demonstrated throughout northern and western Europe.

Clinical features

The most commonly identified manifestations of *C. pneumoniae* infection are pneumonia and bronchitis, which are usually mild but often slow to resolve. Approximately 6–10% of community acquired pneumonia is caused by this organism. Pharyngitis and sinusitis may occur in isolation or together with chest infection, and these together with a usually insidious onset may help to distinguish an outbreak from other causes of atypical pneumonia. Asymptomatic infection is common.

Laboratory confirmation

Diagnosis is usually confirmed by serology or direct antigen detection, as *C. pneumoniae* is difficult to culture. Serology is based on demonstration of a fourfold rise to genus-specific IgG on complement fixation testing which therefore cross-reacts with *C. psittaci* and *C. trachomatis*. Micro-immunofluorescence detection of *C. pneumoniae*-specific antibody, including an IgM test for diagnosis of acute infection, may be more appropriate. IgM rises can be detected after about 3 weeks and IgG 6–8 weeks after onset. Re-infection provides an IgG response in 1–2 weeks without an IgM response. Direct antigen testing on sputum, tracheal aspirate or tissue, and PCR tests may be possible.

Transmission

No zoonotic or environmental reservoir has been discovered. Spread is likely to be person-to-person, presumably via respiratory tract secretions. Transmission appears to be slow, but outbreaks, particularly in closed institutions, do occur.

Pathogenesis

The incubation period is unclear: estimates range from 10 to 30 days.

The infectious period is also unclear, but appears to be prolonged.

Although strong antibody responses occur, re-infection (even within the same outbreak) is reported. Most severe cases or deaths occur in those with underlying disease.

Prevention

General measures for respiratory infection, including:
- stay away from work or school when ill;
- cover mouth when coughing or sneezing;
- sanitary disposal of respiratory secretions;
- handwashing;
- avoid overcrowding.

Surveillance

In common with most other countries, sporadic infection with *C. pneumoniae* is not statutorily notifiable in the UK. However, possible outbreaks or clusters should be reported to local Public Health departments. Laboratories should report all clinically significant infections to national surveillance systems.

Response to a case

- Hygiene advice to cases and advice to stay at home whilst coughing/sneezing.
- Check for links to other cases.

Investigation of a cluster

- Seek microbiological advice to confirm as *C. pneumoniae* infection.
- Look for direct contact between cases or attendance at same functions or institutions.

Control of an outbreak

Likely to be difficult due to asymptomatic infectious cases, re-infection, prolonged infectivity and long incubation period. Could include hygiene measures, case-finding and treatment, but effectiveness not known.

Suggested case-definition for outbreak

Demonstration of *C. pneumoniae*-specific IgM or 4-fold rise in specific IgG.

3.9 *Chlamydia psittaci*

Psittacosis (or ornithosis) is a potentially fatal systemic disease caused by *Chlamydia psittaci*. It is a zoonotic infection particularly associated with avian species.

Suggested on-call action

- If linked cases suspected, institute outbreak plan.
- If not, ensure case investigated promptly on next working day.

Epidemiology

Much of the reported epidemiology of psittacosis is based on a combination of respiratory symptoms and demonstration of *Chlamydia* group antigen on serology; it therefore requires re-examination in the light of the discovery of the more common *C. pneumoniae* (see Chapter 3.8) which also causes disease fitting such a case-definition.

Cases occur worldwide and are more common in those exposed to birds occupationally or as pet owners.

Clinical features

Onset may be insidious or non-specific with fever and malaise, followed by an atypical pneumonia, with unproductive cough, fever and headache, with 20% mortality in the untreated. Other syndromes resemble infectious mononucleosis and typhoid, or asymptomatic infection may occur. Most cases report fever and most eventually develop a cough. Headache, myalgia and chills are each reported in about half of cases. Relapses may occur. Ovine strains may cause serious infection in pregnant women, resulting in late abortion, neonatal death and disseminated intravascular coagulation in the mother.

Laboratory confirmation

Culture is rarely used because of the risk of laboratory-acquired illness, and diagnosis is usually based on serology. As routine complement fixation tests (CFTs) cross-react with *C. pneumoniae*, further testing may be necessary to confirm which species is responsible. Acute and convalescent samples of serum are usually collected about 3 weeks apart.

Microimmunofluorescence (MIF) tests are becoming increasingly available and antigen or genome detection may also be possible in some laboratories if rapid results are required.

Transmission

C. psittaci is a zoonotic disease. Animal reservoirs include psittacine birds such as parakeets, parrots and lovebirds; other birds, particularly ducks, turkeys and pigeons; and less commonly mammals, especially sheep. Infection is transmitted to humans by inhalation of infected aerosols contaminated by droppings, nasal discharges or products of conception (e.g. sheep abortions) in which it may survive for months at ambient temperatures. Birds may be asymptomatic carriers of the organism. *C. psittaci* is destroyed by routine disinfectants such as alcohol, iodine or hypochlorite.

Groups at increased risk of disease include those in the pet trade, bird fanciers, poultry workers, abattoir workers, veterinarians and laboratory workers. Owners of pet birds are also at risk; the increase in psittacosis in the UK and Sweden has been linked to importation of exotic birds for pets.

If human-to-human spread of *C. psittaci* occurs at all (earlier reports may actually have been *C. pneumoniae*) then it is rare.

Pathogenesis

The incubation period has been reported as anything from 4 days to 4 weeks. Most cases probably occur 6–15 days after exposure.

The infectious period in birds may last for months. Human cases are not considered infectious for practical purposes.

Protective immunity to re-infection is short-lived. Those at risk of severe infection include pregnant women (especially to ovine chlamydial infection) and the elderly.

Prevention

• Quarantine and other controls on imported birds.
• Masks, good ventilation and measures to avoid contamination in poultry plants.
• Pregnant women to avoid exposure to sheep, especially during lambing.

Surveillance

Although not statutorily notifiable in most of the UK (local exceptions exist), all cases of psittacosis should be reported promptly to local public health authorities. Psittacosis is notifiable in many European countries, including Germany, Sweden and Norway. Laboratories should report all clinically significant infections to national surveillance systems.

Response to a case

• All cases should be reported by the clinician or microbiologist for investigation by local public health officers (e.g. the CCDC in England and Wales).
• Look for exposure to psittacines, poultry, other birds and mammals. Trace source back to pet shop, aviary, farm, etc. Involve veterinary and microbiological colleagues to test animals for infection. Infected birds should be treated or destroyed, and the environment thoroughly cleaned and disinfected.
• Ensure other potential cases are tested.
• No need for isolation. Cough into paper towel for safe disposal.

Investigation of a cluster

• Discuss further investigation with microbiologist to confirm *C. psittaci* as cause, and to see if typing possible (e.g. MIF).
• Conduct hypothesis-generating study to include pet birds (possibly illegal); pet mammals; hobbies (e.g. pigeon racing); visits to pet shops, farms, bird centres, etc.; occupational exposure to animals. Document less defined exposures, e.g. walking through fields (potentially contaminated pasture?), roofing (exposure to pigeons?), etc. Check if any institution or home visited had a pet bird.

Control of an outbreak

Work with veterinary colleagues:
• Look for infected birds or mammals.
• Treat or destroy infected birds.
• Thoroughly clean and disinfect environment.
• Case-finding to ensure those infected receive treatment.
• Action to prevent recurrence.

> **Suggested case-definition for outbreak**
>
> Because of possibility of asymptomatic infection and cross-reactivity of CFTs with *C. pneumoniae*, it is not possible to give an all-purpose case-definition. An outbreak-specific case-definition should be constructed with the aid of a reference laboratory.

3.10 *Chlamydia trachomatis* (genital)

Chlamydia trachomatis is one of three species of the genus *Chlamydia*. One group of serovars cause genital infection, neonatal ophthalmia, pneumonia and adult ocular infection. Different serovars cause lymphogranuloma venereum and endemic trachoma.

> **Suggested on-call action**
>
> This is not generally applicable.

Epidemiology

Genital *Chlamydia trachomatis* infection is the most commonly diagnosed bacterial sexually transmitted infection in England and Wales and the commonest cause of infertility in women. In recent years there have been increases in diagnosis rates, particularly in men and women aged 16–19. These increases may in part reflect an increase in the number of diagnostic tests that have been performed, but are nevertheless indicative of a considerable burden of infection. Surveys among sexually active women in the UK have found prevalence rates of 4–12%. Similar results have been reported in European and North American studies. Risk factors for infection include age 25 or less, recent change of sexual partner, use of oral contraceptives and low socio-economic status.

Clinical features

Many cases of infection in men and women are asymptomatic. In women there may be a cervicitis and urethritis, which may be complicated by pelvic inflammatory disease, tubal damage, infertility and ectopic pregnancy. In men there is urethritis which may be complicated by epididymitis.

Laboratory confirmation

Infection may be confirmed by enzyme immunoassay, direct fluorescent antibody test, ligase chain reaction (may be used on urine), polymerase chain reaction or culture of cervical or urethral samples.

Transmission and pathogenesis

Transmission is by direct, usually sexual, contact. Adult eye infection can be spread indirectly by fingers contaminated with infected genital discharges. The incubation period is 7–14 days and the case will remain infectious until treated. Only limited short-term immunity occurs and re-infection rates are high.

Prevention

Programmes of opportunistic selective screening, case finding and partner notification are cost-effective in reducing new cases of infection and their complications. Use of condoms during sexual intercourse will reduce individual risk. In the UK, diagnostic testing is recommended for men and women with symptoms of *Chlamydia* infection, and women who have gynaecological surgery involving instrumentation of the uterus. Opportunistic screening has been recommended for men and women attending GUM clinics, women seeking termination of pregnancy and their partners, sexu-

ally active women aged under 25 years and sexually active women aged over 25 years with a new sexual partner or who have had two or more sexual partners in the previous 12 months. Universal population screening is not recommended.

Surveillance

It is not necessary to report individual cases to local public health departments. In the UK, cases who attend GUM clinics are reported through the KC60 returns. However, many cases are treated in general practice. Laboratories should report positive results through the national laboratory reporting system.

Response to a case

Treatment is with a seven-day course of doxycycline or erythromycin or a single dose of azithromycin. During treatment, cases should avoid sexual intercourse. Sexual contacts should be traced and treated. Referral of cases to a GUM clinic for management is recommended.

Investigation of a cluster and control of outbreaks

This is not generally applicable.

Suggested case definition

Cases are defined by the results of appropriate laboratory tests.

3.11 Cholera

Cholera is a life-threatening secretory diarrhoea characterized by numerous large-volume watery stools resulting from infection with toxin-producing *Vibrio cholerae* O1. *V. cholerae* O1 is divided into two biotypes— classical and El Tor. *V. cholerae* O139 has recently been identified as causing epidemic cholera.

Suggested on-call action

- Cases should normally be admitted to an infectious diseases unit and enteric precautions instituted.
- Confirm diagnosis and the toxin production status of the isolate.
- Exclude cases in risk groups 1 to 4 (Box 2.2.1) for 48 hours after the first normal stool.
- Identify household contacts and those with common exposure, place under surveillance for 5 days from last contact and exclude from food handling.

Epidemiology

Importation of cholera into the UK is rare; fewer than 50 cases a year were imported into England and Wales in 1990–99. Cholera has become more widespread worldwide as the virulent El Tor biotype has spread, encouraged by the increase in international migration and the breakdown of public health measures, especially when associated with war, famine and other disasters. European visitors are unlikely to visit areas where cholera is common.

Clinical features

Sudden onset of copious, watery diarrhoea and sometimes vomiting. There may be severe muscle pain as a result of hypokalaemia. This dramatic presentation is distinctive, but mild or subclinical infections are in fact more common. The outcome depends on the amount of fluid and electrolyte loss and replacement; severe untreated cases have 50% case-fatality, but with correct treatment, less than 1% die.

Laboratory confirmation

Vibrios are small, comma-shaped, motile, Gram-negative bacilli, which may be seen on direct microscopy of stools or cultured from stool or a rectal swab. Various media have been described for culture; colonies can be recognized by fermentation reactions or by using antisera or fluorescent antibody tests. Determination of toxin production is important, as non-toxin producing organisms are not of public health significance. More recently the polymerase chain reaction (PCR) and other nucleic acid-based rapid techniques have been described.

Transmission

Infection is faeco–oral, commonly through contaminated water; undercooked seafood can also act as a vehicle. Cholera vibrios are sensitive to acidity; most die in the stomach, achlorhydria increases susceptibility to infection. Following colonization of the small bowel, an enterotoxin that interferes with intestinal epithelial cell metabolism is produced, causing secretion of electrolytes and water into the intestinal lumen. Stool volumes of up to 30 L a day lead to rapid dehydration.

Pathogenesis

- Incubation period: 6–48 h.
- Infectivity: during the period of diarrhoea and up to 7 days after.

Prevention

- Control by sanitation is effective, but may not be feasible in endemic areas.
- A parenteral vaccine of whole killed bacteria has been used widely, but is relatively ineffective and is not generally recommended.
- Antibiotic prophylaxis is feasible for small groups over short periods in high-risk situations.
- Breastfeeding in endemic areas protects infants from disease.

Surveillance

Cholera is a notifiable disease, and the public health authorities should be informed of any case. WHO should be informed by the national contacts. Illnesses caused by strains of *V. cholerae* other than toxigenic *V. cholerae* O1 or O139 should not be reported as cases of cholera.

Response to a case

- See on-call box above.
- Individual cases should be investigated to determine the source.
- Microbiological clearance: When indicated, two consecutive negative stools taken at intervals of at least 24 h are required.
- Hygiene advice to the case and contacts.

Investigation of a cluster

Clusters should be investigated in case there is secondary transmission within the household or community. This is rare in Europe.

Control of an outbreak

Outbreaks are rare in developed countries and are controlled through the provision of safe drinking water supplies.

Suggested case-definition for an outbreak
Clinical: an illness characterized by diarrhoea and/or vomiting in a contact of a case. *Confirmed*: clinical case with isolation of toxigenic *Vibrio cholerae* O1 or O139 from stool or vomitus.

3.12 *Clostridium difficile*

Clostridium difficile (CD) infection is an important cause of potentially severe toxic enteritis in hospitalized patients, particularly the elderly and debilitated. Infection is nearly always associated with, and triggered by, the use of antibiotics prescribed to treat other conditions or given prophylactically.

Suggested on-call action
Community outbreaks are very unusual. Hospital outbreaks will be managed by the Infection Control Doctor. The CCDC should be prepared to participate in meetings of the outbreak control group. The CCDC may be called upon to investigate and manage outbreaks of CD infection in community nursing homes.

Epidemiology

Reports of infections caused by CD have increased dramatically in recent years, from 555 in 1990 to 15 182 in 1999. However, this in part reflects increased investigation and reporting rather than a true increase in incidence. Elderly, hospitalized patients are at greatest risk. There is a background rate of CD infection in most hospitals, and outbreaks occur from time to time. It is estimated that CD infection is responsible for 20% of cases of antibiotic-associated diarrhoea.

Clinical features

CD infection is associated with a spectrum of clinical disease including antibiotic-associated diarrhoea (AAD), antibiotic-associated colitis (AAC) and the potentially fatal pseudomembranous colitis (PMC).

In a typical case, diarrhoea starts within a few days of starting antibiotics, although antibiotics taken 1–2 months previously may still predispose to infection. Abdominal pain and fever may be present. In PMC, tissue damage results in pseudomembranes and there may be serious complications.

Laboratory confirmation

Laboratory diagnosis ideally requires demonstration of toxin in faecal samples. The gold standard is a cytotoxin assay for toxin, but many laboratories use enzyme immunoassay tests. Culture is required if typing is to be performed to establish which strains are present in a ward or hospital. The histological appearance of large-bowel tissue obtained at sigmoidoscopy may be helpful.

Transmission

Between 2–3% of healthy adults and up to 36% of hospital patients have CD in their faecal flora and are asymptomatic carriers. It is only when the organism starts to produce toxin that symptoms occur. This is usually in response to treatment with broad-spectrum antibiotics.

Cases of endogenous CD infection may spread to other patients by the faecal–oral route directly, via the hands of healthcare workers, or through the accumulation of spores in the environment. Spread does not occur from an asymptomatic carrier in the absence of diarrhoea.

Transmission of CD infection to medical and nursing staff has been reported, although this is unusual and the disease is usually mild and short-lived.

Pathogenesis

Risk factors which predispose to CD infection include antibiotic treatment, age, cytotoxic agents, intensive care, naso-gastric intubation, concurrent illness and alteration in gut motility.

Prevention

Prevention of CD infection is achieved by ensuring that patients do not become susceptible through disruption of their normal intestinal flora, through careful measures to control antibiotic usage and by preventing exposure to the organism through standard infection control procedures. Ampicillin, amoxycillin and cephalosporins are the antibiotics most frequently implicated. In hospital there should be strict antibiotic policies.

A high level of diagnostic awareness should be maintained. Any patient with diarrhoea should be isolated with enteric precautions, and faecal samples should be submitted for CD toxin testing. A high level of environmental cleanliness should be observed.

Surveillance

Surveillance of CD infection in England and Wales is through national laboratory reporting of isolates of the organism and detection of toxin.

Response to a case

- Involve hospital infection control nurse.
- Side room isolation with enteric precautions, use of gloves and aprons and attention to handwashing by all staff.
- Treatment with oral metronidazole or oral vancomycin. The advice of a consultant microbiologist should be followed.
- Thorough environmental cleaning, but use of environmental disinfectants is unnecessary.

Investigation of a cluster

- All patients with diarrhoea should be identified, risk factors should be documented and faecal samples submitted for toxin tests and culture.
- In a hospital outbreak, CD typing may help to determine whether all patients are infected with the same strain, whether relapses are due to the original outbreak strain and whether patients are infected with more than one strain at a time.
- Environmental sampling is not recommended as a routine monitoring procedure but may form part of an investigation, especially if isolates can be typed.

Control of an outbreak

- Outbreak control measures include strict adherence to antibiotic policies, case finding through enhanced surveillance, side room isolation, enteric precautions and handwashing, restricting movements and transfers of patients, environmental cleaning, disinfection and sterilization of equipment and correct handling of infected linen.

• Screening for and treatment of asymptomatic patients who are CD carriers is unnecessary. There is no need to screen asymptomatic staff for carriage of CD. Staff who are asymptomatic carriers do not present a risk to patients and they can continue in their normal duties. Staff who are on antibiotics can remain at work even if CD is affecting patients.

Suggested case-definition

CD diarrhoea: diarrhoea not attributable to any other cause at the same time as a positive toxin assay (with or without a positive CD culture) and/or endoscopic evidence of PMC.

An outbreak of CD diarrhoea: two or more related cases satisfying the above criteria with dates of onset in a given time period that is determined locally, based on knowledge of the background rate.

3.13 *Clostridium perfringens*

Clostridium perfringens (formerly *C. welchii*) is primarily a food-borne pathogen, which causes a mild gastrointestinal illness due to an enterotoxin. Although rarely identified as a cause of sporadic illness, *C. perfringens* is a frequently identified cause of outbreaks. These outbreaks are commonly associated with mass catering: institutions serving groups vulnerable to serious illness (e.g. hospitals or nursing homes) need to take particular care.

Suggested on-call action

If you or the reporting laboratory/clinician aware of other potentially linked cases, consult local outbreak plan.

Epidemiology

The incidence of *C. perfringens* food poisoning presenting to general practice in England is about 1.3 per 1000 person-years. *C. perfringens* is identified as the cause of 5% of outbreaks reported to the PHLS Communicable Disease Surveillance Centre. There is little known variation by age, sex, ethnicity, occupation and geography within the UK. Asymptomatic carriage of the organism is extremely common.

Reported cases are higher in autumn and winter months than in summer, perhaps because of seasonal consumption of the types of foods (e.g. stews) often associated with infection. The association of infection with institutions or large gatherings likewise probably reflects patterns of food preparation. Outbreaks often have a high attack rate.

A much more serious form of *C. perfringens* poisoning was identified in postwar Germany ('Darmbrand') and Papua New Guinea in 1964 (enteritis necrotans or 'pigbel'). This form of the disease, caused by a different toxin, occurs in other third world countries and is particularly associated with malnutrition. *C. perfringens* is also the major cause of gas gangrene.

Clinical features

The main features of *C. perfringens* food poisoning are watery, often violent, diarrhoea and colicky, often severe, abdominal pain. Both are usually present, with colic the first to appear. Nausea may occur, but vomiting is rare. Signs of systemic infection are usually not present. Most cases recover within 24h, although elderly or debilitated patients may be more severely affected and occasional deaths are reported.

Laboratory confirmation

Clostridium perfringens can be isolated from anaerobic culture of stool samples. They are divided into five types (A–E) on the basis of toxin production. Those most frequently associated with food poisoning are the A2 strains, which form markedly heat-resistant spores. A1 strains, whose spores are relatively heat-sensitive, may also cause illness.

As carriage of *C. perfringens* is near universal in healthy humans and carriage of heat resistant organisms not uncommon, isolation of the organism from sporadic cases is of little value. However, serotyping (there are 75 serotypes and a number of untypable strains), which allows cases to be linked to each other and to potential food vehicles, is a powerful tool in outbreak investigation. Other factors which may help separate cases from carriers are a quantitative culture of organisms (over 10^6/g faeces usually significant) or the demonstration of enterotoxin in faeces. Several colonies should be sent for serotyping as more than one serotype can be present in the same specimen: failure to do this may confuse epidemiological investigation of an incident.

Transmission

C. perfringens is ubiquitous in soil and in the gastrointestinal tracts of mammals and birds. Many opportunities exist for spores to contaminate food, particularly meat and meat products, but provided contamination remains low illness does not result. *C. perfringens* can grow at temperatures between 20 and 50 °C with optimal growth at 43–45 °C, when a generation time of 10 min can be achieved. Spores, particularly those of the A2 strains, can survive normal cooking, including boiling for longer than one hour. These 'heat activated' spores will then germinate in the protein-rich environment as the food cools; the longer the food remains at the organism's preferred temperature, the larger the number of resulting organisms. If the food is not then reheated to at least 70 °C for two minutes throughout its bulk to kill the vegetative cells before eating, then a potentially infectious dose is ingested. The ingested organisms sporulate in the gut and (probably as a result of the initial heat shock) produce the enterotoxin, as a by-product which causes disease. Bulk cooking of meat/poultry stews, roasts, pies and gravies appears to be particularly vulnerable to this chain of events.

Pathogenesis

- The incubation period is usually 8–18 h, although a range of 5–24 h has been reported.
- *C. perfringens* gastroenteritis is not spread from person to person, and asymptomatic food handlers are not thought to be infectious to others.
- The infectious dose in food is usually greater than 10^6 organisms.
- The role of immunity is not yet understood.

Prevention

Prevention of *C. perfringens* food poisoning is dependent upon adequate temperature control of food after (initial) cooking. Food handlers need to be encouraged to serve meat dishes whilst still hot from initial cooking *or*, if not to be served immediately:

- refrigerate to below 10 °C within two hours of end of cooking;
- reheat with a method shown to achieve 70 °C for at least 2 min throughout the bulk of the food (microwaves, in particular, may not be able to achieve this);
- cook and reheat as small a quantity of food as is practicable—a maximum portion of 3 kg of meat was suggested after one large outbreak; and
- take particular care in large functions, or if consumers likely to include elderly or debilitated people.

Surveillance

Although, as with all cases of food poisoning, this is a notifiable disease in the UK, sporadic infection is rarely recognized. Most reported cases are identified as part of an outbreak.

Response to a case

- As with all cases of diarrhoea, hygiene advice should be given and it is best if the case does not attend work or school until he/she has normal stools.

• Occupational details should be sought: cases in risk groups 1–4 (Box 2.2.1) should be excluded until 48 h after the first normal stool. No microbiological clearance is necessary.
• No action is necessary with asymptomatic contacts of cases.
• Antibiotics are usually not indicated.

Investigation of a cluster

A laboratory-identified cluster is currently a rare event. Should one occur in a group of individuals with a compatible clinical illness, then analysis of person/place/time variables should be followed by a semistructured questionnaire aimed at identifying common foods, especially cooked meat/poultry products.

Control of an outbreak

As secondary spread from cases is unlikely, the aim of the outbreak investigation is to discover how it happened, so that lessons can be learnt. In practice this means trying to identify how an infectious dose resulted in a food presented for consumption. The vehicle of infection is identified by microbiological analysis of remaining food to find the same serotype as the cases (make sure you know how the food was stored after serving but before sampling) or by an analytical epidemiological study to show that cases were statistically significantly more likely to have eaten the food than controls. The environmental investigation will concentrate on how the food was cooked, stored and reheated. It is worth remembering that type A1 spores should not survive adequate initial cooking.

Suggested case-definition for analytical study of *C. perfringens* outbreak

Clinical: diarrhoea or abdominal pain with onset between 8 and 18 h of exposure.
Confirmed: clinical case with isolate of outbreak serotype and/or demonstration of enterotoxin in faeces.

3.14 Coxsackievirus infections

Coxsackieviruses are members of the Picornaviridae virus family. They are small RNA enteroviruses, which cause various diseases in man and other animals. Two groups are recognized, group A (23 serotypes) and group B (6 serotypes). The viruses show a seasonal, sporadic and epidemic pattern of clinical and subclinical infection including vesicular skin rashes, pharyngitis, meningitis, myocarditis and pericarditis.

Suggested on-call action

None generally needed.

Epidemiology

Serological studies indicate that a quarter of adults have serological evidence of recent group B infection and half have evidence of past infection. This suggests that Coxsackievirus infection is common and often subclinical.

In recent years annual laboratory reports in England and Wales of group A isolates have varied between 72 and 453 and of group B between 207 and 1231. Most isolates are from faecal samples or throat swabs, with fewer from CSF. The clinical conditions associated with virus isolation are typically meningitis and other more serious infections. Milder clinical syndromes do not normally merit laboratory diagnosis.

The commonest serotypes are A9 and A16 and B4, B5 and B2. Two thirds of isolates are reported between July and December and isolation rates are highest in infants under one year of age. Cases may be sporadic but outbreaks and clusters are reported.

Some serogroups show secular trends with peaks every two to five years. Outbreaks of A9 were reported in the UK in 1976 and 1985 and

A16 was epidemic in 1981. An outbreak of viral meningitis due to B5 was reported in Cyprus in 1996.

Laboratory data of this sort must be treated cautiously as some groups of patients will be investigated more vigorously, and only certain serotypes are detected by the cell culture method used by most virus laboratories.

Consultations in general practice for hand, foot and mouth disease (usually due to serogroup A16) are reported from spotter practices to the RCGP weekly returns service. Epidemics occur every 2–3 years. The seasonal pattern is bi-modal with incidence peaking in summer and early winter. Children aged 0–4 years are usually affected, and in this age-group weekly consultation rates may reach 148 per 100 000 population.

Clinical features

A range of clinical syndromes is recognized (see Table 3.14.1).

Pharyngitis, orchitis, parotid gland inflam-mation, pancreatitis and disseminated infec-tion in newborn infants may also occur.

Laboratory confirmation

Some serotypes may be isolated from faeces or other clinical specimens in tissue culture. Other serotypes require inoculation in suck-ling mice. Serological tests and PCR can also be used.

Transmission

Human clinical and subclinical cases are the reservoir of infection, and spread is by direct contact with faeces, pharyngeal discharges or respiratory droplets. Spread by food, water, sewage or insects is thought to be unlikely.

Pathogenesis

The incubation period is 3–5 days and a person will be infectious during the acute illness and

Table 3.14.1 Clinical syndromes caused by coxsackievirus infection

Acute haemorrhagic conjunctivitis	Characterized by subconjunctival haemorrhages and lid oedema. Often due to serotype A24
Epidemic myalgia (Bornholm disease)	Chest or abdominal pain, aggravated by movement and associated with fever and headache. Outbreaks have been reported.
Hand, foot and mouth disease	Usually a mild infection characterized by ulcers in the mouth and a maculopapular or vesicular rash on the hands, feet and buttocks. Often due to serotype A16. Systemic features and lymphadenopathy are absent and recovery is uneventful.
Herpangina	Fever, painful dysphagia, abdominal pain and vomiting with vesicles and shallow ulcers on tonsils and soft palate.
Meningitis	Fever with signs and symptoms of meningeal involvement, encephalitic signs may be present.
Myocarditis	Starts with non-specific symptoms such as fever and aches then progresses to breathlessness, palpitations and chest pain. Heart muscle necrosis varies in extent and severity. Heart failure may follow. Serum cardiac enzymes may be elevated; there may be ECG and chest X-ray abnormalities. Most patients with viral myocarditis recover fully. Treatment is largely supportive.
Pericarditis	Presents with retrosternal chest pain, aggravated by movement, fever and malaise. A pericardial rub may be heard on auscultation
Skin rashes	Rashes are common. A wide range of appearances may be seen including a fine pink rubella-like rash or petechial, purpuric, vesicular, bullous or urticarial rashes.

for some time after that, as the virus may persist in the faeces for several weeks.

Prevention

Health education, personal hygiene and reducing overcrowding will reduce the opportunities for exposure. Pregnant women may wish to avoid exposure, as a possible risk of abortion has been suggested.

Surveillance

Sporadic cases will not normally be reported to public health authorities, but clusters of cases and outbreaks should be reported.

Response to a case

Most clinical syndromes are mild and self-limiting. Children with hand, foot and mouth disease (HFMD) do not need to be excluded from school.

Response to a cluster and control of an outbreak

The CCDC may wish to alert local schools and general practitioners if an outbreak of HFMD occurs.

Case-definition

Characteristic clinical appearance with or without laboratory confirmation by electron microscopy or viral culture.

3.15 Cryptosporidiosis

Cryptosporidium parvum is a protozoan parasite, which in normal healthy individuals usually causes an acute self-limiting diarrhoeal illness. Its main public health importance lies in the severe illness caused in immuno-compromised individuals, the lack of an effective specific treatment and the potential for outbreaks, including large water-borne outbreaks.

Suggested on-call action

- If case in risk group for onward transmission (Box 2.2.1), exclude from work or nursery.
- If you or reporting laboratory/clinician aware of other potentially linked cases, consult local outbreak plan.

Epidemiology

Laboratory reports of *Cryptosporidium* have risen steadily in the UK over the last 15 years as the number of laboratories testing for the organism has increased. *C. parvum* is now the fourth most commonly identified cause of gastrointestinal infection with around 4600 isolates reported in England and Wales per annum. Evidence of past infection is common, with seroprevalence rates of 20–35% reported in Europe.

Diagnosed infection rates are highest in children aged 1–5 years and rare in those over 45 (Table 3.15.1), although in Finland most cases are reported as occurring in adults, due to travel abroad. Cases are usually equally distributed by sex.

Table 3.15.1 Age-distribution of sporadic cryptosporidiosis

Age-group (years)	% of total cases
Under 1	6
1–4	39
5–14	17
15–24	13
25–34	13
35–44	7
45–54	3
55–64	1
65 plus	2

Source: PHLS Study Group, 1990.

Cryptosporidiosis has a marked seasonal pattern: in western Europe peaks occur in the spring and late autumn (Fig. 2.2.2), although one or both may be absent in some localities or in some years.

Groups at particular risk of infection include animal handlers, travellers abroad (particularly to developing countries), contacts of cases, homosexual men and the immunosuppressed. Rates may also be higher in rural areas. The reported incidence of cryptosporidiosis in some AIDS centres is as high as 20%, although this is not universal and appears to be decreasing. The age-profile of cases in immunosuppressed patients is higher than that shown in Table 3.15.1.

Clinical features

The main presenting symptom is diarrhoea, which in immunocompetent individuals may last from 2 days to 4 weeks, with an average of two weeks. The diarrhoea may contain mucus but rarely blood, may be profuse and may wax and wane. The diarrhoea is often preceded by anorexia and nausea, and accompanied by cramping abdominal pain, loss of weight and offensive-smelling stools. Headache, myalgia, fever or vomiting may occur in a proportion of cases. Asymptomatic excretors are rarely found, although excretion may outlast symptoms in recovering cases.

Immunosuppressed patients have difficulty in clearing the infection, particularly HIV-infected individuals with CD4 T-lymphocyte counts below 200cells/mm^3. Many such individuals have a prolonged and fulminant illness which may contribute to death.

Laboratory confirmation

The mainstay of diagnosis is microscopy of stool samples to detect cryptosporidia oocysts. It is important that such microscopy be undertaken by experienced personnel, both to maximize ascertainment and because a wide variety of microscopic structures (e.g. yeasts) can be confused with *Cryptosporidium* oocysts. Individual cases are sometimes diagnosed by intestinal biopsy, and serological methods

have been used in epidemiological studies, including the huge Milwaukee outbreak.

Genotyping techniques are under development. One system becoming available in the UK splits *C. parvum* into 'genotype 1', found only in man (approximately one-third of cases) and 'genotype 2', found in animals and humans (two-thirds).

Transmission

Cryptosporidium parvum has been demonstrated in a wide variety of animals including cattle, sheep, goats, horses, pigs, cats, dogs, rodents and humans. Clinical disease and most oocyst excretion are thought to occur mainly in young animals. Transmission to humans is by faeco–oral spread from animals or other humans. The main routes of spread are as follows.

1 *Person to person*: cryptosporidiosis can be transmitted by cases to family members, nursery contacts, carers and sexual partners. Spread can be direct faeco–oral or via contaminated items such as nappies. Aerosol or droplet spread from liquid faeces may also occur. Secondary spread in households is common and may occur after resolution of clinical symptoms in the index case. Many outbreaks have been reported in nurseries.

2 *Animal to person*: human infection may occur from contact with farm or laboratory animals and, occasionally, household pets. In addition to agricultural and veterinary workers, those at risk include children visiting farms on educational or recreational visits where they may handle lambs or calves. A number of outbreaks associated with such visits have been reported from the UK.

3 *Drinking water*: contamination of drinking water may occur from agricultural sources or human sewage contamination. Oocysts passed in faeces can survive in the environment for months. They are resistant to chlorination and their removal relies on physical methods of water treatment such as filtration, coagulation and sedimentation. Over 20 drinking water—related outbreaks have been reported in the UK. The largest water-borne outbreak worldwide occurred in Milwaukee, USA in 1993 when an estimated 400000 people became ill. A review of the UK outbreaks found a common thread of an inadequacy in the treatment provided or of the operation of the treatment process.

4 *Other*: infection has been reported via food and milk. Swimming-pool outbreaks are being increasingly reported, usually as a result of faecal contamination of water and inadequate pool maintenance. Transmission has been reported from healthcare workers to patients (both immunosuppressed and immunocompetent) and between patients. The source of much cryptosporidiosis in the UK remains unclear. Vertical transmission has not been documented.

Pathogenesis

The incubation period is unclear: 7–10 days would seem to be average, but a range spanning 1–28 days has been reported.

The infectious period commences at onset of symptoms and may continue for several weeks after resolution. Asymptomatic infection has been reported, but is not thought to be common.

The infective dose appears to be very small, perhaps as low as 10 oocysts in some cases, with an ID_{50} of 130 oocysts. The UK Expert Group found it was not possible to recommend a health-related standard for *Cryptosporidium* in drinking water.

In immunocompetent individuals the immune response successfully limits the infection. AIDS patients are at increased risk of acquisition and increased severity, particularly those with CD4 T-lymphocyte counts under 200 cells/mm^3. Relative immunosuppression due to chickenpox and malnutrition has also been associated with infection, but renal patients do not appear to be at increased risk. Oocyst excretion may be very high in the immunosuppressed.

Prevention

• Handwashing after contact with faeces, nappies and animals.
• Safe disposal of sewage, taking particular care to avoid water sources.

• Risk assessment for water supplies, protection against agricultural contamination, adequate water treatment (e.g. coagulation-aided filtration) and monitoring of water quality, particularly turbidity.
• Enteric precautions for cases (Chapter 1.2) and exclusion of those in at-risk groups (Box 2.2.1).
• Immunosuppressed patients to boil water (both tap and bottle) before consumption and avoid contact with farm animals and infected humans.
• Guidelines for farm visits by children have been developed and can be adapted for local use (Health and Safety Executive, UK). Guidelines have also been developed for swimming pools (Pool Water Advisory Group, UK).
• *Cryptosporidium* is resistant to many common disinfectants. Ammonia, sodium hypochlorite, formalin, glutaraldehyde and hydrogen peroxide may be effective.

Surveillance

All clinically significant infections should be reported to local public health authorities (notifiable as suspected food poisoning in the UK) and to national laboratory surveillance systems.

The most important function of surveillance of cryptosporidiosis is the detection of outbreaks, particularly water-borne outbreaks. All diarrhoeal samples should be examined for oocysts and all positives reported. Home postcode should be collected on all cases to be plotted on water supply zone maps, which can be provided by water providers and need regular updating. Trigger levels can be calculated for districts and regions: a seasonal baseline can be set, based on historical data with 95% or 99% confidence intervals calculated from Poisson distribution tables. High figures for one week only may be the result of reporting bias. The age-distribution of cases should also be monitored.

Water utilities should also undertake appropriate monitoring of water quality and inform the CCDC of potentially significant failures, e.g. levels of one oocyst per 10L of water (see Box 3.15.2).

Box 3.15.1 Selected recommendations of Bouchier report

1.2.6 Water utilities to develop local liaison arrangements with Health and Local Authorities for rapid appraisal of potential health risk.

1.2.8 Water utilities to provide CCDC with water supply zone maps. HA to make early contact with water utility if outbreak of cryptosporidiosis suspected.

1.2.9 Human cryptosporidiosis to be laboratory reportable disease.

1.2.10 HA to make postcode of cases available to water utilities for mapping.

1.2.40 Criteria should be in place for identifying outbreaks and activating control teams.

1.2.55 All parties to simulate incident/outbreak events to rehearse emergency procedures.

1.2.61 Outbreak Control Team to use guidance on epidemiological investigation of outbreaks of infection (Appendix A4 of report).

1.2.63 All water to be used by immunocompromised persons should be boiled first.

Further reading: I.T. Bouchier (Chairman). *Cryptosporidium in Water Supplies*. Third report of the group of experts to Department of Environment, Transport, and the Region and the Department of Health. London: DETR, 1998.

Response to case

- Enteric precautions for case (see Chapter 1.2).
- Exclude if in risk group (Box 2.2.1) until 48 h after first normal stool. No microbiological clearance necessary.
- Investigate illness in family or other contacts.
- Obtain history of raw water consumption (including postcodes of premises on which consumed and any consumption from private water supplies), contact with other cases, contact with animals, nurseries, swimming pools, travel and milk consumption in previous 14 days.

Investigation of cluster

- Check to see if neighbouring areas, particularly those sharing a water supply, have an increase.
- Check age-range of affected cases: an increase in cases in adults could suggest water-borne infection, or link with immunosuppressed patients. If most cases in school age children, consider visits to farms or swimming pools.
- Epidemic curve may suggest point source, continuing source or person-to-person spread.

- Check with water utility whether any recent evidence of increased contamination or failure of treatment.
- Plot cases by water supply zones. Check with water company how cases relate to water sources (e.g. reservoirs, treatment centres) during relevant period: supply zones are not fixed and some areas may also receive water from mixed sources.
- Collect and review risk factor details from individual cases for hypothesis generation and further investigation as appropriate (see Chapter 4.3). Case finding may also be necessary.
- Organize confirmatory testing and genotyping by reference laboratory.

Control of an outbreak

- If a water-borne outbreak is likely, then the following action should be taken:

  Issue 'boil water' notice if contamination likely to be ongoing. A communications plan should already exist for public information. Water needs only to be brought to the boil; prolonged boiling is not necessary.

  Organize Outbreak Control Team to include relevant water company specialists/ managers and local authority. If potentially

Box 3.15.2 Response to detection of oocysts in water supply

The relationship between oocyst counts and the health risk to those who drink the water is unclear. However the water companies in the UK will inform health authorities of breaches in water quality standards. An appropriate response would be (based on Hunter, 2000):
Collect the following information for risk assessment.
- When and where sample taken.
- Number of oocysts detected and results of any viability testing.
- Results of repeat testing (should be done urgently).
- Source and treatment of affected water supply.
- Any recent changes in source or treatment.
- Distribution of water supply.
- Any treatment failure or high turbidity identified?
- How long water takes to go through distribution system.
- History of *Cryptosporidium* sampling and results for this supply.
- Any previous outbreaks associated with this supply.
For a low oocyst count in a supply in which oocysts frequently detected and not associated with previous outbreaks, further action may not be necessary.
Call Incident Management Team. Significant exposure is likely if there is:
- unusually high oocyst count or demonstration of viability;
- evidence of treatment failure or increased turbidity;
- a groundwater source; or
- an association with previous outbreaks.
Possible actions include the following.
- None.
- Advice to particular groups.
- Enhanced surveillance for human cases.
- Provision of alternative water supply.
- Boil water notice to affected area.
Boil water notices are issued if risk is thought to be ongoing, for example if:
- repeat samples are positive;
- treatment or turbidity problems continue; or
- contaminated water has not yet cleared from the distribution system.

serious, add CDSC, PHLS and Environment Agency (England and Wales) or their equivalents in other countries. The addition to the team of an individual who has dealt with such an outbreak before should be considered.

Consult Bouchier report (see Box 3.15.1) for more detailed advice.
- Exclude symptomatic cases in risk groups (Box 2.2.1).
- Advise public on how to prevent secondary spread.
- Institute good practice guidelines at any implicated nursery, farm, swimming pool or hospital.

Suggested case-definition for analytical study of outbreak

(a) Cohort study (e.g. nursery, school class)
Clinical: diarrhoea within 2–14 days of exposure.
Confirmed: diarrhoea and oocysts see in faecal specimen.
(b) Case–control study (e.g. general population)
Diarrhoea plus oocysts (of correct genotype, if known) in faeces, with no other date of onset since commencement of increase in cases.

3.16 Cyclosporiasis

Cyclospora cayetanensis is a protozoan, which causes human gastroenteritis. Less than 100 cases are diagnosed annually in the UK, almost all aged over 15 years. Infection occurs worldwide. In the UK over half of cases are reported to have contracted the infection abroad: risk areas include the Americas (Mexico, Peru), the Caribbean, China, the Indian subcontinent (including Nepal, where outbreaks occur during the rainy season), south-east Asia, Turkey and Yemen.

Cyclosporiasis presents with watery diarrhoea, often associated with weight loss, nausea and abdominal cramps. Diarrhoea may be prolonged but is self-limiting. Diagnosis is confirmed by detection of oocysts in faeces. Laboratories with little experience of *Cyclospora* should refer putative positives to more experienced laboratories for confirmation, as pseudo-outbreaks have occurred.

Humans are so far the only host species identified for *C. cayetanensis*. Oocysts are excreted in a non-infective unsporulated form; sporulation takes about a week in the environment and human infection results from ingestion of mature sporulated oocysts. Spread is therefore indirect via vehicles such as drinking water, swimming pools and food: outbreaks have been associated with fresh raspberries, basil and lettuce. Prevention and control in developed countries relies on sanitary disposal of faeces.

3.17 Cytomegalovirus

Cytomegalovirus (CMV), a herpes virus, causes a variety of infections. Its major impact is in the newborn and the immunocompromised.

On-call action
No person-to-person spread under normal conditions, therefore no need for urgent action.

Epidemiology

The prevalence of CMV rises with age; 60–90% of adults have antibodies.

Clinical features

Congenital infection may cause stillbirth, perinatal death, present as cytomegaloviruria in an otherwise normal infant or as a disease with fever, hepatitis, pneumonitis, and severe brain damage.

Infection acquired postnatally or later in life is often asymptomatic, or an acute febrile illness, cytomegalovirus mononucleosis, may occur.

CMV is a major cause of morbidity in immunocompromised patients. Disease may result from reactivation of latent infection. There may be pulmonary, GI, or CNS involvement, CMV causes retinitis and ulcerative disease of the GI tract in the terminal phase of AIDS.

A post-transfusion syndrome, which resembles infectious mononucleosis, can develop following transfusion with blood containing CMV.

Laboratory confirmation

CMV may be isolated from urine, other body fluids, or tissues. However, CMV may be excreted by individuals without active disease; a positive culture must be interpreted with caution. The demonstration of active disease may require biopsy. New techniques for rapid diagnosis demonstrating CMV antigens or DNA are being developed.

Transmission

CMV is transmitted through body fluids, blood, or transplanted organs. In the newborn infection may have been acquired transplacentally or during birth.

Pathogenesis

The incubation period for transfusion CMV mononucleosis is 2–4 weeks. Infectivity of body fluids may persist for many months.

Prevention

Screening of transplant donors for active disease.

Ganciclovir i.v. has been proposed for the prophylaxis of CMV disease in transplant recipients at risk for developing CMV disease. Oral ganciclovir has been used for the prevention of CMV disease in HIV-positive individuals.

Surveillance

No need to report individual cases, other than through routine laboratory surveillance.

Response to a case

No public health response usually necessary.

Investigation of a cluster and control of an outbreak

Investigate to ensure that it is not caused by exposure to contaminated blood or blood products.

Suggested case-definition

Neonatal: clinically compatible disease with isolate or PCR positive.

Adult: clinically compatible disease with isolate or CMV DNA detection or antigen detection or specific IgM-positive or fourfold rise in antibody titre.

3.18 Dengue fever

Dengue is a febrile disease caused by a flavivirus with four distinct serogroups, transmitted by the bite of *Aedes* mosquitoes.

Suggested on-call action

None usually necessary.

Epidemiology

Endemic throughout the tropics and subtropics; dengue haemorrhagic fever is most common in children less than 10 years old living where dengue is endemic.

Clinical diagnosis

Dengue presents with an abrupt onset of fever, chills, headache, backache and severe prostration. Aching in the legs and joints occurs during the first hours of illness. Fever and symptoms persist for 48–96 h, followed by rapid defervescence; after about 24 h a second rapid temperature rise follows (saddleback temperature). Typical dengue is not fatal.

In dengue haemorrhagic fever, bleeding tendencies occur with shock 2–6 days after onset. Mortality for dengue haemorrhagic fever ranges from 6 to 30%; most deaths occur in infants less than 1 year old.

Laboratory confirmation

Serologic diagnosis may be made by haemagglutination inhibiting and complement fixation tests using paired sera.

Transmission

Spread by mosquito bites (e.g. *Aedes aegypti*).

Pathogenesis

Incubation period of 3–15 days.

Prevention

• Avoidance of mosquito bites, e.g. with bed nets and insect repellent.
• Control or eradication of the mosquito vector.
• To prevent transmission to mosquitoes, patients in endemic areas should be kept under mosquito netting until the second bout of fever has abated.

Surveillance

Public health officials should be informed.

Response to a case

Human-to-human spread of dengue has not been recorded, therefore isolation is not required. Specimens should be taken using universal precautions and the laboratory informed.

Investigation of a cluster and control of an outbreak

Not relevant to European countries.

Suggested case-definition

A clinically compatible case confirmed by
• growth from or demonstration of virus in serum and/or tissue samples by immunohistochemistry or by viral nucleic acid detection; *or*
• demonstration of a fourfold or greater rise in IgG or IgM antibody titres to one or more dengue virus antigens in paired serum samples.

3.19 Diphtheria

Diphtheria is an infection of the upper respiratory tract, and sometimes the skin. It is caused by toxin-producing (toxigenic) strains of *Corynebacterium diphtheriae*, and occasionally by toxigenic *C. ulcerans*. It is a rare infection, although when a case does occur it tends to generate significant work for the public health team, as it is potentially fatal if untreated.

Suggested on-call action

• Obtain full clinical details, travel and vaccination history.
• Liaise with both local and reference labs to ensure rapid diagnosis and toxogenicity testing.
• Prepare list of close contacts.
• If diagnosis strongly suspected, arrange for immediate swabbing, chemoprophylaxis and vaccination of close contacts.
• Ensure case is admitted to specialist unit.

Epidemiology

Diphtheria is rare in countries with well established immunization programmes. In the UK, where immunization was introduced in 1940, there are about four cases a year. Most of these are imported from the Indian subcontinent and many are mild cases in vaccinated individuals. The case fatality rate is 5–10%. Indigenous cases are very rare, although there are a few UK-acquired cases every year due to toxigenic *C. ulcerans*. There has been a rise in infections due to non-toxigenic strains of *C. diphtheriae* in recent years; these cases have presented with a mild sore throat only.

The epidemiology is similar in other countries of western Europe, although there was a small outbreak among alcoholics in Sweden during the 1980s. A large epidemic of diphtheria occurred in countries of the former USSR during the 1990s; at its peak in 1995 there were approximately 52000 cases and 1700 deaths.

Clinical features

Diphtheria is rarely recognized on clinical grounds, as many cases are in vaccinated individuals. In classical respiratory diphtheria there is sore throat, fever, enlarged cervical lymph nodes and swelling of the soft tissues of the neck—the 'bull neck' appearance. The pharyngeal membrane, which is not always present, is typically grey, thick, and difficult to remove. There may be hoarseness and stridor. Nasal diphtheria usually presents with a blood-stained nasal discharge. Cutaneous diphtheria causes small ulcers, often on the legs.

The disease is caused by a toxin that particularly affects the heart and nervous system. The effects of this toxin are irreversible and so late treatment (with antitoxin) is ineffective.

Laboratory confirmation

It is usually the identification of a *Corynebacterium* sp. from a nose or throat swab or skin ulcer that alerts the public health physician to the possibility of diphtheria. Any isolate of a potentially toxigenic corynebacterium should be referred promptly to the national reference laboratory for confirmation and toxigenicity testing. Where the diagnosis seems likely, an acute serum specimen should be obtained before giving antitoxin, and any skin lesions should be swabbed.

Transmission

Man is the only reservoir and carriers are rare in vaccinated populations, so an infectious case is the usual source. Transmission is usually by airborne droplets or direct contact with infected respiratory discharges or skin ulcers; rarely from contact with articles contaminated by discharges from infected lesions. Diphtheria is not highly infectious, although exposed cutaneous lesions are more infectious than nasopharyngeal cases.

Pathogenesis

The incubation period is two to five days, occasionally longer.

Cases are no longer infectious after three days of antibiotic treatment. Untreated cases are infectious for up to four weeks.

The infectious dose is not known.

Natural immunity usually (although not always) develops after infection.

Prevention

Diphtheria is preventable by immunization. The UK schedule is three doses of diphtheria toxoid (combined with tetanus, pertussis and Hib) at 2, 3 and 4 months of age, with boosters at 3–5 years and 13–18 years (NB the second booster is with a low-dose adult formulation). Boosters are also recommended for travellers to countries where diphtheria is endemic or epidemic. Levels of immunity are low in the elderly because of waning immunity.

Surveillance

All forms of the disease are notifiable in most European countries, including the UK. Diphtheria should immediately be reported to the public health authorities on suspicion. Laboratory reporting should specify whether the organism is a toxin producer.

Response to a case

Secure confirmation from reference laboratory. All cases must be assessed by a suitably experienced physician. Unless there is strong clinical suspicion, other control measures can await confirmation. No control measures are required for infections due to non-toxigenic strains. Confirmation of toxigenicity can be obtained within a few hours by PCR.

For confirmed or strongly suspected toxigenic infections:

Measures for the case

1 Arrange strict barrier nursing until microbiological clearance demonstrated (minimum two negative nose and throat swabs, at least 24 h apart, the first at least 24 h after stopping antibiotics).
2 Secure microbiological clearance with a seven-day course of erythromycin (or other macrolide antibiotic).
3 Give a booster or primary vaccination course (depending on vaccination status).
4 The effects of diphtheria toxin are irreversible, so early diagnosis and treatment with antitoxin is vital. It is important to know how

to access supplies of diphtheria antitoxin out of hours.

Measures for close contacts

Close contacts include household and kissing contacts; this may be extended further, e.g. to school contacts if many of these less close contacts are unvaccinated.

1 Obtain swabs from nose and throat, and any skin lesions, for culture.

2 Monitor for seven days from last contact with case (daily measurement of temperature and examination of throat).

3 Exclude food handlers and those with close contact with unvaccinated children from work until all swabs shown to be negative.

4 Give a seven-day course of erythromycin (or other macrolide antibiotic).

5 Obtain further nose and throat swabs after course of antibiotics, and repeat course if still positive.

6 Give a booster or primary vaccination course (depending on vaccination status).

Infections due to toxigenic *C. ulcerans* should be treated the same as *C. diphtheriae*, as there is some evidence that person-to-person transmission may occur.

No public health action is required for infections due to non-toxigenic *C. diphtheriae*, although the patient should be treated with penicillin or erythromycin if symptomatic.

Response to a cluster/outbreak

As for an individual case, but in addition consider the need for a community-wide vaccination programme.

Suggested case-definition for an outbreak
Laboratory evidence of infection due to toxigenic *C. dipltheriae* or *C. ulcerans*, in a patient with compatible symptoms. Sore throat only in a vaccinated individual is a compatible symptom.

3.20 Encephalitis, acute

Suggested on-call action
The causes of acute encephalitis are unlikely to cause outbreaks and do not require public health action unless rabies is suspected.

Acute encephalitis is inflammation of the brain, caused by a variety of viruses. The commonest cause in western Europe is herpes simplex type 1 (about 30 cases a year in the UK) which is a severe infection mainly affecting adults; the case fatality rate may be as high as 70%. Herpes simplex encephalitis is intrinsically acquired, so no public health action is required in response to a case.

Tick-borne encephalitis (see Chapter 3.75) occurs in many European countries, and there are several mosquito-borne encephalitides in the USA. Other causes of acute encephalitis are Japanese B encephalitis (Chapter 3.39) and rabies (Chapter 3.60). Encephalitis also occurs as an acute complication of measles and chickenpox. Acute encephalitis is notifiable in England, Wales and Northern Ireland.

3.21 Enterococci, including VRE

Enterococci, including the species *E. faecalis* and *E. faecium*, are normally present in the gastrointestinal tract. They are of low virulence but can cause a range of infections in immunocompromised hospital patients, including wound infection, urinary tract infection, septicaemia and endocarditis.

Enterococci readily become resistant to antibiotics. By the mid-1980s resistance to commonly used antibiotics was widespread, leaving only glycopeptides (vancomycin and teicoplanin) available for treatment. In 1987 vancomycin-resistant enterococci (VRE) were reported and have since spread to many hospitals. Vancomycin resistance may be coded by transferable plasmids and there is concern that it may transfer to other more pathogenic bacteria. Transfer to MRSA has already been reported.

On-call action

Offer assistance to the control of infection team.

Epidemiology

In the UK laboratory reports of enterococci (VRE and non-VRE) positive blood cultures are collated by CDSC. There are about 3300 reports per year. VRE have been reported from 93 hospitals in England and Wales and there have been reports of 25 hospital outbreaks. VRE have also been reported from USA, Canada, Sweden, Italy and Germany.

Diagnosis

Enterococcal infection should be suspected in any case of sepsis in critically ill hospitalized patients, particularly those with severe underlying disease or immunosuppression. Appropriate microbiological investigation is essential to accurately identify enterococci and detect vancomycin resistance. Typing of strains is available.

Transmission

Most enterococcal infection is endogenously acquired, but spread can occur from infected or colonized patients, either directly or indirectly via the hands of medical and nursing staff, contaminated equipment or environmental surfaces.

Prevention

Infection and colonization with VRE may be reduced by prudent use of vancomycin, less use of cephalosporins, prompt diagnosis of VRE by the microbiology laboratory and implementation of appropriate control of infection measures. Periodic antibiotic sensitivity surveys have been introduced by some hospitals.

Surveillance

Cases should be reported to national surveillance, and isolates may be submitted to the PHLS Antibiotic Reference Unit (or equivalent in other countries).

Response to a case

Treatment is with a combination of antibiotics usually involving an aminoglycoside, a beta-lactam and a glycopeptide. Resistance to all combinations may be seen. Cases should be nursed in a side room with source isolation precautions.

Investigation of a cluster and control of an outbreak

A search for other cases of infection and colonization should be made by requesting microbiological samples from other patients on the same ward or unit. Cases should be isolated. Staff are rarely the source of infection but may be considered for screening with hand and rectal swabs. Infection control measures should be reviewed and reinforced, particularly handwashing and environmental cleaning. Environmental microbiology samples may be requested. Movement of staff and transfers of patients should be minimized.

Case-definition

Cases are defined microbiologically, based on the results of culture and antibiotic sensitivity testing.

3.22 Epstein–Barr virus

Epstein–Barr virus (EBV), a member of the herpes virus group, is the cause of infectious mononucleosis (glandular fever), an acute viral syndrome characterized by the presence of atypical mononuclear cells in the peripheral blood. After recovery, EBV persists in lymphoid tissue of the oropharynx and possibly the salivary glands and is associated with intermittent viral excretion in saliva. EBV is also associated with Burkitt's lymphoma in African patients, and other neoplasias.

On-call action
Not generally applicable.

Epidemiology

In countries where there is overcrowding and poor hygiene 90% of children have serological evidence of EBV infection by the age of 2 years. In developed countries infection is delayed until adolescence and early adult life.

Diagnosis

The features of infectious mononucleosis are fever, tonsillitis, lymphadenopathy, splenomegaly and hepatitis. Treatment with ampicillin leads to a temporary erythematous maculopapular skin rash. Young children generally have a mild illness.

Diagnosis is confirmed by the finding of atypical mononuclear cells in the peripheral blood. A range of serological tests are available.

Transmission

Most cases are spread from asymptomatic carriers. Spread is by the oro–pharyngeal route as a result of contact with saliva, either directly during kissing or indirectly on hands or fomites. Attack rates may be as high as 50%. EBV can also be spread in blood transfusions.

Pathogenesis

The incubation period is 4–6 weeks. A person may remain infectious for a year or more. Life-long immunity follows infection, although latent infection can reactivate.

Prevention

Health education and hygienic measures where practical to reduce exposure to saliva, especially from infected persons.

Surveillance

Reporting of cases is not generally necessary.

Response to a case

No exclusion necessary.

3.23 *Escherichia coli* O157 (and other *E. coli* gastro-enteritis)

Many different strains of *E. coli* are associated with gastrointestinal illness, which can be classified into six main syndromes. The most serious illness that is caused by verocytotoxic *E. coli* (VTEC), also know as enterohaemorrhagic *E. coli*, which is the focus of this chapter. The other syndromes are summarized in Table 3.23.1.

The most common VTEC strain is *E. coli* O157:H7, an organism identified as a human pathogen only in the last 20 years. *E. coli* O157 has the potential to cause haemolytic uraemic syndrome (the commonest cause of acute renal failure in children) and death. It may be food-borne and can cause large outbreaks, with the potential for secondary spread.

Table 3.23.1 *E. coli* other than VTEC

Designation	Epidemiology	Illness	Incubation	Sources	Main 'O' serogroups
Enterotoxigenic (ETEC)	Major cause of travellers' diarrhoea Dehydrating diarrhoea in children in developing countries	Watery diarrhoea Abdominal pain Lasts 1–5 days	10–72 hours	Food and water contaminated by humans Direct person-to-person spread rare	6, 8, 15, 20, 25, 27, 63, 78, 80, 114, 115, 128ac, 148, 153, 159, 167.
Enteropathogenic (EPEC)	Sporadic cases and outbreaks in children, usually aged less than 2 years	Watery diarrhoea, vomiting, fever Lasts up to 2 weeks	9–12 hours	Faeco–oral, especially in nurseries Contaminated infant foods in developing countries	18, 26, 44, 55, 86, 111, 114, 119, 125, 126, 127, 128, 142.
Enteroinvasive (EIEC)	Occasional cause of travellers' diarrhoea or outbreaks	Watery diarrhoea, often blood Abdominal pain Lasts up to 2 weeks	10–18 hours	Probably contaminated food	28ac, 29, 112ac, 124, 136, 143, 144, 152, 164, 167.
Enteroaggregative (EAggEC)	Common in infants in developing countries (inc. Indian subcontinent) Also reported rarely in UK and Germany	Diarrhoea, often watery Often blood or mucus Often chronic	20–48 hours	Probably contaminated food and water	–
Diffuse-adherence (DAEC)	Preschool children in developing countries	Diarrhoea	Unclear	Unclear	–

Control
Enteric precautions for cases, personal hygiene
Exclude risk groups until 48 hours after first normal stool
Advice to travellers abroad
Handwashing and environmental cleaning in nurseries

Table 3.23.2 Causes of haemolytic uraemic syndrome

Typical ('post-diarrhoeal', 'epidemic', 'D+')
   E. coli O157:H7 and O157:H—
   Other *E. coli* (e.g. O111, O26, O103, O104, O119)
   Viruses, e.g. coxsackie
   Shigella dysentery
   Streptococcus pneumoniae

Atypical ('sporadic', 'D—')
   Inherited disorders
   SLE
   Cancer
   Drugs, e.g. mitomycin C, cyclosporin, quinine, crack cocaine
   Pregnancy
   Oral contraceptives

Epidemiology

There were about 1100 laboratory-confirmed cases of *E. coli* O157 infection reported in England and Wales in 1999, a crude annual incidence rate of 20 per million population. Around 20 outbreaks are reported each year. The highest age-specific incidence of diagnosed infection is in children under five, and there is a slight male preponderance. Infection is more common in summer and early autumn (Fig. 2.2.2). There is marked regional variation within the UK, with the highest rates in rural areas, particularly in Scotland.

Approximately 80% of reported cases in the UK are sporadic, but a large outbreak in central Scotland associated with contaminated meats from a butcher's shop caused 20 deaths in elderly people in 1996. An outbreak in Japan in the same year, associated with mass-produced lunches for schoolchildren, led to 6300 identified cases. About 10% of UK cases acquire their infection abroad.

Clinical features

Infection with *E. coli* O157 may cause no symptoms; a diarrhoeal illness; haemorrhagic colitis with bloody diarrhoea and severe abdominal pain but usually no fever; haemolytic uraemic syndrome (HUS) with renal failure, haemolytic anaemia and thrombocytopaenia, particularly in children; and thrombocytopenic purpura, particularly in adults, which may add neurological complications to the features of HUS. The case fatality rate of severe infection (HUS or TTP) is reported as 3–17%.

HUS may occur 2–14 days after the onset of diarrhoea (usually 5–10 days). It affects 2–8% of reported cases and is more common if diarrhoea is bloody. Other risk factors for HUS include child under five years of age, elderly patient, high white blood cell count and use of antidiarrhoeal agents. VTEC causes the more common glomerular ('typical') form of HUS (Table 3.23.2).

Laboratory confirmation

Diagnosis is usually based on stool culture. Because most *E. coli* O157 differ from the majority of *E. coli* in not fermenting sorbitol, they show up as pale colonies when plated on sorbitol—McConkey agar. This plate should be used as a routine screen for all diarrhoeal specimens, irrespective of history of blood in stool. Biochemical and serological tests can then confirm the isolate as O157. VTEC strains produce one or both of two verocytotoxins (VT1 and VT2): tests for these toxins are available at reference laboratories. Phage typing and genotyping are available to aid epidemiological investigations. Twenty-nine different phage types were identified from human cases in a recent European study, with the predominant type varying by country of origin: two-thirds of cases in England and Wales were due to three phage types (PT2, PT21/28 and PT8); PT2 and PT8 predominate in Germany, PT4 and PT8 in Sweden, PT32 in Ireland, and PT2 in Finland. Serology can be used for retrospective diagnosis, and salivary testing may be available. Methods exist for examining food, water, environmental and animal samples for *E. coli* O157.

Transmission

The natural reservoir of *E. coli* O157 is the gastrointestinal tract of animals, particularly cattle, but also sheep, goats, deer, horses, dogs, birds and flies. Humans are infected via the following.

1 Contaminated foods: carcasses may become contaminated through contact with intestinal contents at slaughter. Mincing beef compounds the problem, as the contaminating organisms may be introduced into the interior of food such as beefburgers, where they will survive inadequate cooking. Other food vehicles may be cross-contaminated in the kitchen from raw food (e.g. cooked meats) or in the field by animal faeces (e.g. 'windfall apples' and radish sprouts). Milk (and other dairy products), either unpasteurized or contaminated postpasteurization, has been implicated in some outbreaks. The organism is relatively resistant to acid, fermentation and drying.

2 Infection may be transmitted by direct contact with animals, e.g. at farm visitor centres. Excreting animals are usually asymptomatic.

3 Secondary faeco–oral spread from infected cases is common, particularly in families and institutions. Routes may include sharing towels and contaminating food. Asymptomatic excretion is common in family contacts of cases.

4 Other: drinking and bathing in contaminated waters have both been linked with incidents of infection. Nursing and laboratory staff have acquired infection through occupational exposure.

Pathogenesis

The incubation period ranges from 1 to 9 days between exposure and onset of diarrhoea, with a median of 3–4 days. HUS may follow after a further 5–10 days.

The infectious period is unclear. One third of children under five excrete the organism for at least three weeks, but prolonged asymptomatic carriage appears to be unusual. Microbiological clearance is usually viewed as two consecutive negative faecal samples, taken at least 48 h apart.

The infectious dose is low, probably under 100 organisms.

Children under five and the elderly are at particular risk of serious infection.

Prevention

• Minimize contamination of carcasses at slaughter.

• Adopt the hazard analysis critical control point (HACCP) approach in both food processing and food service industries to prevent survival of or contamination by *E. coli* O157.

• Good kitchen practices including separation of raw and cooked foods and storage of foods below 10 °C.

• Cook beef, lamb and venison products so that any contaminating organisms are subjected to minimum of 70 °C for two minutes. Cook beefburgers until juices run clear and no pink bits remain inside.

• Pasteurize all milk.

• Adequate hygiene and toilet facilities in nurseries and schools. Supervised handwashing in nurseries and infant schools.

• Precautions during farm visits by children, including:

Handwashing after touching animals.

Avoid eating and drinking whilst visiting animals.

Keep face away from animals.

Do not put hand to mouth.

Do not touch animal droppings.

Clean shoes after visit.

Surveillance

All cases of *E. coli* O157 infection or unexplained HUS should be reported to the local public health authority as a matter of urgency. In the UK, cases should be notified as 'suspected food poisoning' to the CCDC.

Laboratories should test all samples from cases of diarrhoea or bloody stools for *E. coli* O157 and report positives to the appropriate surveillance system. In England and Wales this should include same day report to the CCDC plus CDR reports to CDSC, preferably via CoSurv.

Clinicians should report individual cases of 'typical' HUS and any cluster of bloody diarrhoea to local public health departments as a matter of urgency, even if the causal agent is unknown.

Response to a case

• If in high-risk group for further transmission (Box 2.2.1) exclude from work or nursery until asymptomatic and two consecutive negative faecal specimens taken at least 48 hours apart. This is a potentially serious infection with a low infectious dose.
• Consider cases in infant school children as risk group 4 (Box 2.2.1) and exclude until microbiological clearance.
• Household contacts in high-risk groups to be screened. Exclude those in risk groups (Box 2.2.1) until two negative faecal specimens obtained and, for risk groups 3 and 4 only, until the index case becomes asymptomatic.
• Enteric precautions during diarrhoeal phase.
• Hygiene advice to cases and contacts, particularly handwashing. Suggest remaining off work/school until normal stools for those in non-high-risk groups.
• Food and water history from all cases covering all 10 days before onset.

Investigation of a cluster

• Organize phage-typing, toxin-typing and, if possible, genotyping with reference laboratory. In England and Wales, the relevant laboratory is the Laboratory of Enteric Pathogens at the Central Public Health Laboratory, Colindale.
• Undertake hypothesis generating study to cover all food and water consumed in 10 days before onset of illness, and all social, school and work activities and visits undertaken. Include exposure to farm animals, pets and cases of gastro-enteritis. Ask specifically about minced beef or lamb products, cooked meats and milk.
• Investigation of social networks may reveal potential for person to person spread via common (possibly asymptomatic) contacts.

Control of outbreaks

• Hygiene advice to all cases and contacts.
• Exclude cases as detailed above.
• Enhanced cleaning in all institutional outbreaks.
• Supervised handwashing for children in affected nurseries and infant schools.
• Exclude all cases of diarrhoea from affected (non-residential) institutions, until normal stools and two consecutive negative samples taken at least 48 h apart received.
• In day-care establishments for children under five (high risk of HUS and poor hygiene) screen all attenders. Exclude all positives until microbiological clearance achieved. Adopt similar approach for confused or faecally in-continent elderly attending day-care facilities.
• In residential accommodation for children under five or the elderly, screen all residents. Maintain enteric precautions for all positives until microbiological clearance achieved. Preferably nurse in private room with own washbasin and exclusive use of one toilet whilst diarrhoea continues.
• Institute **urgent** withdrawal of any implicated food. If local supplier involved, ensure personally that this is done: in UK use local authority powers under Food Safety Act (1990) to seize food. If national or regionally distributed food, contact relevant government department: in UK, the Food Standards Agency is responsible for activating the Food Hazard Warning System.
• Ensure adequate precautions taken at any

implicated farm open to public. In UK, take advice of Health and Safety Executive.

Suggested case-definition for outbreak

Confirmed: diarrhoea with demonstration of *E. coli* O157 of outbreak strain in stools.
Presumptive: HUS occurring after diarrhoea with no other cause identified.
Clinical: diarrhoea in person epidemiologically linked to outbreak (e.g. onset within nine days of consuming vehicle) with further investigations awaited.

3.24 Giardiasis

Giardia lamblia, also known as *G. intestinalis* or *G. duodenalis*, is a protozoan parasite that causes intestinal infection throughout the world. In developed countries the illness is particularly associated with water-borne outbreaks, nurseries and other institutions, and travellers abroad.

Suggested on-call action

• Exclude symptomatic cases in risk groups.
• If other cases, consult outbreak control plan.

Epidemiology

Prevalence rates (including asymptomatic excretion) of between 2% and 7% have been demonstrated in developed countries, although a recent study in England and Wales found an annual community incidence of disease of 0.5 per 1000, of which about one-fifth were reported to national surveillance. Reports to CDSC have fallen by a third over the 1990s, resulting in 4240 reports in 1999. The most commonly affected age groups are children under five and adults aged 25–39. A seasonal peak in July to October is reported. Groups with higher rates of infection include residents of institutions, travellers abroad, gay men and the immunocompromised.

Clinical features

About a quarter of acute cases are asymptomatic excretors. Symptomatic diarrhoea may be accompanied by malaise, flatulence, foul-smelling greasy stools, abdominal cramps, bloating, nausea and anorexia. Prolonged diarrhoea, malabsorption and weight loss are suggestive of giardiasis.

Laboratory confirmation

Giardia infection is usually confirmed by microbiological examination of fresh stool samples for cysts. A single stool sample will identify only about 60% of those infected but three samples (preferably taken on non-consecutive days) will identify over 90%. They may not yet be positive at the onset of symptoms.

Antigen assays are reported to be highly sensitive and specific, although they are not yet universally accepted in the UK. They may have a role in cohort screening during outbreaks.

Transmission

Giardiasis results from faeco–oral transmission of *Giardia* cysts. This can occur directly or via food or water. Humans appear to be the main reservoir for *G. lamblia* infection, but other animals including dogs, cats, rodents and domesticated ruminants are commonly affected by this organism. *Giardia* cysts are environmentally resistant and survive well in cold water. Giardiasis is the most frequently diagnosed water-borne disease in the United States, and water-borne outbreaks have been reported from Europe. Recreational contact with water may also be a risk. Person-to-person spread is increasingly recognized as important, both in institutions and from children in the community and within families.

Pathogenesis

• The median incubation period is 7–10 days but extremes of 3–25 days have been reported.
• Cyst excretion may persist for up to six months and may be intermittent.
• As few as 25 cysts may cause infection.

Prevention

Prevention of giardiasis is dependent on:
• Adequate treatment of water supplies; standard chlorination is not sufficient to destroy cysts and should be supplemented by filtration.
• Adequate control of infection and food hygiene practices in institutions, especially those dealing with children.
• Handwashing after toilet use and before preparing food.
• Advice to travellers abroad on safe food and water.

Surveillance

Diagnosed cases should be reported to local public health departments (notify as 'food poisoning' in UK) and to national laboratory reporting systems.

Response to a case

• Hygiene advice should be given. Ideally, the case should not attend work or school until he/she has normal stools.
• Cases in risk groups 1–4 (Table 2.2.1) should be excluded until 48 h after the first normal stool. Microbiological clearance is not necessary before return.
• A number of effective drugs are available for treatment, e.g. metronidazole or tinidazole. Treatment of individual cases of giardiasis forms the basis of control in the UK.
• Screening of household contacts may identify individuals needing treatment.

Investigation of a cluster

Enquiries should include water consumption (compare to water supply zones), food sources, swimming pools, contact with day centres (especially for children) or other institutions, travel and (if cases mainly adult men) sexual contact.

Control of an outbreak

Water-borne outbreaks are usually due to use of untreated surface water, inadequate water treatment (e.g. ineffective filtration) or sewage contamination. Geographic mapping of cases will help the local water company identify areas for further investigation.

Outbreaks in nurseries and other institutions are controlled by enhanced infection control, especially supervised handwashing for all children, and exclusion and treatment of all symptomatic children. Some would also recommend treatment of asymptomatic carriers: while this will help control the outbreak and prevent spread to community and family contacts, the benefit to the asymptomatic individual is unclear.

Suggested case-definition for an outbreak
Demonstration of cysts plus either: • diarrhoea *or* • link to outbreak group.

3.25 Gonorrhoea, syphilis and other acute STIs

Sexually transmitted infections (STIs) are defined by their route of transmission. They are transmitted by direct sexual contact. For HIV infection, see Chapter 3.36. For genital chlamydia infection, see Chapter 3.10.

On-call action
The public health team may be alerted to clusters of cases of STI (e.g. syphilis or gonorrhoea) and should be prepared to initiate or assist with an investigation.

Epidemiology

In recent years in the UK, annual totals of diagnoses of genital warts, genital herpes, gonorrhoea and bacterial vaginosis have increased. This is evidence of a substantial burden of STI morbidity particularly among teenagers. Diagnoses of syphilis and congenital syphilis are uncommon. Diagnoses of lymphogranuloma venereum, chancroid and granuloma inguinale, while common in subtropical and tropical countries, are rare in the UK. More detail is given in Table 3.25.1.

Clinical features and laboratory confirmation

See Table 2.7.1.

Transmission

STIs are spread by direct, usually sexual, contact with infectious discharges or lesions. Syphilis may also be spread *in utero* and via blood transfusions.

Prevention

The prevention of STIs depends on the following.
• Health and sex education to discourage multiple sexual partners and casual sexual activity and to promote correct and consistent use of condoms.
• Early detection of cases and prompt effective treatment.
• Identification, examination and treatment of the sexual partners of cases.
• Opportunistic or routine screening and treatment of certain subgroups of the population who may be at increased risk of STIs or their complications. An example is the routine use of syphilis serological tests in pregnancy, to prevent congenital syphilis.

Surveillance

Individual cases of STIs are not generally reported to the CCDC. However the CCDC is informed of cases of acute hepatitis A and hepatitis B, *Campylobacter*, *Entamoeba histolytica* and *Shigella*, which may be sometimes be sexually transmitted.

Response to a case

The case should receive prompt effective treatment and should refrain from sexual intercourse until treated. Sexual contacts should be identified, examined and treated as appropriate.

Box 3.25.2 Non-venereal treponemes

Bejel, pinta and yaws are three diseases that may be confused with syphilis but are not spread venereally or congenitally. They are caused by *Treponema pallidum endemicum*, *T. carateum* and *T. pallidum pertenue*, respectively, and are serologically indistinguishable from syphilis and from each other. They also respond to the same treatment as syphilis. Their clinical patterns, including the primary cutaneous lesions, can, however, be distinguished.

Bejel is found in poor areas of the Eastern Mediterranean, Asia and Africa; pinta in tropical areas of America; and yaws in the tropics worldwide. Spread is through direct or indirect contact with exudate from skin lesions: yaws is highly infectious, but pinta requires extended close contact. The incubation period is from 2 weeks to 3 months. Control is by treatment of cases and hygienic measures.

Table 3.25.1 Surveillance of acute STIs in England and Wales

Gonorrhoea	The number of cases of uncomplicated gonorrhoea has risen steadily since 1994. Increases have been seen in most areas and in most age groups in both males and females. Male cases outnumber females by more than 2 : 1 and recent studies have shown a disproportionately high incidence of gonorrhoea in young people, homosexual and bisexual men and in those of black-Caribbean ethnic origin.
	In 1998 12 393 cases were reported. The largest numbers of diagnoses were in men aged 25–34 and in women 16–19. Just under half the diagnoses were made in London. Gonorrhoea diagnoses have risen again sharply between 1998 and 1999, by 26% in males and 30% in females. These increases have affected almost all age groups but those aged 16–19 years have been particularly affected, with increases of 52% in males and 39% in females. The largest rises were seen outside London.
	The reasons for these increases remain unclear. A 20% increase in gonorrhoea between 1995 and 1996 occurred in various demographic and behavioural risk groups. The number of isolates that are resistant to penicillin is declining, but there has been an increase in strains that are resistant to ciprofloxacin. It is possible that a rise in treatment failures could enhance transmission of gonorrhoea. Most of the resistant strains are in those of white ethnic origin and are acquired in the UK. This contrasts with earlier years when nearly half of resistant isolates were homosexually acquired. Rectal isolates of gonorrhoea have declined recently. Gonorrhoea diagnoses remain commoner in men than women, even after excluding infections among homosexual men. This highlights the importance of identifying and notifying female contacts, who are more likely to have asymptomatic infection and are more vulnerable to long-term sequelae.
Infectious syphilis	During 1997 a rise was noticed in diagnoses of primary and secondary infectious syphilis, largely explained by an outbreak of infectious syphilis in Bristol. Before this outbreak, most cases of infectious syphilis were acquired abroad, notably in eastern Europe, and a sizeable proportion were acquired homosexually. In the Bristol outbreak all cases acquired their infection heterosexually, mostly in the Bristol area. In 1998 in England and Wales there were 126 cases of infectious syphilis (83 males, 43 females). The largest number of diagnoses was in men and women aged 25–34 years. About 40% of diagnoses were made in London. Between 1995 and 98 there has been little change in either the regional or age distribution of cases.
	In 1999 GUM clinics serving Manchester reported 25 cases of infectious syphilis, compared with only 1–2 cases in each of the preceding three years. This will almost certainly lead to an increase in the national total of cases for 1999. In contrast to the Bristol incident, transmission is reportedly associated with sex between men rather than heterosexual exposure.
Genital warts	Genital warts is the commonest STI diagnosed at GUM clinics in England. Between 1995 and 1998 diagnoses rose to a total of 59 973 (30 914 males, 29 059 females). Diagnoses in 1998 were most numerous in men aged 25–34 and in women aged 20–24. Between 1995 and 98 there were significant increases in all regions and in all age groups except those aged 15 and under.
Genital herpes simplex virus infection	Between 1996 and 1998, diagnoses rose slightly to a total of 15 706 (6087 males, 9619 females). Most diagnoses were in the 25–34 years age group in both males and females. Between 1995 and 98 there were few changes in the regional or age distribution of diagnoses.
	Much of the long-term rise in genital warts and genital herpes simplex infection are due to changes in health-seeking behaviour as well as in incidence. There has been a recent sharp increase in genital wart infection amongst homosexual men and teenagers.

Investigation of a cluster and control of an outbreak

Clusters of cases of STIs may occur. The CCDC should be prepared to initiate or assist with an epidemiological investigation in collaboration with staff from the local GUM clinic.

3.26 Hantavirus

Hantavirus infection is an acute zoonotic viral disease.

Suggested on-call action
None usually required.

Epidemiology

Hantavirus infections are found where there is close contact between people and infected rodents. In Europe, foci are recognized in the Balkans, the Ardennes and Scandinavia.

Clinical features

The clinical picture depends upon the subtype causing the infection and is characterized by haemorrhagic fever with renal syndrome (HFRS), or acute pulmonary oedema (HPS). HFRS manifests as fever, thrombocytopenia and acute renal failure, and HPS as fever with respiratory difficulty. A number of different subtypes exist, each of which is associated with a particular rodent species. Of the two European subtypes, Puumala tends to cause milder disease (nephropathia epidemica), but Dobrava HFRS is often severe (Table 3.26.1).

Laboratory confirmation

Demonstration of specific antibody (IgM or IgG) by ELISA or IFA. IgM is often present on hospitalization. PCR for specific RNA may be available.

Table 3.26.1 Some hantavirus subtypes

HFRS	
Dobrava	Balkans
Puumala	Northern Europe
Hantaan	Asia
Seoul	Worldwide
HPS	
Sin Nombre	North America
New York-1	US
Bayou	US
Black Creek	US

Transmission

Aerosol transmission from rodent excreta. Human to human transmission has been reported in HPS.

Control

- HFRS is not transmitted from person to person, and there is no need for urgent public health action.
- In areas that are known to be endemic, rodents should be excluded from living quarters.
- In view of the possibility of person-to-person spread in HPS suspected cases should be nursed in isolation.

Suggested case-definition
HFRS or HPS confirmed by IgM or PCR.

3.27 Head lice

Head lice (*Pediculus humanus capitis*) are wingless arthropods that infest the head and feed by sucking blood.

On-call action
None.

Epidemiology

Few surveillance data on head lice are available in Europe; nevertheless it is a common public health problem and excites great public interest. In England and Wales no national statistics have been published since 1989. Anyone with head hair can get head lice but the most commonly affected groups are primary school–age children and their families and contacts. After puberty, girls seem to have higher infestation rates than boys. People of any social class and ethnic group can be affected.

The point prevalence is said to be up to 10% but during outbreaks this may rise to 50–70% within certain population groups. Spread within the population is sustained by a reservoir of undetected cases. Nearly six million pesticide treatments were used in the UK in 1994/95.

Clinical features

Many early infestations are asymptomatic. Itching and scratching of the scalp may appear 2–3 weeks after the onset of infestation. There may be enlargement of cervical lymph nodes due to secondary bacterial infection, or a rash on the nape of the neck due to an allergic reaction to lice faeces.

Diagnosis depends on finding live lice on the head. Empty eggshells (nits) are not proof of active infestation.

Lice move rapidly away from any disturbance, and examination of dry hair is unreliable. Lice can only be reliably detected by combing wet lubricated hair with a fine toothcomb. If lice are present they fall out or are stuck to the comb.

Laboratory confirmation

If necessary, lice and nymphs can be examined with a magnifying glass or low-power microscope to confirm their presence.

Transmission and pathogenesis

Biology and life cycle

Lice are obligate parasites. They have three pairs of legs that end in a single claw used for grasping the hair shaft. Lice require a temperature of 31 °C or greater and therefore live close to the scalp where they feed by biting and sucking blood. The female head louse produces on average 56 eggs after a single insemination, at the rate of approximately six eggs per day. The eggs are tear-shaped, 1 mm long and are securely glued to the hair shaft close to the scalp. The eggs hatch after 7–10 days and the emerging nymphs moult three times before reaching maturity in 6–12 days. The full-grown louse is 3 mm long and lives for about 20 days. Empty egg sacks are white and shiny, and may be found further along the hair, as the hair grows out. Although there may be large number of lice on an affected head, the average number is about 10.

Spread

Head lice clamber from shaft to shaft in dry hair and move readily from person to person when heads touch. It is not clear how long a period of head-to-head contact is required for transmission to take place. Some commentators state 30 seconds, but others have argued that common sense and experience dictates a much shorter period of contact.

Head lice can also spread when personal items (combs, brushes, etc.) and bedding are shared, but this is not an important route of transmission. Head lice will dehydrate and die within 48 h of being removed from the scalp. Head lice cannot jump from person to person but they are occasionally flicked from one head to another during combing or brushing.

Transmission occurs in schools, at home and in the wider community. A person will remain infectious for as long as there are adult lice on the head. Anyone with hair can be affected, and re-infestation may occur. Humans are the only source of head lice, which are host-specific and do not spread from or to animals.

Prevention

There is no evidence that any individual or community intervention has any other than the most transient effect on the prevalence of head lice in the community. Efforts to reduce

Table 3.27.1 Head lice: suggested responsibilities

Parents	Parents are responsible for brushing or combing their children's hair daily and using the detector comb each week to detect infestation. They are also responsible for telling all contacts of infested family members about the infestation, as well as warning any school, nursery or playgroup attended by their children that their child has head lice. Parents are also responsible for ensuring that the recommended treatment has been carried out. Treatment should only be used on the member of the family who has an infestation.
Health visitors and school health nurses	Health visitors and school health nurses are involved with the education of parents about head lice. Emphasis should be placed on the parents' responsibility to prevent, detect and treat infestations as well alerting contacts. In cases of recurrent or apparently resistant outbreaks in schools, nurseries, etc., health visitors and school nurses should ensure the policy is being correctly followed, offer advice to families with recurrent problems and consider further measures in conjunction with school doctors, General Practitioners and the CCDC.
Head teacher	The head teacher will inform the parents of pupils about any outbreaks of head lice. If a child is found to have an infestation, a letter may be sent to the child's parents, advising on treatment, contact tracing and prevention measures, incorporating the advice of the school nurse. A standard letter may be sent to all parents of pupils in the same class as the affected child, advising them to check their child's hair. Preventative measures will be emphasized in this letter. Children need not be sent home from school on the day when an infestation is found. If treatment is started that evening the child may continue at school.
Consultant for Communicable Disease Control and Community Infection Control Nurses	To receive notifications of particular head lice problems in community settings and to advise on management. To involve other carers, such as District Nurses, health visitors or school health nurses, GPs and teachers as appropriate. To make available information on head lice for the public and professionals.
General practitioners and practice staff	General practitioners should be able to explain the use of a detection comb and wet combing to confirm active infestation and discuss the two treatment options. A patient information leaflet should be available. If appropriate they may prescribe pediculocides. Only those with confirmed infestations should be treated.
Pharmacists	Pharmacists should be able to explain the use of a detection comb and wet combing to confirm active infestation and discuss the two treatment options. They should offer for sale wet combing materials or pediculocides as appropriate. Shampoos should not be offered for sale. A patient information leaflet should be provided with all prescriptions and sales of head lice treatment. Detector combs should be available.

the burden of head lice in any given population depend therefore on case finding by regular diagnostic wet combing followed by prompt treatment of cases if active infestation is found. Contacts of cases must also be examined and treated if appropriate.

Regular combing of dry hair even with an electronic comb does not reliably prevent or clear infestation, although it is often recommended. Repellents and alternative remedies are widely promoted, but evidence for their effectiveness is limited.

Surveillance

If head lice are causing particular problems in community settings such as schools, the CCDC should be informed.

Response to a case

It is not necessary to exclude children with head lice from school or nursery. There are two methods of treatment.

Chemical pediculocides

A number of chemical pediculocides are available, but because of resistance and concerns about safety they must be used with care. Pediculocides may not kill all unhatched eggs and so single applications are usually insufficient. Shampoo formulations have contact times that are too short, and are not recommended. After treatment, wet combing should be carried out to check for lice. Pediculocides should only be used if live lice are confirmed, and should never be used prophylactically.

Mechanical removal of lice

Lice and larvae as they hatch can be mechanically removed by wet combing well lubricated hair with a detector comb every four days for two weeks. This breaks the life cycle of the head louse.

All contacts of a case should be examined for head lice by wet combing and treated if necessary.

Investigation of a cluster

Clusters of cases of head lice are usually reported from schools or other institutional settings. The school health nurse is usually the most appropriate person to investigate and advise on control measures.

Control of an outbreak

Parents should be alerted and asked to carry out case finding by wet combing. They should be advised to treat their child promptly if live lice are discovered, using one of the two treatment options. Accurate information, explanation and sympathetic reassurance will be required.

3.28 *Helicobacter pylori*

Helicobacter pylori infection occurs throughout the world; prevalence in developed countries is 20–50% (up to 75% in socially deprived areas) and, in general, increases with age, with an acquisition rate of 1–3% p.a. Most infection is asymptomatic, but it may cause gastritis and both gastric and duodenal ulceration. Infection is also associated with gastric adenocarcinoma and perhaps ischaemic heart disease. The annual incidence of peptic ulcer disease is 0.18%, and over 90% of patients will have *H. pylori* infection. Diagnosis is by serology, breath testing with urea, culture from gastric biopsy/aspirate, or antigen testing of faeces. Treatment is with a mix of antibiotics and antisecretory drugs.

Transmission is unclear but most likely to be via the gastro–oral route (e.g. from vomiting) although oral–oral or faeco–oral are also possible. Spread via contaminated gastric tubes and endoscopes is recorded. There is some evidence that *H. pylori* is a zoonosis, with food a possible vehicle of infection for humans.

Infectivity is assumed to be lifelong and to

be higher in those with achlorhydria. Other than routine hygiene and disinfection precautions, there is insufficient evidence at present to recommend further preventative interventions.

3.29 Hepatitis A

Hepatitis A virus (HAV) is an enterically transmitted acute infection of the liver, which is primarily spread faeco–orally.

Suggested on-call action

- If a case in risk group for further transmission (Box 2.2.1) exclude from work or nursery.
- Exclude any contacts in risk groups who are known to be unwell.
- Refer household contacts for vaccination.
- If you or referring clinician/microbiologist aware of potentially linked cases, refer to local outbreak plan.

Epidemiology

The incidence of hepatitis A has been decreasing in developed countries over the last 50 years. A cyclical pattern with peaks every 6–10 years is demonstrable in many countries: the last such peak in the UK was in 1990 when over 7500 laboratory-confirmed cases were reported in England and Wales. By 1997–99 reports had fallen to around 1300 p.a. Incidence of HAV is less in Scandinavia (where the cyclical pattern has disappeared) and higher in Mediterranean countries (Table 3.29.1). The majority of confirmed cases in the UK occur in those aged 5–44 years, although younger cases are more likely to be asymptomatic and therefore less likely to be diagnosed. A marked excess of males has become apparent in the last few years. Around 14% of UK cases are known to have travelled abroad, mostly to the Indian subcontinent. Other groups at increased risk include those in contact with a case of HAV (e.g. family or nursery), homosexually active men, intravenous drug users, haemophiliacs and residents and workers in institutions for the mentally handicapped.

Clinical features

The clinical picture may range from no symptoms to fulminant hepatitis and is greatly

Table 3.29.1 General patterns of HAV infection in European countries

Endemicity	Countries	Age of cases	Most common transmission
Very low	Scandinavia	Over 20	Travel abroad
Low	Germany Netherlands Switzerland UK	5–40	Common source outbreaks, person to person, and travel abroad
Intermediate	Austria Belgium France Greece Italy Portugal Spain	5–24	Person to person, contaminated food/water, common source outbreaks, and travel abroad

influenced by age. Less than 10% of those aged under 6 develop jaundice but 40% have fever and dark urine and 60% symptoms such as nausea/vomiting, malaise and diarrhoea. Around half of older children and three quarters of adults develop jaundice after a 2–3 day prodrome of malaise, anorexia, nausea, fever and dark urine. Overall case fatality is around 0.5% but is raised (to nearly 2%) in the over-50s. Those with pre-existing liver disease and/or existing hepatitis C infection may suffer more severe disease.

Laboratory confirmation

Confirmation of acute HAV is dependent upon demonstration of specific IgM antibodies, which appear 5–10 days into the illness and persist for around 3 months. IgG antibody persists for life and so in the absence of IgM, a fourfold rise in titres in paired samples would be required, although patients rarely present in time for this to this to be demonstrable. Persistent IgG may be taken as evidence of immunity due to past infection (or immunization). Salivary IgM (and IgG) testing is available at specialist laboratories and may be useful in outbreak investigations.

Transmission

HAV infection is spread primarily by the faeco–oral route from other humans. Up to 10^8 infectious units per millilitre are excreted in faeces during the late incubation period and the first week of symptoms. Viraemia also occurs during the prodromal phase of the illness but at much lower levels than in stool. Saliva and urine are of low infectivity.

Faeco–oral spread is likely to be responsible for secondary transmission to household and nursery contacts, perhaps aided by transmission via fomites. Infection in illicit drug users has been reported in several western European countries and is likely to be due to poor hygiene, although contamination of drugs and needle sharing may contribute. Travellers to endemic countries risk exposure via food or water: this includes children of immigrants from such countries. HAV can survive for 3–10 months in water, suggesting that even in Europe, shellfish harvested from sewage-contaminated waters are a potential source; shellfish concentrate viruses by filtering large quantities of water and are often eaten raw or after gentle steaming which is inadequate to inactivate HAV. Infected food handlers with poor personal hygiene may also contaminate food.

Many cases of HAV do not have a recognized risk factor: it is likely that many of these contracted their infection from an undiagnosed or asymptomatic child case in their household. Such cases may be a factor in community outbreaks that evolve slowly over several months.

Pathogenesis

The incubation period is reported as 15–45 days (mean 28 days) and appears to be less for larger inocula of the virus.

The infectious period is from 2 weeks before onset of jaundice until one week after. Infectivity is maximal during the prodromal period.

Immunity to previous infection is lifelong.

Prevention

• Personal hygiene, especially toilet hygiene in nurseries and schools.
• Sanitary disposal of sewage and treatment of water supplies.
• Vaccination of travellers to countries outside of northern or western Europe, North America or Australasia, at least 2 weeks before the date of departure. If time permits those over 50 years of age or born in high endemicity areas or with a history of jaundice can be tested for immunity before vaccination. Immunoglobulin (HNIG) may be available for late-presenting travellers.
• Vaccination of other risk groups, including patients with chronic liver disease or haemophilia, sexually active homosexual men, and certain laboratory staff. Illicit drug users should also be considered depending on local epidemiology. Local risk assessment may suggest that vaccine should be offered to staff and residents of certain institutions where

good hygiene standards cannot be achieved. Sanitation workers who come into direct contact with untreated sewage may also be considered for vaccine.

• Travellers to developing countries should take the usual precautions over food and water.
• Shellfish should be steamed for at least 90 seconds or heated at 85–90 °C for 4 min before eating.

Surveillance

Confirmed or suspected cases of hepatitis A should be reported to local public health authorities (notifiable as 'viral hepatitis' in the UK). All laboratory-confirmed acute cases (e.g. IgM-positive) should be reported to national surveillance systems.

Response to a case

• Clinicians and microbiologists to report all acute cases to local public health authorities.
• Enteric precautions until one week after onset of jaundice (if no jaundice, precautions until 10 days after onset of first symptoms).
• Exclude all cases in groups with increased risk of further transmission (Box 2.2.1) until 7 days after onset of jaundice.
• Exclude household and sexual contacts with symptoms as for cases.
• Personal hygiene advice to case and contacts. Asymptomatic contacts that attend nursery or infant school should have handwashing supervised.
• Vaccination should be offered to relevant family, sexual, household and other close contacts. The best prophylactic strategy is as yet unclear, but we would suggest the following:
  Presenting within 7 days of exposure: give vaccine.
  7–14 days: give HNIG if available, otherwise give vaccine.
  2–6 weeks: give HNIG to adults and others at risk of severe disease.
• Collect risk factor data for 2–5 weeks before onset: contact with case, travel abroad, mental handicap or other institution, seafood, meals out of household, blood transfusion, occupation.

Investigation of a cluster

• Confirm that cases are acute (clinical jaundice and/or IgM positive).
• Describe by person, place and time. Does epidemic curve suggest point source, ongoing transmission (or both) or continuing source? Are there cases in neighbouring areas?
• Collect risk factor data as for individual case and interview cases sensitively regarding sexuality, sexual activity and illicit drug use. Obtain full occupational and recreational history, e.g. exposure to faeces, nappies, sewage, untreated water, etc. Obtain as full a food history as patient recall allows for 2–5 weeks before onset.
• Discuss with microbiologist use of salivary testing for case finding and availability of genotyping to confirm cases are linked.

Control of an outbreak

• Try to define population at risk suitable for vaccination, e.g. staff and pupils at a nursery.
• Hygiene advice to cases, contacts and any implicated institution. Ensure that toilet and hygiene facilities are adequate.
• For community outbreaks, reinforce hygiene measures in nurseries and schools and vaccinate contacts of cases.
• For prolonged community outbreaks with disease rates of over 50 per 100 000 p.a., discuss further interventions with relevant experts.

Suggested case-definition for an outbreak

Confirmed: demonstration of specific IgM in serum or saliva.
Suspected: case of acute jaundice in at risk population without other known cause. (confirmation important in groups at risk of other hepatitis viruses, e.g. drug users).

3.30 Hepatitis B

Hepatitis B is an acute viral infection of the liver. Its public health importance lies in the severity of disease, its ability to cause long-term carriage leading eventually to cirrhosis and hepatocellular cancer, its transmissibility by the blood-borne route and the availability of vaccines and specific immunoglobulin.

Suggested on-call action (next working day)

- Arrange for laboratory confirmation.
- Identify likely source of infection.
- Arrange for testing and vaccination of close household/sexual contacts.

Epidemiology

Acute hepatitis B is uncommon in the UK and western Europe. The annual incidence is the UK is less than 1 per 100 000 (about 500 cases a year), although the true incidence is higher, as about 70% of infections are subclinical. Most cases are in adults at high risk of infection (see Table 3.30.1). The carriage rate in the general population is about 0.5%, although there is considerable geographical variation with higher rates in inner cities amongst those of black and minority ethnic origin. Some ethnic groups have high rates of carriage, notably

Table 3.30.1 Risk groups for hepatitis B in western Europe

Intravenous drug users
Homosexual and bisexual men who frequently
   change sex partners
Close family and sexual contacts of cases and
   carriers
Haemophiliacs
Renal dialysis patients
Healthcare workers
Staff and residents of mental institutions
Morticians and embalmers
Prisoners
Long-term travellers to high prevalence countries
Babies born to acutely infected or carrier mothers

---

those from countries in south-east Asia and the Far East.

The UK and Scandinavian countries have among the lowest rates of acute infection and carriage in the world; many developing countries have carriage rates above 10%, and there are an estimated 350 million carriers worldwide.

Clinical features

Hepatitis B is clinically indistinguishable from other causes of viral hepatitis. After a non-specific prodromal illness with fever and malaise, jaundice appears and the fever stops. The course of the disease is very variable and jaundice may persist for months. Liver failure is an important early complication.

Laboratory confirmation

The diagnosis and stage of infection can be determined from the antigen and antibody profile in the blood (Fig. 3.30.1). Patients with detectable hepatitis B antigen at six months (surface antigen (HBsAg) and/or e antigen (HBeAg)) are considered to be carriers.

Transmission

Man is the only reservoir. Transmission is from person to person by a number of blood-borne routes (Table 3.30.2).

In low-prevalence countries transmission occurs mainly through shared syringes, needlestick injuries, sexual contact, bites and scratches. In high prevalence countries, perinatal transmission is the most important route; ulcerating skin disease and biting insects also play a role in developing countries.

Pathogenesis

The incubation period is 3–6 months. Carriers of hepatitis B surface antigen who are also e antigen positive and/or e antibody negative are much more infectious than those who are e antibody positive. Patients who do not become carriers and develop natural immunity are immune for life.

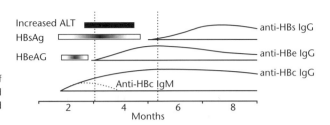

Figure 3.30.1 Occurrence of hepatitis B virus markers and antibodies in the blood of infected patients.

Table 3.30.2 Common routes of transmission for hepatitis B

Drug users who share injecting equipment.
Receipt of blood transfusions or clotting factor concentrate for haemophilia and other blood disorders.
Injury from a needle or sharp instrument contaminated with blood from an infected person.
By acupuncture, tattooing, earpiercing or electrolysis with inadequately sterilized equipment.
Vertical transmission from a mother to her baby before birth, during birth or after birth.
Through sexual intercourse.

Approximately 10% of patients with acute hepatitis B become chronic carriers. Long-term complications of being a carrier include cirrhosis and hepatocellular carcinoma.

Prevention

Hepatitis B can be prevented by ensuring that all blood and blood products are screened and not derived from donors at risk of infection. Universal procedures for the prevention of blood-borne virus transmission should be adopted in hospitals and all situations where needles and other skin-piercing equipment are used. Infected healthcare workers should be prevented from performing exposure-prone procedures. Use of condoms will prevent sexual transmission of hepatitis B. These general measures for the prevention of blood-borne virus infections are covered in detail in Chapter 2.11.

Hepatitis B vaccines are genetically engineered preparations. In the UK and some other

European countries selective vaccination is recommended only for high-risk groups (see Table 3.30.1); in many other countries a universal strategy of vaccinating either newborns or adolescents has been adopted.

The UK schedule is three injections at 0, 1 and 6 months. Where more rapid protection is required (e.g. for travellers or for postexposure prophylaxis) this schedule can be accelerated to 0, 1 and 2 months (or to 0, 7 and 21 days), in which case a fourth dose should be given at 12 months. The vaccine should not be given in the buttock as efficacy may be reduced.

Protection is probably lifelong in a healthy adult who responds to the primary course. Healthcare workers and babies born to hepatitis B carrier mothers should, however, have their antibody status checked 4–6 months after immunization. Poor responders (anti-HBs 10–100 miu/mL) should receive a booster dose and in non-responders (anti-HBs < 10 miu/mL) a repeat course should be considered. Adults over 40 years of age and those with immunodeficiency are more likely to be non-responders.

All women should be screened in pregnancy. Babies born to mothers who are HBsAg-positive and anti-HBe-positive (i.e. low infectivity) should receive an accelerated course of vaccine. Babies whose mothers are e antigen-positive, or who have had acute hepatitis B in pregnancy, or who have no e markers, or whose e markers are not known, should in addition to a course of vaccine receive hepatitis B-specific immunoglobulin (HBIG) 200 iu intramuscularly as soon as possible after birth.

Postexposure prophylaxis should also be offered for significant exposures (inoculations, cuts, abrasions, eye splashes) to a known or suspected HBsAg source (see Table 3.30.3). A

Table 3.30.3 HBV prophylaxis for reported exposure incidents. With permission from S. Handysides (1992) *Exposure to Hepatitis B Virus: Guidance on Post-Exposure Prophylaxis*. CDR Review. PHLS Communicable Disease Surveillance Centre

HBV status of person exposed	Significant exposure			Non-significant exposure	
	HBsAg positive source	Unknown source	HBsAg negative source	Continued risk	No further risk
≤1 doses HB vaccine pre-exposure	Accelerated course of HB vaccine*. HBIG × 1	Accelerated course of HB vaccine*	Initiate course of HB vaccine	Initiate course of HB vaccine	No HBV prophylaxis Reassure
≥2 doses HB vaccine pre-exposure (anti-HBs not known)	One dose of HB vaccine followed by second dose one month later	One dose of HB vaccine	Finish course of HB vaccine	Finish course of HB vaccine	No HBV prophylaxis Reassure
Known responder to HB vaccine (anti-HBs ≥ 10 miU/ml)	Booster dose of HB vaccine	Consider booster dose of HB vaccine	Consider booster dose of HB vaccine	Consider booster dose of HB vaccine	No HBV prophylaxis Reassure
Known non-responder to HB vaccine (anti-HBs < 10 miU/mL 2–4 months post-vaccination)	HBIG × 1 Consider booster dose of HB vaccine	HBIG × 1 Consider booster dose of HB vaccine	No HBIG Consider booster dose of HB vaccine	No HBIG Consider booster dose of HB vaccine	No HBV prophylaxis Reassure

* An accelerated course of vaccine consists of doses spaced at 0.1 and 2 months. A booster dose is given at 12 months to those at continuing risk of exposure to HBV.

significant exposure is one in which HBV transmission may occur. This may be:
• An injury involving a contaminated needle, blade or other sharp object.
• Blood contaminating non-intact skin or eyes.

HBV does not cross intact skin. Exposure to vomit, faeces and sterile or uncontaminated sharp objects poses no risk. Transmission is not known to have occurred as a result of spitting or urine splashing.

The dose of HBIG is 200 iu for children aged 0–4 years, 300 iu for children aged 5–9 years and 500 iu for adults and children aged 10 years or more.

Surveillance

Acute hepatitis B is notifiable in most European countries. Surveillance should ideally be based on laboratory reports, as the disease is clinically indistinguishable from other causes of viral hepatitis.

Response to a case

Laboratory confirmation should be obtained. Determine possible source of infection: obtain history of i.v. drug abuse, sexual orientation, occupation, recent surgery/blood transfusion, and travel. Identify sexual and close household contacts and arrange to have their hepatitis B markers checked to see if they have already been infected before vaccinating them. Contacts who are HBsAg, anti-HBs or anti-HBc positive do not need to be vaccinated, although for sexual partners the first dose of vaccine should be given while awaiting test results and the use of condoms advised until immunity is established.

Investigation of a cluster and response to an outbreak

Look for a common source. If an infected healthcare worker (HCW) is the source, a lookback investigation should be conducted to identify other cases associated with the HCW (see Chapter 4.6).

Suggested case-definition for an outbreak
Jaundice plus presence in serum of HBsAg, or HBeAg, or anti-HBc IgM.

3.31 Hepatitis C

Hepatitis C virus (HCV) is an important public health problem. Large numbers of people are chronically infected and many will go on to develop chronic liver disease in the future. HCV is blood-borne: in western Europe sharing of injecting equipment by drug users has replaced transfusion of contaminated blood or blood products as the main route of transmission.

On-call action
Only rarely will HCV cases, clusters or incidents be notified outside normal office hours. Local circumstances will dictate what immediate action can usefully be taken at that time.

Epidemiology

HCV was first identified in 1989 and a test became available in 1990. Laboratory reports of HCV infection are influenced by awareness among healthcare professionals and the availability and extent of testing and reporting of results. Current tests do not differentiate between present and past infection and most acute infections are asymptomatic so it is difficult to distinguish incident from prevalent cases.

In England and Wales, there were 4563 reports of positive anti-HCV tests in 1998 and 5572 in 1999. Of the reports that included risk factor information, 80% identified injecting drug use as the main route of transmission.

Worldwide it is estimated that 200 million people may be infected with HCV.

In the UK, Belgium and other western European countries 0.1–1% of the general population has HCV infection. Infection is more prevalent in subgroups that have been exposed to the virus in the past, such as injecting drug users and those who have had multiple transfusions including haemophiliacs.

Immigrants from some African countries have a level of HCV infection of around 2–6%, but the reported prevalence in India is low.

Clinical features

Acute hepatitis C is a mild infection and three quarters of those infected have no clinical symptoms. Often the only evidence of infection is elevated liver enzymes. Jaundice, a common sign of other forms of hepatitis, is unusual. Serious liver disease early in the course of the infection is rare. Of those infected with HCV at least 80% continue to be infected with the virus and are said be carriers.

Of those with HCV infection, 80% will develop histological features of chronic hepatitis within 2–3 years of infection, 10–20% will progress to cirrhosis over a period of 6–40 years and of these 1% will go on to develop liver cancer each year.

Laboratory confirmation

HCV is a small (<50 nm) enveloped single-stranded RNA virus distantly related to the flavivirus family. Antibodies to HCV are detected by enzyme immunoassay (EIA) and confirmed by a recombinant immunoblot assay (RIBA) test. A positive antibody test is evidence of previous exposure to HCV but gives no indication of whether the virus is still present. Following exposure antibody tests should be positive by six months. Infection can be detected earlier by PCR testing for the presence of HCV RNA.

Transmission

HCV is spread by contact with blood or body fluids from an infected person in the following ways.

1 Drug users who share injecting equipment.

2 Receipt of blood transfusions or clotting factor concentrate for haemophilia and other blood disorders.

3 Injury from a needle or sharp instrument contaminated with blood from an infected person. Some healthcare workers become infected in this way. There have also been reports of infected surgeons passing infection to their patients while operating.

4 By acupuncture, tattooing, earpiercing or electrolysis with inadequately sterilized equipment.

5 Vertical transmission from a mother to her baby before birth, during birth or after birth. A number of studies have given estimates ranging from 0 to 10% of babies born to HCV-infected mothers who develop chronic HCV infection. The risk of transmission through breastfeeding is minimal.

6 HCV can be transmitted sexually but this is uncommon. When infection spreads between partners this may be due to sharing of personal items such as razors and toothbrushes. Spread via other body fluids such as saliva is also rare.

HCV cannot be passed by sharing food, utensils, baths or toilets with someone with the infection and it cannot be passed on by coughing, sneezing or touching. Horizontal spread within families does not seem to be an important route of transmission.

Pathogenesis

The incubation period is 1–2 months. A person will remain infectious for as long as they are infected with the virus.

Control of HCV infection

Unlike hepatitis A and hepatitis B, at present no vaccine is available for hepatitis C and developing a vaccine will be difficult because of the variability of the virus. Current HCV treatments are not very effective and so for

Table 3.31.1 Target groups for HCV prevention

Injecting drug users	Needle and syringe exchange schemes, low threshold methadone maintenance programmes and education have been shown to reduce transmission of HIV but are less effective in reducing transmission of HCV. There is evidence that HCV transmission occurs without sharing of needles and syringes. Any equipment used in the injecting process such as spoons, filters, water and tourniquets can spread infection.
	Educational programmes should be targeted at younger drug injectors and people injecting drugs for the first time. Hygienic injecting practices should be promoted. Alternative drug administration routes such as smoking and snorting should be encouraged.
	Alcohol and hepatitis B are important cofactors in the production of liver disease. Both are common amongst injecting drug users. Established IDUs and ex-IDUs should have access to advice, counselling, testing and referral if appropriate either through primary care or specialized services.
People infected with and affected by HCV	People with HCV infection and their sexual partners and household contacts need access to high quality information, authoritative advice, counselling, testing and referral if appropriate. They should be familiar with the steps they should take to reduce the risk of further transmission (see Chapter 1.2, universal precautions for blood-borne infections).
Health and social care workers including staff of alcohol and drug agencies	Staff should have a good knowledge of HCV and other blood-borne viral infections so that they can implement infection control measures, including universal precautions.
Prisoners, prison staff and Probation Service staff	Prisoners must have access to information and professional advice, including counselling, testing and referral if appropriate. There should be a national debate about the provision of injecting equipment in prison.
General population especially adolescents	There must be widespread awareness of HCV infection and its transmission. Universal precautions should be promoted particularly with respect to the management of bleeding and blood spillages in the community.
Blood Transfusion Service, organ and tissue donation	People with HCV and those who may have been exposed to HCV should not give blood or carry a donor card. Testing and heat treatment should be used where appropriate.
HCV infection in mothers and infants	Universal antenatal screening for HCV is not recommended. However, pregnant women at risk of HCV infection should be offered hepatitis C screening. Breast feeding should be discouraged only if the mother is viraemic.

the foreseeable future HCV will be controlled by:

• preventing further transmission of HCV (Table 3.31.1);

• advising and managing those people who are already infected;

• setting up public health information systems which will allow the occurrence and distribution of infection to be tracked and which will evaluate the costs and effectiveness of existing and new treatments as they become available.

Surveillance

Most cases of HCV infection are chronic cases that are detected as a result of serological testing because of a possible past exposure. The laboratory will report these cases to CDSC for national surveillance purposes. Occasionally acute cases are diagnosed and these should be reported to the CCDC. The CCDC should enquire about possible routes and circumstances of exposure. The CCDC should take particular care to rule out the possibility of infection as a result of healthcare, acupuncture or other alternative therapy and blood transfusion.

Response to a case

• The cases should receive information about the infection and advice on preventing further spread. This should be accompanied by a written advice sheet.
• Refer for investigation and possible treatment if indicated and longer-term support and counselling. The current treatment is with interferon alpha and ribavarin.

Investigation of an HCV incident or outbreak

All those who have potentially been exposed

Table 3.31.2 Hepatitis C case definitions

Prevalent case	Anti-HCV positive by: Two different ELISAs or ELISA and RIBA or HCV RNA by PCR
Acute hepatitis C	an illness with: a discrete date of onset jaundice or elevated serum AST/ALT anti-HAV IgM negative anti-HBc IgM negative (if done) or HBsAg negative and HCV RNA positive by PCR
Seroconversion	Documentation of a previous serum antibody test which was anti-HCV negative by either EIA-3, RIBA-3, or both EIA-2 and RIBA-2 and a recent serum which is anti-HCV positive by: two different EIA-3 assays, or by EIA-3 and RIBA-3, or positive for HCV RNA by PCR

should be identified and offered testing. Those with evidence of infection will need sympathetic counselling and should be offered long-term follow in conjunction with a liver specialist who can advise on treatment options. If a healthcare worker who has performed exposure prone procedures is found to have HCV infection a look back exercise may be required (see Chapter 4.6).

3.32 Hepatitis, delta

Delta hepatitis is caused by a satellite virus that only infects patients during the antigen-positive stages of acute hepatitis B or long-term HBsAg carriers. The epidemiology is thus similar to that of hepatitis B (see Chapter 3.30). Transmission is by the same routes as hepatitis B. The incubation period is 2–8 weeks. General control measures for blood-borne viruses will prevent spread of delta hepatitis. There is no specific vaccine or immunoglobulin.

3.33 Hepatitis E

Although rare in north-west Europe, hepatitis E virus (HEV) is the main cause of enterically transmitted non-A non-B hepatitis worldwide. HEV causes an illness similar to hepatitis A (abdominal pain, anorexia, dark urine, fever, hepatomegaly, jaundice, malaise, nausea and vomiting) without chronic sequelae or carriage. Case-fatality is low, except in women infected in the third trimester of pregnancy, when it may reach 20%. Specific IgM testing is available in specialist laboratories, although a positive result should be treated with caution in those without risk factors.

Outbreaks of HEV have occurred in many developing countries of Asia, Africa and Central America, including India, Pakistan and Bangladesh. HEV is also responsible for around half of acute sporadic hepatitis in many developing areas. Most clinically reported cases occur in young or middle-aged adults.

HEV is transmitted faeco–orally, with most outbreaks linked to faecally contaminated drinking water. Person-to-person spread is inefficient (2% secondary attack rate reported), but nosocomial spread is described. Virus excretion in stools occurs at around clinical onset and lasts up to 14 days. The incubation period is reported as 15–60 days (mean=40 days).

Prevention relies primarily on provision of safe water supplies: European travellers to developing countries, particularly if pregnant, should take care with food and water. Confirmed or suspected cases should be notified to local public health authorities.

3.34 Herpes simplex

Infection with herpes simplex viruses (HSV) is characterized by a localized primary infection, latency and localized recurrence. HSV 1 is typically associated with gingivostomatitis and HSV 2 with genital infection, which is covered in Chapter 3.25. However, either may affect the genital tract and HSV 2 can cause primary infection of the mouth.

On-call action

This is not generally applicable.

Epidemiology

The incidence of HSV 1 infection peaks first in preschool-aged children. There is a second lower peak in young adults. It is rare in infancy because of passive maternal antibody. It is estimated that 50–90% of adults have antibodies to HSV 1.

Clinical features

Primary infection produces a painful ulcerating vesicular eruption in the mouth with fever and other systemic symptoms. Lesions may develop at other sites such as the nose, eye, finger (herpetic whitlow) and perineum as a result of autoinoculation. The illness resolves after 10–14 days. Complications are rare but herpetic encephalitis has been reported. Following primary infection, HSV persists in a latent form in the sensory nerve ganglion and at a later date may reactivate and cause a painful local skin eruption, usually on the lip (cold sore). Reactivation may affect 45% of persons who had a primary infection and is provoked by fever, sunlight, trauma, menstruation and emotional stress. The risk of reactivation declines with age.

Laboratory confirmation

HSV are typical large DNA herpes viruses. The diagnosis is usually made clinically, but vesicle fluid or scrapings can be examined for virus particles by electron microscopy. Monoclonal antibodies or viral culture are required to distinguish HSV from varicella-zoster virus infection.

Transmission

Humans are the only reservoir of infection. The virus may be shed from the mouth of people who have never had secondary lesions.

Infection is spread by direct contact with contaminated saliva, often by kissing but also as a result of wrestling (herpes gladiatorum) or other contact sports. Airborne transmission is unlikely. The virus does not survive for long periods in the environment and cannot penetrate intact skin. Following exposure 80% of non-immune subjects will be infected. Medical and nursing staff may get lesions as a result of carrying out procedures with ungloved hands.

Pathogenesis

The incubation period is 2–12 days and a person may remain infectious for several weeks as a result of intermittent shedding of virus in the saliva. Patients with impaired cellular immunity, skin disorders and burns are at risk of severe and persistent HSV infections.

Prevention

Health education and attention to personal hygiene may reduce exposure. Gloves should be available for health and social care staff in contact with potential infection. Patients with HSV infection should avoid contact with infants, burns patients, and people with eczema or impaired immunity.

Response to a case/cluster

Patients with extensive infection should be nursed with source isolation. Children with cold sores do not need to be excluded from school.

Case-definition

Characteristic lesions with or without laboratory confirmation by electron microscopy or viral culture.

3.35 *Haemophilus influenzae* type b (Hib)

Haemophilus influenzae type b (Hib) is a bacterial infection of young children, which causes meningitis and other bacteraemic diseases including pneumonia, epiglottitis, facial cellulitis and bone and joint infections. Its importance lies in the high rate of disease complications and the availability of a vaccine.

Suggested on-call action

- Seek laboratory confirmation.
- Obtain vaccination history.
- Arrange for chemoprophylaxis and vaccination of contacts.

Epidemiology

The disease is commonest in children under 5. Before vaccination was introduced in the UK, Hib was the second most common cause of bacterial meningitis overall, and the commonest in young children. One in 600 children developed invasive Hib disease before the age of 5. The case fatality rate is 4–5% (higher in infants) and up to 30% of survivors have permanent neurological sequelae, including deafness, convulsions and mental impairment.

Hib is now rare in most of western Europe. There were 29 cases of Hib meningitis notified in England and Wales in 1999, of which about half were in unvaccinated adults. The remainder were either vaccine failures or in unvaccinated children.

Other serotypes of *H. influenzae* occasionally cause invasive disease and non-encapsulated *H. influenzae* sometimes cause ear infections or acute exacerbations of chronic bronchitis.

Clinical features

Hib meningitis typically has a slower onset than meningococcal meningitis, with symptoms developing over 3 or 4 days. There is progressive headache, drowsiness, and vomiting with intermittent fever. Photophobia may be present. A haemorrhagic rash is sometimes present, but is unusual. In soft tissue, bone and joint infections there is swelling of the affected area. Hib epiglottitis presents with acute respiratory obstruction.

Laboratory confirmation

This is important as the clinical features are variable and non-specific; also to ascertain vaccine failures. A positive culture may be obtained from blood or CSF. Alternatively Hib antigen can be demonstrated by latex agglutination or PCR. All strains should be sent to the national reference laboratory for confirmation and typing.

Transmission

Man is the only reservoir. Transmission is by droplet infection and direct contact with nose and throat secretions. In unvaccinated populations carriage is common in young children; about 4–5% of unvaccinated 3-year-olds are carriers. Vaccination prevents carriage.

Pathogenesis

The incubation period is not known, but is probably only 2–4 days. Cases are non-infectious within 48h of starting effective antibiotic treatment. Disease usually results in lifetime immunity, although repeat infections have been described. Immunity is also derived from carriage, from infection with cross-protective antigens such as *E. coli*, and from vaccination.

Prevention

Hib vaccines are protein-polysaccharide conjugates that provide over 95% protection in infants from two months of age. The UK schedule is three doses at 2, 3 and 4 months of age, given at the same time as diphtheria/tetanus/pertussis and polio vaccines. Coverage is currently 94% by two years of age. Children over 12 months require only a single dose. No boosters are given in the UK (although many countries in Europe give a booster in the second year of life). The only contraindication is a severe reaction to a previous dose.

Surveillance

Hib meningitis is notifiable in most countries of western Europe, although this does not apply to other forms of invasive Hib disease. Surveillance of Hib should always be based on laboratory reports. Any case in a vaccinated child should be reported to the national surveillance unit.

Response to a case

Laboratory confirmation must be sought. Check vaccination status of the case and of household contacts. Household contacts do not require chemoprophylaxis if all children in the household have been vaccinated. If there are any unvaccinated children under five in the household, they should be vaccinated and all household members (including adults, who may be the source of infection) should be given chemoprophylaxis (Box 3.35.1). The case should also receive chemoprophylaxis and vaccine. Nursery contact should be given chemoprophylaxis (and vaccine, if unvaccinated) if there are two or more cases within 120 days. Patients should be warned of the adverse effects of rifampicin (red staining of urine, sputum, tears and contact lenses, interference with the oral contraceptive pill).

There is no need to exclude siblings or other close contacts of cases from nursery or school.

Investigation and control of a cluster

In addition to the measures described for a case, there may be a need to conduct a local vaccination programme if coverage is low.

Suggested case-definition for an outbreak

Confirmed: clinically compatible illness with an isolate or antigen detection of Hib from a normally sterile site.

Clinical: meningitis or epiglottitis with no other cause in:

(a) an unvaccinated child under five years of age *or*

(b) an unvaccinated individual with links to confirmed case(s).

Box 3.35.1 Chemoprophylaxis for invasive Hib disease

Rifampicin, orally, 20 mg/kg daily for 4 days (maximum 600 mg daily).

3.36 HIV

The acquired immune deficiency syndrome (AIDS) was first described in 1981 in the USA when cases of *Pneumocystis carinii* pneumonia (PCP), other opportunistic infections and cancers such as Kaposi's sarcoma were reported in young homosexual men with impaired immunity. Haemophiliacs, recipients of blood transfusions and injecting drug users were also affected. With the discovery of the human immunodeficiency virus (HIV-1) in 1983 came the recognition that AIDS was the result of advanced HIV-1 infection. The development of laboratory tests for HIV-1 infection followed.

HIV-1 is a member of the lentivirus genus of the Retroviridae family of RNA viruses. There is a second human immunodeficiency virus, HIV-2, which is endemic in western Africa. It causes a spectrum of disease similar to that produced by HIV-1 although progression to AIDS is uncommon.

On-call action

The public health doctor should be prepared to advise on the management of HIV-related incidents, particularly exposure incidents (see Box 3.36.1).

Epidemiology

Effective surveillance of HIV infection is particularly important because of its enormous public health significance. In the UK a range of different sources of surveillance data are avail-

Table 3.36.1 Main sources of UK surveillance data: HIV and AIDS

Clinicians' reports of cases of HIV infection (with or without AIDS) and deaths in people with HIV infection
Laboratory reports of newly diagnosed HIV infections
Unlinked anonymous HIV prevalence monitoring
Survey of prevalent HIV infections diagnosed (SOPHID)
Mortality reports
Laboratory reporting of CD4 counts
Results of voluntary HIV testing
Reporting of HIV infection in pregnancy and in children
Surveillance of tuberculosis and other AIDS indicator diseases
Behavioural surveys and monitoring
Reports from genitourinary medicine clinics (KC60 returns)
Reporting of results of screening blood donations
Reports of occupational exposure

---

able (Table 3.36.1). Similar surveillance data sources are used in most western European countries. Particular importance is attached to determining the most likely route of exposure for each case. This has allowed the progress of the epidemic to be defined and the most appropriate control measures to be implemented.

HIV infection is now found throughout the world but prevalence and incidence in different countries varies widely and depends on the methods of surveillance that are used. Infection is prevalent in central Africa, the Caribbean area, the Indian subcontinent and some South American countries.

By December 1999 the World Health Organization estimated that 33.6 million people were living with HIV infection throughout the world and there had been 5.6 million new infections in 1999 alone. The steepest increases in reports of HIV infection have come from the newly independent states of the former Soviet Union, particularly Ukraine, where transmission is mainly among injecting drug users.

At the end of 1998, it was estimated that there were 4 million cases of HIV infection in

India, spread mainly through injecting drug use. The pattern of HIV infection in other parts of Asia is variable.

Sub-Saharan Africa remains the region most affected by HIV infection, particularly southern Africa. In these areas sexual transmission among heterosexual individuals is common and approximately equal rates of infection are observed in men and women. In some areas up to 30% of all adults age 15–49 years are infected. The prevalence of HIV infection in West Africa is increasing, and this may have implications for European countries including the UK, which has large numbers of migrants of Nigerian and Ghanaian origin.

Compared with European neighbours, the UK has a relatively low prevalence of HIV infection. This is due to targeted interventions among behaviourally vulnerable groups, the early introduction of public education campaigns, the availability of free and open access GUM clinics and the widespread provision of needle exchange schemes.

Back calculation suggests that the first cases of HIV infection appeared in the UK in the late 1970s. HIV infection is now found in all population groups and in every region. However, the highest levels of HIV infection are in those groups whose behaviour puts them at particular risk namely homosexual and bisexual men, people attending GUM clinics (a group of people with an increased risk of STIs) and injecting drug users attending agencies. The current epidemiology of HIV infection in the UK is summarized in Table 3.36.2.

Clinical features

HIV-1 binds to CD4 receptors on helper T-lymphocytes or macrophages. The virus is internalized and viral RNA is transcribed into DNA by a reverse transcriptase and integrated into the host cell genome. The cell is then permanently infected. Virions may bud from the cell surface to infect another cell, or infection may be spread when cells divide. There is much heterogeneity of DNA sequences among HIV isolates. Eventually the infected cell is killed by the virus.

HIV infection leads to a depletion of T4 cells in the peripheral blood and eventually there is a fall in the T4/T8 ratio and total lymphocyte count. A T4 (CD4) count of less than 200 cells/mm^3 indicates severe immunosuppression and is usually associated with opportunistic infections, neoplasia and full-blown AIDS.

The acquisition of HIV infection is quickly followed by a period of viraemia, with or without symptoms, during which the individual is very infectious. Antibodies against HIV develop and the infection may remain apparently dormant for many years, but infected individuals do not clear the infection, and remain potentially infectious to others.

The clinical manifestations of HIV infection extend from the initial acute retroviral syndrome to full-blown AIDS characterized by life-threatening opportunistic infections and neoplasms (Table 3.36.3). Most individuals are asymptomatic for several years after the initial acute retroviral infection.

Laboratory confirmation

Diagnosis of HIV infection is usually made by detection of antibodies in serum by enzyme immunoassay (EIA). A positive EIA test should be repeated and then confirmed by Western blot test. HIV ('p24') antigen is detectable in the blood 1–4 weeks after infection; antibodies usually appear within 3–12 weeks of infection and nearly all individuals remain seropositive for life. Atypical lymphocytes may be seen on a blood film, HIV plasma viral load may increase and the CD4 count will fall from the normal value of 600–1400 cell/mm^3.

Transmission

HIV is spread from person to person as a result of exposure to infected blood or tissues, usually as a result of sexual contact, sharing needles or syringes or transfusion of infected blood or blood components. Normal social or domestic contact carries no risk of transmission. Transmission is especially efficient between male homosexuals in whom receptive anal intercourse and multiple sexual partners are particular risk factors. In countries where

Table 3.36.2 Summary of the current epidemiology of HIV infection in the UK

Women and children	By the end of 1998, 6082 women had been diagnosed with HIV. There were 555 new diagnoses in 1998, of these heterosexual exposure (75%) and injecting drug use (15%) were the main routes of exposure. In 1997 there were 2738 prevalent cases in females, of these approximately half were of Black-African ethnic origin and most were resident in London. Of the 1628 infants born to HIV-infected mothers 38% are known to be infected. There have been reports of 952 children with HIV infection; vertical transmission and blood factor receipt are the main routes of exposure.
	The level of HIV infection amongst women giving birth in London has continued to increase and is now 1 in 450. The level among women having terminations of pregnancy is almost 1 in 120. Nearly half of these infections remain undiagnosed. In 1998, 330 births occurred to HIV-infected women in the UK resulting in an estimated 58 infected babies.
Homosexual and bisexual men	There is evidence of high risk behaviour and continuing HIV transmission amongst homosexual and bisexual men: there are substantial levels of HIV infection among young homosexual and bisexual men attending GUM clinics, homosexual and bisexual men aware of their HIV infection continue to acquire other STIs, there are significant numbers of reports of gonorrhoea due to homosexual exposure and there is no suggestion from age and CD4 count at HIV diagnosis of an ageing cohort of those infected through sex between men.
	It is estimated that there are 1500 new HIV infections amongst homosexual and bisexual men each year. This is probably lower than the peak seen in the early 1980s. Around 28% of infections in this group remain undiagnosed.
Heterosexuals	Transmission of HIV infection in non-injecting heterosexuals in the UK is continuing to occur at low levels with little change in prevalence in the last year. However, the rising level of acute sexually transmitted infections and the higher HIV prevalence among GUM clinic attenders indicate continuing high-risk behaviour. A substantial number of HIV infections remain undiagnosed and so those who are infected are unable to benefit from recent new treatments. Most cases of heterosexually acquired HIV infection are linked to Africa. There is, as yet, little evidence of any links with South Asia.
Injecting drug users	Although the prevalence of HIV infection in IDUs is generally stable there is some evidence that the proportion of injecting drug users who report recent sharing of injecting paraphernalia has increased. Also cases of acute hepatitis B infection attributed to injecting drug use have increased recently. There is continuing potential for HIV transmission to occur amongst injecting drug users along with other blood-borne viruses such as hepatitis B and hepatitis C.

heterosexual spread is common, sexually transmitted infections causing genital ulceration and multiple partners are associated with the highest rates of transmission. HIV is present in saliva, tears and urine but transmission as a result of contact with these secretions is uncommon. HIV infection is not thought to be transmitted by biting insects.

Between 15 and 30% of infants born to HIV infected mothers are infected with HIV as a result of vertical transmission either before, during or shortly after birth due to breast-feeding.

Pathogenesis

Following exposure HIV antigen or viral nucleic acid sequences may be detected in the blood within 1–4 weeks and HIV antibodies can be detected within 4–12 weeks. Half of those with HIV infection will develop AIDS

Table 3.36.3 Clinical manifestations of HIV infection

Acute retroviral syndrome	About 1–6 weeks after exposure there may be fever, sweats, malaise, myalgia and a rash. HIV (p24) antigen is usually detectable in serum but the EIA antibody test is often negative.
AIDS-related complex (ARC)	ARC includes persistent generalized lymphadenopathy (PGL), immune thrombocytopenic purpura (ITP), oropharyngeal candidiasis, herpes zoster, chronic diarrhoea, hairy leukoplakia and the constitutional wasting syndrome.
Common AIDS infections	• *Pneumocystis carinii* pneumonia • Oesophageal or bronchial candidiasis • Cytomegalovirus infection • Extrapulmonary cryptococcosis • *Mycobacterium avium-intracellulare* infection
AIDS: neoplasms	• Kaposi's sarcoma • Non-Hodgkin's lymphoma • Brain lymphoma
Other conditions associated with HIV infection	• Tuberculosis • Perianal and genital condyloma acuminata • Seborrhoeic dermatitis • Psoriasis • Molluscum contagiosum • HIV encephalopathy • Peripheral neuropathies

within 7–10 years and of these 80–90% will die within 3–5 years. In developed countries in recent years highly active antiretroviral therapy (HAART) has dramatically reduced the number of AIDS cases and AIDS deaths.

A person with HIV infection will be infectious to others from shortly after the onset of the HIV infection throughout the rest of his or her life. It is thought that infectiousness increases with the degree of immunosuppression, viral load and the presence of sexually transmitted infections. Susceptibility to HIV infection is universal. Sexually transmitted infections producing genital ulceration may increase susceptibility. It is not known whether there is any immunity to HIV infection. Recovery from HIV infection has never been convincingly described.

Prevention

The variability of HIV-1 makes the development of an effective vaccine very difficult and therefore unlikely in the near future.

Most HIV prevention programmes rely on public health education about the need to avoid activities that carry a risk of HIV transmission, particularly high-risk sexual activity and injecting drug use. The main HIV preventative measures are summarized in Table 3.36.4.

Surveillance

In the UK the CCDC may maintain a confidential, anonymized database of local residents with HIV infection for epidemiological and service planning purposes. Data on local cases are sought from the microbiologist and the GUM, infectious disease and haematology consultants and should be updated at least every year. The data can be compared with central databases held by CDSC.

Response to a case

There is no cure for HIV infection but a growing number of antiviral drugs are available which slow the progression of disease. Treatment is aimed at reducing the plasma viral

Table 3.36.4 HIV preventative measures

Sexual transmission can be reduced by promoting sexual abstinence or completely monogamous relationships between two uninfected partners or by reducing the number of sexual partners and minimizing exposure to body fluids during intercourse by using latex condoms.

Services for diagnosing and treating sexually transmitted infections including voluntary confidential testing for HIV infection and HIV counselling.

Transmission among intravenous drug users can be reduced by appropriate educational efforts and treatment programs including needle and syringe exchange schemes and drug substitute prescribing programmes.

Perinatal transmission can be reduced by counselling and testing for HIV infection for all pregnant women as a routine part of antenatal care combined with interventions to reduce the risk of vertical transmission from mother to infant including antiviral treatment, caesarean section and advice to refrain from breast-feeding.

Healthcare workers and others should be advised to take particular care when handling blood or sharp instruments and to adopt universal precautions for the prevention of blood-borne viral infections when caring for any patient with HIV infection. Treatment with antiviral drugs may be appropriate following occupational exposure to HIV-contaminated material.

Transmission by blood and blood products can be prevented by serological testing of blood and plasma and by heat treatment of clotting factors. Persons who have engaged in behaviours that place them at increased risk of HIV infection should be advised to refrain from donating blood, organs or tissues, including semen.

load and is started before the immune system is irreversibly damaged.

Hospital patients with HIV infection should be nursed with universal precautions for blood-borne viral infections. Side room isolation is unnecessary unless there is a risk of haemorrhage. The person with HIV infection should be offered advice on preventing further spread and should be encouraged to identify sexual and needle sharing contacts so that counselling and HIV testing can be arranged.

Investigation and control of an HIV incident or cluster

Clusters of cases of HIV infection are uncommon but may be detected when contact tracing is carried out in sexual or drug using networks. Occasionally a local increase in the incidence of HIV infection may occur. Standard outbreak investigation methods should be adopted. Particular care is needed to preserve patient confidentiality. Colleagues in the local GUM clinic or drug team should be able to assist with case finding, interviews and blood tests.

HIV-related incidents occur more commonly and may include: a healthcare worker with HIV infection, a percutaneous injury involving exposure to material from an HIV-infected person or a person with HIV infection who will not reliably follow advice to prevent further spread.

Guidelines on how to respond to these incidents are available. Generally public health legislation has not proved to be helpful in controlling spread from a person with HIV infection.

Suggested case-definition

HIV infection is defined by a positive test for antibody to HIV.

AIDS is defined as the development of one or more of the specific infections or neoplasms accepted as markers of immunodeficiency in severely immunocompromised patients with no inherited, iatrogenic, or environmental cause for the observed immune suppression. A CD4 count of less than 200 cells/mm^3 has been incorporated into the AIDS case definition in the USA.

Box 3.36.1 HIV postexposure prophylaxis

• The risk of acquiring HIV infection following a needlestick injury or other occupational exposure to HIV is small but can be reduced by the use of antiretroviral drug combinations for postexposure prophylaxis (PEP).

• Use of PEP may also be considered following HIV exposure in non-occupational settings.

• The risk of acquiring HIV infection following a needlestick injury from a patient with HIV infection is 3 per 1000 injuries. The risk of acquiring HIV infection through mucous membrane exposure is less than 1 per 1000.

• Some needlestick injuries carry a higher risk than others. These include injuries with hollow needles, deep injuries, source patients who are terminally ill and injuries with needles that are visibly blood-stained or which have been in an artery or vein.

• Combination antiretroviral prophylaxis to healthcare workers occupationally exposed to HIV infection is associated with an 80% reduction in the risk of occupationally acquired HIV infection.

Action following an HIV exposure

• A risk assessment should be carried out by someone other than the exposed person. It may be appropriate for the exposed person to take the first dose of PEP pending the outcome of a more thorough risk assessment.

• PEP should be considered whenever there has been a significant exposure to material known to be or strongly suspected to be infected with HIV infection.

• A significant exposure would be percutaneous exposure, exposure of broken skin or mucous membrane exposure. High-risk body fluids are blood, semen, vaginal secretions, amniotic fluid, human breast milk, CSF, fluid from body cavities and joints, blood-stained saliva, tissues and organs. Urine, vomit, saliva and faeces are low-risk materials unless visibly blood-stained. The HIV status of the source patient may be known. If not, a designated doctor should approach the patient and ask for their informed agreement to HIV testing. This course of action should be universally adopted with all significant exposures.

• With unknown sources the risk assessment will be informed by consideration of the circumstances of the exposure and the epidemiological likelihood of HIV in the source. In most such exposures in the UK it will probably be difficult to justify the use of PEP.

• Most exposures requiring PEP will take place in an acute hospital setting, particularly in hospitals which regularly care for people with HIV infection. Appropriate psychological support should be available. PEP should normally be continued for four weeks. There should be weekly follow-up by an experienced occupational health practitioner. All healthcare workers occupationally exposed to HIV should have follow-up counselling, postexposure testing and medical evaluation whether or not they have received PEP. All should be encouraged to seek medical advice about any acute illness that occurs during the follow-up period. Pending follow-up, and in the absence of seroconversion, healthcare workers need not be subject to any modification of their working practices. They should, however, be advised about safer sex and avoiding blood donation during the follow-up period. At least six months should elapse after cessation of PEP before a negative antibody test is used to reassure the individual that infection has not occurred.

• For optimal efficacy, PEP should be commenced as soon as possible and ideally within an hour of the incident. However, it may still be worth considering starting PEP even if up to two weeks have elapsed since the exposure.

• Starter packs containing a three-day course should be readily available at strategic locations including the occupational health department, pharmacy, accident and emergency department and selected wards or departments.

Continued

Box 3.36.1 *Continued.*

UK healthcare workers seconded overseas
• Employers should consider making seven-day starter packs of PEP drugs available to workers and students travelling to countries where antiretroviral therapy is not commonly available. In circumstances where it has been considered necessary to start PEP, expert advice by phone will be required to help the student or healthcare worker to decide whether or not PEP needs to be continued for four weeks and if so, whether urgent repatriation is required.
• On return from working abroad in countries of high HIV prevalence, healthcare workers, including students, should be asked to complete a questionnaire about possible significant exposures. This will alert their occupational health departments for the need for a more detailed de-briefing. Of the eight probable occupationally acquired HIV infections reported in the UK, seven were associated with exposure in high-prevalence areas abroad.

Exposure outside the healthcare setting
• Exposure outside the healthcare setting may include sexual exposure, sharing drug-injecting equipment and significant exposure to HIV-infected material in other circumstances.
• Such exposures may give rise to request for PEP or the need to consider it. There is insufficient evidence at present to make a recommendation either in favour of the use of PEP in these circumstances, or against its use. Benefit is more likely when:
The risk of transmission is considered high.
Such exposure is considered unlikely to be repeated.
PEP can be started promptly.
Good adherence to the regime is considered likely.

Pregnancy
PEP can be used in pregnancy; however, expert advice should be sought. Urgent pregnancy testing should be arranged for any female healthcare worker who cannot rule out the possibility of pregnancy before starting PEP.

The choice of drugs for PEP
• PEP currently comprises:
Zidovudine 200 mg tds or 250 mg bd;
plus lamivudine 150 mg bd;
plus nelfinavir 750 tds or 1250 bd (or soft-gel saquinavir).
• PEP should be started within an hour and continued for four weeks.

3.37 Human transmissible spongiform encephalopathies

Human transmissible spongiform encephalopathies (TSEs) are a group of conditions characterized by progressive fatal encephalopathy with typical spongiform pathological appearances in the brain. They include classical Creutzfeldt–Jakob disease (CJD), variant Creutzfeldt–Jakob disease (vCJD), and kuru. The causal agent of vCJD is PrP, a prion protein.

Suggested on-call action
• None usually necessary.
• May need to prepare for media interest

Epidemiology

CJD in its classical form is the commonest of the human TSEs but is still rare, with an annual incidence worldwide of 0.5–1.0 cases per million population. In the UK there are about 35 cases per year, with an average age of onset of 55–75 years.

The first case of vCJD came to the attention of the CJD Surveillance Unit in 1995. At the time of going to press, 79 cases had been reported in the UK, two in France and two in Ireland. The number of reported cases may be increasing slightly at present. The future course of the epidemic is unknown: mathematical modelling has predicted the number of future cases to be between zero and 136 000. The age distribution of vCJD is younger than in classical CJD (range 14–53 years, mean of 28), and cases have a different symptom profile and a different appearance of brain tissue on postmortem. There may be genetic differences in susceptibility: all cases of vCJD tested to date are homologous for methionine at codon 129 of the prion protein gene, this is similar to cattle, where codon 129 codes for methionine—about 38% of the UK population are of this genotype. No relationship with occupation is apparent.

Kuru is a disease that occurs exclusively in Papua New Guinea; it has now almost disappeared.

Clinical features

The onset of vCJD is with variable psychiatric symptoms. This is typically followed by abnormal sensation at 2 months, ataxia at 5 months, myoclonus at 8 months, akinetic mutism at 11 months, with death at 12–24 months.

Laboratory confirmation

The diagnosis of vCJD is made on the basis of typical clinical features (see case definition) and postmortem findings of spongiform change and extensive PrP deposition with florid plaques throughout the cerebrum and cerebellum.

Transmission

Most cases of classical CJD are sporadic, about 15% are inherited and around 1% are iatrogenic, transmitted from human pituitary derived growth hormone injections, corneal transplants and brain surgery involving contaminated instruments. Classical CJD is not thought to be transmissible via blood transfusion.

The most likely source of vCJD in humans is cattle infected with bovine spongiform encephalopathy (BSE). The PrP causing vCJD and BSE are indistinguishable from each other, but are different to those causing classical CJD or scrapie. The route of spread is unknown although consumption of infected bovine neural tissue is thought to be the most likely. Such exposure is likely to have been at its greatest before the introduction of effective control measures in 1990. In addition to the CNS tissues (including eye and pituitary) that are infectious in all types of TSE, vCJD also involves the lymphoreticular system and so tissues such as tonsils, appendix, thymus, lymph nodes, spleen, Peyer's patches and possibly bone marrow could all be infectious. Iatrogenic transmission from contaminated surgical instruments and blood transfusions are both theoretically possible. Although scrapie, the main TSE of sheep, is not thought to be transmissible to man, it is possible that sheep infected with BSE could have entered the food chain.

Kuru is transmitted by cannibalistic consumption of infected human brain tissue.

Pathogenesis

The incubation period for vCJD is unknown, but is probably several years; for iatrogenic CJD and kuru the mean incubation is 12 years. The infective dose is unknown, but is likely to be affected by route of exposure. Cattle under 30 months of age are thought to be significantly less likely to be infectious.

Prevention

Steps should be taken to prevent BSE in cattle and transmission of infected tissues to man.

These include banning consumption of potentially infected feed to cattle, avoiding human consumption of nervous and lymphoreticular tissues, safe preparation of carcasses and slaughter of affected herds.

Measures to reduce the risk of iatrogenic illness include:
• adequate cleaning and sterilization of surgical instruments before re-use (may still be some residual risk);
• avoiding re-use of instruments used on known CJD cases and high-risk groups (e.g. received cadaver-derived growth hormone);
• where possible, not re-using surgical instruments after operations on high-risk tissues (official UK guidance awaited at time of writing);
• use of leukodepleted blood for transfusions;
• use of non-UK-sourced plasma and blood products;
• avoiding transplant donations from certain high-risk groups.

Further information is available from http://www.open.gov.uk/doh/coinh.htm.

Pentosan polysulphate is under evaluation as a potential postexposure prophylactic.

Surveillance

In the UK, suspected cases of vCJD should be reported to the national CJD Surveillance Unit in Edinburgh. This unit is responsible for surveillance, advising on diagnosis, and identification of certain control measures, e.g. to withdraw any blood donations made by the case. Surveillance is based on direct referral from targeted professionals (e.g. neurologists), unsolicited referrals from other professionals and review of death certificates with certain causes of death coded.

European level surveillance occurs through two EU-funded schemes, 'EUROCJD' and 'NEUROCJD'.

Response to a case

Report to national CJD Surveillance Unit. Check for recent surgery or blood donation. A lookback exercise should be considered in any case of vCJD who has undergone an invasive procedure, particularly if involving nervous or lymphoid tissue. This should be based upon a risk assessment considering the type of exposure and how long previously the exposure occurred. Advice is available from an expert panel contactable via the Department of Health. Those at highest risk are probably those exposed to instruments on the first few occasions of use after the potential contamination.

Investigation of a cluster

The uncertain and prolonged incubation period make the identification and investigation of clusters difficult. Look for common exposures over a wide period of time, particularly common sources of beef and bovine products since 1980. Expert advice should be sought.

Suggested case-definition

Confirmed: progressive neuropsychiatric disorder and neuropathological confirmation of vCJD on postmortem.

Probable: progressive neuropsychiatric disorder, lasting more than 6 months, with routine investigations not suggesting an alternative diagnosis and no history of iatrogenic exposure *and* either (a) or (b):

(a) Four from following list:
Early psychiatric symptoms; persistent painful sensory symptoms; ataxia, myoclonus *or* chorea *or* dystonia; dementia.
And EEG does not show changes typical of sporadic CJD.
And bilateral pulvinar high signal on MRI scan.

(b) Positive tonsil biopsy.

3.38 Influenza

Influenza virus is a highly infectious cause of acute respiratory infection. It is a major cause of morbidity during epidemics and can be life-threatening in the elderly and chronically unwell.

Epidemiology

Influenza causes both annual winter epidemics of varying size and severity, and occasional more severe pandemics. All age-groups are affected, with highest incidence in children but most hospitalizations and deaths in the elderly. Between 3000 and 20000 excess winter deaths per year are attributed to influenza in the UK depending on the size of the epidemic. Community outbreaks in the winter tend to last 6–10 weeks, peaking at around the fourth week.

Influenza A and B viruses may alter gradually by 'antigenic drift': every few years this will result in a significant epidemic with rapid spread and a 10–20% attack rate. Influenza A may also change abruptly by 'antigenic shift' producing a subtype to which there is little existing population immunity and causing a major pandemic, usually with severe disease in all ages: these have occurred in 1918 (causing 20 million deaths worldwide), 1957, 1968 and 1977.

Clinical features

About half of cases will have the classic 'flu picture of a sudden onset of fever, chills, headache, muscle aches, myalgia and anorexia. There may also be a dry cough, sore throat, or runny nose. Up to 25% of children may also have nausea, vomiting or diarrhoea if infected by influenza B or A (H1N1). The illness lasts 2–7 days and may include marked prostration. Up to 10% of these cases progress to tracheobronchitis or pneumonia. Those at particular risk of complications are those with underlying chronic chest, heart or kidney disease, diabetes or immunosuppression.

20% of infections are asymptomatic and 30% have upper respiratory symptoms but no fever.

Laboratory confirmation

Confirmation of diagnosis is dependent upon laboratory tests, usually by direct immunofluorescence (DIF), virus isolation or serology. The virus may be detected from nasopharyngeal aspirates, nasal swabs or throat swabs: these must be collected early in the disease and require special transport media. Results can be available in 2–3 days, although one week is usual for routine samples. Serology requires 2 specimens, 10–21 days apart, and is about 80% sensitive: it is useful for retrospective diagnosis. In outbreaks, PCR testing (highly sensitive in early infection) or same day DIF results may be available.

Influenza virus has 3 types (A, B, C) of which influenza C produces only sporadic infections. Subtyping of influenza A is based on a combination of H antigen (15 subtypes) and N antigen (9 subtypes), e.g. H1N1 or H3N2. All recent common human pathogens are combinations of H1, H2 or H3 with N1 or N2. Strains may be further differentiated by serology and named after the place and years of their identification (e.g. A/Sydney/97): these can be compared to current vaccine strains.

Transmission

Influenza in humans is transmitted via the respiratory secretions of cases, mainly by airborne droplet spread. Transmission is facilitated by overcrowding and enclosed spaces, particularly by the number of susceptibles sharing the same room as the case. Spread in such circumstances is usually rapid and attack rates high.

Transmission may also occur via direct or indirect contact: this may occasionally cause a slowly evolving outbreak with low attack rates. Many outbreaks have occurred in hospitals.

The reservoir for influenza A is zoonotic, particularly aquatic birds: transmission to humans is rarely direct but the spread of new strains may occur via intermediaries such as pigs. Influenza B only affects humans.

Pathogenesis

The incubation period is short, usually 1–3 days, occasionally up to 5 days.

The infectious period lasts from one day before until 3–5 days after onset of symptoms in adults. Studies in children have found virus excretion from 3 days before onset to up to 9 days after: in practice, they can return to school when clinically well. Those with severe illness may also excrete for longer periods and at higher levels.

The infectious dose is low.

Immunity develops and protects against clinical illness with the same strain for many years. Cross-immunity to related strains occurs. It is not clear why outbreaks often cease before exhausting the pool of susceptibles.

Prevention

• Basic personal hygiene to reduce transmission by coughing, sneezing or contaminated hands.
• Immunization reduces the risk of hospital admissions and death and has a good safety record. Annual immunization with WHO recommended vaccines should be offered to all those with an increased risk of serious illness from influenza. Current UK recommendations are that this should include those with:
   chronic respiratory disease, including asthma;
   chronic renal disease;
   immunosuppression due to disease or treatment;
   diabetes mellitus;
   age of 65 years or more.
• In addition, people in long-stay residential care should also be vaccinated because of the risk of rapid spread. As efficacy in elderly people may be lower than the 70–90% in younger adults, indirect protection in this group may also be valuable. Immunization is sometimes offered to healthcare workers both to protect patients and maintain staffing levels: however, uptake is often poor.

• Uptake of immunization in disease-based risk groups has been poor in the UK and other countries. Primary care staff can increase uptake by compiling an at-risk register from chronic disease, computerized patient or prescription records, or as patients are seen during the year. A letter should be sent to each of these patients, preferably from their family doctor, recommending vaccination. Education on the benefits of vaccination is required both for the target population and for healthcare workers. Health Authorities should appoint a coordinator to lead on improving influenza immunization uptake locally.
• The antiviral drug amantadine hydrochloride can be used during epidemics of influenza A for:
   individuals in at-risk groups for whom immunization is unavailable or contraindicated;
   unimmunized patients in at-risk groups for two weeks while the vaccine takes effect;
   healthcare workers and other key personnel to prevent disruption of services during a major epidemic.
• National and local planning prior to occurrence of a pandemic (see Box 3.38.1 for local plan).

Surveillance

• Influenza activity can be monitored via a combination of clinical surveillance for 'influenza-like illness' and laboratory data.
• At the international level, WHO coordinates a global network covering 83 countries and publishes information in the Weekly Epidemiological Record. Eight European countries (including the UK) participate in the European Influenza Surveillance Scheme (www.eiss.org).
• At the national level, data are available from:
   General practice consultations (e.g. RCGP Research Unit spotter practices).
   Illness in schoolchildren (e.g. Medical Officers of Schools Association).
   Mortality statistics (e.g. Office of National Statistics).
   Collaborative studies (e.g. surveillance sam-

Box 3.38.1 Main features of a district pandemic influenza plan

Objectives
1 Reduce mortality and morbidity.
2 Care for large numbers at home, in hospital and dying.
3 Maintain essential public services.
4 Provide up to date reliable information to staff and public.

Administrative
1 Pre-pandemic planning.
2 Constitution for Pandemic Co-ordinating Committee.
3 Roles and responsibilities for individuals.
4 Arrangements for updating.

Calculate vaccine requirements
1 Frontline healthcare staff.
2 Other essential public services.
3 Individuals at high risk of severe disease.
4 Residents of long-stay facilities.
5 Rest of population by age-bands.

Contingency plans
1 Communications
2 Surveillance
3 Immunization services
4 Local outbreak plans (hospital and community)
5 Maintaining health services (increased workload)
6 Mortuary arrangements
7 Essential public services
8 Social services
9 Treatment protocols, e.g. antiviral drugs

Table 3.38.1 Thresholds for influenza clinical activity

Consultation rate (per 100 000)	Status
Up to 50	Baseline
50–199	Normal winter
200–399	Above average
400 plus	Epidemic

be useful. Clinical data can be obtained from computerized GPs or other primary care providers. Participating GPs and local laboratories should ideally co-operate to obtain representative virological surveillance data.
• Some countries set thresholds for clinical activity, indices, e.g. for the RCGP scheme in England and Wales, see Table 3.38.1. These levels differ for each country.

Response to a case

• Although spread may occur before diagnosis, symptomatic cases should ideally not attend work or school until recovered.
• Avoid contact with those at increased risk of severe illness. In hospital, isolate or cohort during acute illness.
• Handwashing and safe disposal of respiratory secretions.

Response to a cluster

Only of concern if cases have links to institutions containing individuals at increased risk of severe disease and/or rapid spread.

Control of an outbreak

For outbreaks in institutions containing individuals at risk of severe disease:
• Organize typing of virus to compare to vaccine.
• Immunize anyone not yet protected.
• Consider amantadine cover for at risk patients for two weeks until vaccine induced protection present (if influenza A).
• Exclude staff and visitors with respiratory illness.

ples collected from primary care patients with influenza-like illness).
Laboratory surveillance of routine samples (e.g. CoSurv). However, these samples are heavily biased in terms of age (particularly children) and severity (hospitalization).
UK data from these sources are available on the PHLS website (www.phls.co.uk).
• Regional or district monitoring may also

- Isolate or cohort those with acute symptoms.
- Reinforce hygiene measures.

3.39 Japanese B encephalitis

This is a mosquito-borne viral encephalitis caused by a flavivirus. It occurs throughout south-east Asia and the far east. Most infections are inapparent, although the illness can be severe with high mortality and permanent neurological sequelae in survivors.

The reservoir is pigs, and occasionally birds. Transmission to man is via a mosquito that lives in rice-growing areas. Transmission rates are highest in the rainy season.

Travellers to endemic countries are only at risk if they spend long periods (more than a month) in rural areas where pig farming and rice growing coexist. An unlicensed, inactivated vaccine is available. The schedule is three doses at days 0, 7–14 and 28; two doses at days 0 and 7–14 gives short-term protection in about 80% of vaccinees. The usual precautions against mosquito bites should be taken (see Chapter 3.46).

3.40 Kawasaki syndrome

Kawasaki disease (KD), also known as Kawasaki syndrome or 'mucocutaneous lymph node syndrome', is a generalized vasculitis of unknown aetiology, possibly caused by an infectious agent. 20–25% of untreated children develop coronary artery abnormalities.

Suggested on-call action
None.

Epidemiology

KD has been reported throughout the world and is being increasingly recognized. KD occurs more often in boys than in girls (1.5 : 1); about 80% of cases are less than five years old. Incidence rates in North America are highest in children of Asian (especially Japanese or Korean) ethnicity. The disease occurs year-round; a greater number of cases are reported in the winter and spring. Several regional outbreaks have been reported since 1976 in North America.

Clinical features

In the absence of a specific diagnostic test, Kawasaki disease is a clinical diagnosis based on the characteristic history and physical findings. Features may include conjunctivitis; swollen, fissured lips; strawberry tongue; cervical lymphadenopathy; erythematous rash; peeling of fingers and toes. Clinical criteria have been developed by the Japanese Kawasaki Disease Research Committee.

Consideration of measles is important as appropriate control measures cannot be taken if measles is misdiagnosed as KD.

Risk factors for coronary artery aneurysms include male, age less than one year, recurrence of fever after an afebrile period of 24 h and other signs, such as arrhythmias, of cardiac involvement.

Transmission

Unknown.

Pathogenesis

Unknown.

Prevention

Initial therapy is directed at reducing fever and other inflammatory features to prevent the development of coronary arteritis using intravenous immunoglobulin and oral acetylsalicylic acid.

Surveillance

Cases of KD should be reported to any specific KD reporting system, such as that run by the British Paediatric Surveillance Unit in the UK. Clusters should be reported to local public health departments.

Response to a case

Report to surveillance system.

Investigation of a cluster and control of an outbreak

Seek specialist advice. A cluster of KD cases should be used as an opportunity for detailed investigation to learn more about the aetiology.

Case-definition
Seek advice form KD reporting system.

3.41 Legionellosis

Infection with *Legionella pneumophila* can cause a potentially life-threatening atypical pneumonia (Legionnaires' disease) or a milder febrile illness (Pontiac fever).

Suggested on-call action
• If linked to other cases, or if in hospital during incubation period, consult outbreak control plan. • Otherwise, organize investigation of case on next working day.

Epidemiology

The true incidence of Legionnaires' disease (LD) is not known: estimates range from 2 to 20/100 000. Outside of outbreaks, LD appears to be responsible for between 0.5 and 5% of community acquired pneumonias. Approximately 200 cases are reported in England and Wales each year, of which over 70% are in males and over 90% are aged over 30 years. Cases peak from June to October.

Travel abroad is a major risk factor for LD: nearly half of UK cases are contracted abroad. Within Europe those most commonly affected are residents of northern European countries visiting southern countries: the highest number of cases occur in travellers to Spain, followed by Turkey, France, Italy and Greece. The highest rate (per traveller) is in visitors to Turkey. About 15% of UK cases are linked to local outbreaks (predominantly due to 'wet cooling systems' or hot water systems) and about 2% are hospital-acquired. Many cases are, however, sporadic and from an unidentified source. Large outbreaks have recently occurred in the Netherlands and Belgium.

Cigarette smoking, advanced age, chronic lung or kidney disease, immunosuppression and excess alcohol intake are risk factors for identified infection.

Clinical features

Both Legionnaires' disease and Pontiac fever (PF) commence with non-specific 'flu-like symptoms such as malaise, fever, myalgia, anorexia and headache, often with diarrhoea and confusion. Pontiac fever is self-limiting but LD progresses to pneumonia which, in an individual patient, is difficult to differentiate clinically from other causes of atypical pneumonia. In an outbreak, diagnostic clues might be 25–50% of cases with diarrhoea, confusion, high fever, a lack of upper respiratory symptoms and poor response to penicillins or cephalosporins.

Laboratory diagnosis

Almost all legionellosis in immunocompetent individuals is due to *L. pneumophila*, of which serogroup 1 is responsible for the large majority of diagnosed infections. Legionellae are not usually identified in routine culture of sputum, although special media can be deployed. Serogroup 1 antibody may be tested for in most laboratories but takes 3–6 weeks to rise to diagnostic levels. Serogroup 1 antigen may be detected in urine samples at a much earlier stage of the illness. Reference laboratories may be able to diagnose infection due to other serogroups if routine samples are negative in epidemiologically suspected Legionnaires' clusters. Genotyping (e.g. RFLP) is available to support epidemiological investigation of culture positive cases.

Legionellae are common contaminants of warm water and so routine environmental testing is not helpful. However, culturing is useful in investigating suspected water sources for identified cases: five litres of water is necessary for culture.

Transmission

The reservoir for the organism is environmental water, in which it occurs in low concentrations. Transmission to humans occurs via inhalation of aerosols or droplet nuclei containing an infective dose of the organism. Legionellae grow at temperatures between 25 °C and 45 °C (preferably 30–40 °C) and so the highest risk occurs with water systems which lead to the aerosolization of water which has been stored at these temperatures. Such systems include hot water systems (especially showers), wet cooling systems (e.g. cooling towers and evaporative condensers), whirlpool spas, indoor and outdoor fountain/sprinkler systems, humidifiers, respiratory therapy equipment and industrial grinders.

Wet cooling systems may contaminate air outside the building.

Legionellae can survive in water stored between 0 °C and 60 °C. They survive normal levels of chlorination and are aided by sediment accumulation and commensal microflora in the water. Temperatures above 63 °C are bactericidal, as are many common disinfectants (e.g. phenol, glutaraldehyde, hypochlorite).

Pathogenesis

The incubation period for Legionnaires' disease is 2–10 days (average 5.5 days) and for Pontiac fever it is 5–66 h (average 36 h).

Legionella is not communicable from person to person.

The infectious dose is unknown, but certainly low. Attack rates are higher in PF (>90%) than LD (<5%).

Prevention

• Design and maintenance of water systems: store hot water above 60 °C and deliver above 50 °C; store and deliver cold water below 20 °C. Eliminate stagnant water.
• New air-conditioning systems to be air-cooled.
• Maintenance and hygiene of wet cooling systems in line with national recommendations (e.g. Health and Safety Executive guidance). Drain when not in use.
• Regular cleaning, disinfection and changing of water in indoor fountains and whirlpool spas.
• Use sterile water for respiratory therapy devices.

Surveillance

Although not formally notifiable in many countries (including England and Wales) cases of laboratory-confirmed legionellosis should be reported to local public health authorities on the day of diagnosis. Clusters of respiratory infection should be reported without waiting for confirmation. Cases should also be reported to the relevant national surveillance scheme.

Legionellosis should be included in hospital infection surveillance schemes, especially for higher-risk patients.

Cases associated with travel to other European countries are reported to the European Working Group for Legionella Infection (EWGLI) collaborator in the presumed country of infection by the project co-ordinating centre at CDSC, Colindale (UK).

Response to a case

• Ensure appropriate laboratory confirmatory tests undertaken.
• Report to local public health authority.
• Obtain risk factor history for 2–14 days (LD) or 0–3 days (PF) before onset of symptoms: details of places of residence and work; visits for occupational or leisure reasons; exposure to industrial sites, hotels, hospitals, leisure/sport/garden centres; air conditioning, showers, whirlpools/jacuzzis, fountains, humidifiers, nebulizers, etc.
• If recognized risk factor identified (e.g. cooling tower at work) discuss inspection of possible source, examination of maintenance records and sampling with environmental health and microbiology colleagues. Enquire about respiratory illness in others exposed to potential source.
• Report travel outside district to relevant public health authority and travel outside country to national surveillance centre.
• If case likely to have acquired infection in hospital, convene incident control team. Isolation is unnecessary.

Investigation of a cluster

• Undertake hypothesis generation exercise of risk factors as identified for individual cases including day by day analysis of movements in 14 days before onset.
• Further case-finding: ensure all cases of community or hospital-acquired pneumonia are tested for legionellosis. If serogroup 1 disease, encourage urine antigen testing for rapid diagnosis. Where possible, also encourage culture so that typing may be performed.
• Use geographical analysis of home, work and places visited of cases to look for links. Have cases been within 1 km of each other?
• If cases have been to same area, identify all potential sources. Consider inspection and sampling of all cooling towers in area.
• In nosocomial outbreaks, test all water sources (hot and cold) and relevant environmental samples (e.g. showerheads) in suspect wards. Obtain specialist engineering advice on plumbing and heating systems.
• Compare typing results from cases and suspected source.

Control of an outbreak

• Shutdown of suspected source whilst expert engineering advice obtained.
• Drainage, cleaning, disinfection, maintenance and re-evaluation of suspected source. Occasionally major redesign or closure necessary.
• Warn clinicians of increase and of appropriate antibiotics.

Suggested case-definition for use in an outbreak

Confirmed: case of pneumonia (LD) or flu-like illness (PF) with *Legionella* infection diagnosed by culture, urine antigen or four fold rise in serum titres (to 1 : 64 by IFAT or 1 : 16 by RMAT).

Presumptive: pneumonia or 'flu-like illness with single high serum titre (1 : 128 by IFAT, 1 : 32 by RMAT).

Clinical: case of pneumonia epidemiologically linked to confirmed LD *or* case of 'flu-like illness linked to confirmed PF, awaiting final confirmation (including six-week serology).

3.42 Leprosy

Leprosy is a chronic inflammatory disease caused by *Mycobacterium leprae*.

Epidemiology

Leprosy occurs in almost all the tropical and warm temperate regions. It becomes less common as living standards rise and is associated with overcrowding. All cases in North Europe are imported.

Clinical features

The organism has a predilection for the skin and nerves. Nerve involvement results in an area of anaesthesia and or muscle weakness/wasting; tissue damage occurs secondarily to the anaesthesia.

The clinical appearance of the disease depends upon the degree of cell mediated immunity (CMI). In tuberculoid (TT) disease there is a high degree of CMI, and disease is localized whereas in lepromatous (LL) there is little CMI and skin and nerves are heavily infiltrated with bacilli.

Immunologically mediated reactions usually occur during treatment as CMI returns. These may include erythema nodosum leprosum and tender enlarging nerves.

Laboratory confirmation

The diagnosis can usually be made following a careful examination. This is then confirmed by identifying mycobacteria in slit skin smears or histological preparations. In lepromatous patients, nodules should be biopsied and the nasal mucosa should be scraped. In tuberculoid patients the edge of a lesion should be biopsied.

Transmission

The major source of infection is patients with lepromatous leprosy who shed large numbers of bacilli in their nasal secretions. The portal of entry is probably the respiratory tract.

Pathogenesis

The incubation of the disease is from a few months to many years. Lepromatous patients may be infectious for several years.

Prevention

Identification and treatment of lepromatous patients is the mainstay of prevention.

Surveillance

Leprosy is a notifiable disease in most countries. In the UK there is a leprosy register of all cases.

Response to a case

Cases should be referred to a specialist unit for treatment. Lepromatous cases should be isolated until treatment has been initiated.

Investigation of a cluster

A cluster should be investigated for misdiagnosis or laboratory contamination.

Case-definition

A clinically compatible case that is laboratory-confirmed by demonstration of acid-fast bacilli in skin or dermal nerve.

3.43 Leptospirosis

Leptospirosis is rare cause of septicaemia caused by the zoonotic genus *Leptospira*, which occurs worldwide.

Epidemiology

Leptospirosis is an occupational hazard to farmers and sewage workers and a recreational hazard to swimmers, canoeists, divers, sailors, etc. Worldwide it is seen in areas of poverty, where there can be epidemics. In the UK the most commonly identified serovars are *L. hardjo* and *L. icterohaemorrhagiae*, associated with cattle and rats, respectively. Fewer than 50 cases a year have been reported in England and Wales during 1989–99.

Clinical features

The clinical spectrum of disease is wide; any serovar can cause many clinical presentations. Classically there is an abrupt onset with headache, myalgia, conjunctival suffusion and fever. Following a week of illness the fever may settle only to rise again. During the later phase, meningism, renal and vasculitic manifestations may occur. The combination of leptospirosis with jaundice and uraemia is sometimes known as Weil's disease. Death is usually associated with renal failure; however, it may be due to myocarditis or massive blood loss.

Laboratory confirmation

The organism *L. interrogans* comprises 130 serovars in 16 serogroups. During the first phase organisms may be visualized in (under dark field illumination) and cultured from blood, CSF or urine. The organism may persist in urine. As the immune response develops, a significant rise in antibodies may be detected using ELISA.

During the first phase of the illness there may be a leukopenia, although jaundice may be associated with neutrophilia. About one quarter of cases will have an elevated urea.

Transmission

Leptospirosis affects many wild and domestic animals worldwide. Humans acquire the infection by contact with water, soil, or other material contaminated with the urine of infected animals. Leptospires are excreted in the urine of infected animals and infection in man is due to contact with urine or urine-soaked soil. The organism probably enters through mucosa or broken skin.

Pathogenesis

Incubation period: usually 7–13 days (range 4–19 days).

Infectious period: Patients continue to excrete leptospires for many months but person-to-person spread is rare. Urine-contaminated soil can remain infective for as long as 14 days.

Previous infection protects against re-infection with the same serovar—but may not protect against other serovars.

Prevention

- Control rodent populations.
- Education of those at risk to avoid contaminated areas and cover cuts and abraded skin.
- Providing those at risk (e.g. sewage workers) with alert/information cards.
- Adequate occupational clothing.
- Immunization of those with occupational exposure to specific serovars has been carried out in some countries (e.g. Italy, France and Spain).

Surveillance

Leptospirosis is notifiable in many countries, including the UK. Cases should be reported to public health authorities so that areas of risk can be identified.

Response to a case

- Treatment with intravenous antibiotics (e.g. benzyl penicillin) in the first 4 days probably

reduces the severity of the attack, though the response may not be dramatic.
• Obtain risk factor information.

Investigation of a cluster

• Clusters should be investigated to determine areas of risk—such as particular water sports locations—so that the public can be informed.
• Laboratory typing may help identify risk factors.

Control of an outbreak

• Outbreaks usually occur in areas of poverty, particularly following flooding and disasters that have increased the rodent population. Rodent control is the main activity.
• Outbreaks resulting from occupational exposure—for example to cattle—should be reported to the veterinary authorities.
• Antibiotic prophylaxis (e.g. doxycycline) may be considered.

Case-definition

Clinical: presence of fever plus at least two clinically compatible features, particularly in the presence of known risk factor(s).
Confirmed: isolation of *Leptospira* spp. from clinical specimen or fourfold or greater rise in antibody titre or demonstration of *Leptospira* spp. in a clinical specimen by immunofluorescence or silver staining

---

3.44 Listeria

Infection by *Listeria monocytogenes* is usually food-borne but presents as septicaemia or meningitis. Although rare, infection in vulnerable groups has high case-fatality, with fetuses, neonates, the elderly and the immunocompromised particularly at risk.

Suggested on-call action

If you or reporting clinician/microbiologist know of associated cases consult outbreak control plan.

Epidemiology

Slightly over 100 cases of listeriosis are reported in the UK each year, in line with a typical incidence in Europe of 2 per million per annum. UK incidence was more than twice this level for a three-year period in 1987–89, and a food-borne outbreak affecting 1500 people occurred in Italy in 1997. Infection occurs worldwide.

Reported infection is highest in those under 1 month of age, followed by those over 70. Approximately 20% of reported cases occur in pregnant women. These observations are likely to be due to ascertainment bias because of severity of infection. In contrast to the low reported incidence, the high case-fatality means that 10–15 deaths are recorded yearly in the UK. Human infection peaks in late summer and early autumn, whereas animal listeriosis peaks in spring.

Clinical features

Infection in immunocompetent adults is usually asymptomatic or a mild 'flu-like illness, although it may occasionally cause meningitis and/or septicaemia, particularly in the elderly or immunocompromised. Infection in pregnant women is also usually mild but transplacental spread before the first trimester usually results in fetal death; fetal infection during the third trimester may result in stillbirth or neonatal septicaemia and/or meningitis within 48h of delivery. A red papular rash often accompanies this 'early-onset' neonatal infection. Neonates are also susceptible to 'late-onset' sepsis approximately 10 days after delivery. Case fatality is approximately 50% in early-onset and 25% in late-onset neonatal sepsis. Case-fatality is also high in those aged over 60 years.

Laboratory confirmation

Diagnosis is usually by blood or cerebrospinal fluid culture, which usually takes 48 h, plus another 24 h for confirmation. In *Listeria* meningitis, approximately half of cases have organisms demonstrable on CSF microscopy, accompanied by polymorphs or lymphocytes, increased protein and normal or decreased glucose.

There are 13 serovars of *L. monocytogenes*, of which 4b, 1/2a and 1/2b cause 90% of clinical cases. Serovar 4 was particularly associated with the increase and subsequent fall in cases in 1987–89 and is also associated with late-onset neonatal disease. Serovar 1/2 is particularly associated with early-onset sepsis. Phage typing is also obtainable on 80% of serovar 4 and 37% of serovar 1/2 strains.

Transmission

L. monocytogenes is widespread in the environment and can be found in soil, surface water, vegetation and a wide range of wild and domestic animals. It is extremely hardy and survives drying, freezing and thawing, remaining viable in soil or silage for more than 2 years.

The main route of infection for humans is consumption of contaminated food. The organism can grow at temperatures as low as 0 °C (although optimum growth is 30–37 °C), is relatively tolerant of salt and nitrates, and does not 'spoil' or taint food even at high levels of contamination.

Many foods have been associated with transmission of infection but most have some or all of the following features: highly processed, refrigerated, long shelf life, near-neutral pH and consumed without further cooking. Implicated vehicles have included paté, unpasteurized soft cheese, 'cook-chill' meals and unwashed salads. Some outbreaks have been explained by long-term colonization of difficult-to-clean sites in food processing facilities. Infected cattle can contaminate milk.

Other sources of infection include direct transmission from animals, which may cause cutaneous infection, often with obvious occupational exposure; transplacental transmission in pregnant women; exposure to vaginal carriage during birth or hospital cross-infection for late-onset neonatal sepsis; and nosocomial transmission in hospital nurseries.

Pathogenesis

The incubation period has been variously reported from 1 day to over 3 months. Averages quoted for adults are 3 weeks, for neonates a few days, and for intrauterine infection 30 days. The long incubation period renders a search for the source of infection in sporadic cases extremely difficult.

Human excreters with normal hygiene are unlikely to be an important source of infection, except for neonates.

The infectious dose is uncertain (possibly 100–1000/g food) and it is unclear what level is 'safe' for immunocompromised patients.

In addition to fetuses, neonates and the elderly, those at risk of severe infection include patients with malignancy, cirrhosis, diabetes and the immunosuppressed, including those on corticosteroid therapy.

Prevention

• Hazard analysis in food processing to reduce the risk of contamination and multiplication.
• Pasteurization of dairy produce effectively kills *Listeria*.
• Limiting the length of storage of at-risk refrigerated food, e.g. cook-chill meals.
• Advice to pregnant women and immunosuppressed to avoid certain soft cheeses, paté and prepacked salads.
• Thorough reheating of cook-chill/microwave foods.
• Pregnant women to avoid contact with pregnant or newborn animals and silage.
• Thoroughly wash raw vegetables before eating.
• Adequate infection control in delivery rooms and neonatal units.

Surveillance

• Listeriosis should be reported to local public health departments: can notify as 'suspected

food poisoning' in UK. Meningitis is also notifiable in many countries.
• Laboratories should report all clinically significant infections to regional and national surveillance: these may detect outbreaks not apparent at local level.
• Consider as a cause of two or more cases of 'late-onset' neonatal meningitis/septicaemia.

Response to a case

• Report to local and national/regional public health department to aid detection of cluster.
• Collect data on consumption of risk foods in last month.
• No exclusion required, although enteric precautions sensible for hospitalized patients.

Response to a cluster

• Discuss with microbiologist further investigation such as serotyping and phagetyping. Genotyping methods are being developed.
• Institute case-finding with microbiologists and relevant clinicians to ensure adequate microbiological investigation of meningitis/septicaemia in neonates and elderly.
• Undertake a hypothesis-generating study to include all foods consumed, particularly those at increased risk of high level *Listeria* contamination, e.g. unpasteurized dairy produce, soft cheeses, paté, raw vegetables, salads, highly processed foods and cook-chill or microwave products. The prolonged incubation will make accurate recall difficult: 'food preference' questions may also be useful. Consider direct exposure to animals (e.g. farms).
• If cases predominantly neonatal, look at age in days at onset: could this be nosocomial?

Control of an outbreak

• Consider product withdrawal of any implicated food. In the UK, this should be done in conjunction with the Food Standards Agency.
• Obtain specialist environmental health advice to investigate and modify suspect food processes.

> **Suggested case-definition for an outbreak**
>
> 'Flu-like illness, septicaemia or CNS infection, associated with isolate of the outbreak strain of *L. monocytogenes* from blood or CSF.

3.45 Lyme disease

Lyme disease (Bannwarth syndrome, erythema chronicum migrans, borreliosis) is a multisystem illness resulting from exposure to *Ixodes* ticks infected with *Borrelia burgdorferi*.

> **On-call action**
>
> As there is no person-to-person transmission, no on-call action is required.

Epidemiology

Lyme disease is common in North America and northern Europe in areas of heathland, affecting ramblers and campers. Geographic distribution of disease in Europe is associated with the known range of *I. ricinus*. The true incidence of disease is unknown in the UK; reported infection is uncommon (mean 50 cases p.a. in England and Wales) but increasing.

Clinical features

Following a tick bite, which may be inapparent, a rash (erythema chronicum migrans) develops; the appearance is of an expanding erythematous circle with central clearing. Other manifestations include large joint polyarthritis (usually asymmetrical), aseptic meningitis, peripheral root lesions, radiculopathy, meningo-encephalitis and myocarditis. These features may occur without the rash.

The symptoms may persist over a prolonged period. The clinical manifestations seen in Europe and North America differ, with milder disease often reported in Europe.

Laboratory confirmation

Confirmation is by demonstrating elevated IgM antibody. The low sensitivity of serologic testing early in the disease means it is unhelpful; it may be more useful in later disease. Positive or equivocal results on an ELISA or IFA assay require confirmatory testing with a Western immunoblot. Some chronic patients may remain seronegative.

Transmission

Lyme disease is caused by a spirochete, *B. burgdorferi*, transmitted by the bite of *Ixodes* ticks. Deer are the preferred host for adult ticks in the USA; sheep in Europe. Other mammals (e.g. dogs) can be incidental hosts and may develop Lyme disease.

Pathogenesis

Incubation period: erythema migrans, the best clinical indicator of Lyme disease, develops between 3 and 32 days after a tick bite.

Lyme disease is not transmissible from person to person.

Prevention

The main method of prevention is avoidance of tick bites through wearing long trousers. Transmission of *B. burgdorferi* does not usually occur until the tick has been in place for 36–48h; thus, screening and removing ticks after exposure can help prevent infection.

A vaccine has been developed in the US; indications for use are uncertain, and it would not be effective against European variants.

Surveillance

Cases should be reported to the public health authorities so that assessments of risk can be made.

Response to a case

No public health response.

Investigation of a cluster and control of an outbreak

Clusters should be investigated to determine areas of high risk, so that those who might be exposed can be informed.

Suggested case-definition
Clinical diagnosis: Presence of erythema migrans in someone who has been exposed to tick bites.

3.46 Malaria

Malaria is a potentially fatal plasmodial infection. Increasing numbers of patients presenting to healthcare facilities in Europe will have travelled to places where they have been exposed to malaria. There is also a risk of airport malaria.

On-call action
None required unless transfusion-associated malaria suspected, in which case identify other units and individuals exposed urgently.

Epidemiology

Malaria is endemic in more than 100 countries throughout Africa, Central and South America, Asia and Oceania; more than two billion people are exposed to the risk of malaria infection. *P. falciparum* and *P. vivax* are the most common species. *P. falciparum* is the predominant species in Africa and Papua New Guinea. *P. vivax* dominates in South America and Asia; *P. malariae* is widely distributed but is much less common. *P. ovale* is mainly found in Africa. Between 1000 and 1700 cases of malaria have been reported in each year, in England and Wales 1989–99, with 3–12 deaths p.a.

Clinical features

Malaria may present with almost any clinical pattern. The most classical symptom is the malarial rigor; the periodic nature of the attacks of fever may give a clue as to the diagnosis. The disease must be considered in anyone who has been exposed to the parasite, by travel, blood transfusion, or the rare airport malaria.

Delay in diagnosis of *P. falciparum* malaria is associated with increased mortality; the course may be rapidly progressive, with a high mortality in non-immune subjects. The rise in chloroquine resistance means that there are few areas in the world where chloroquine can be relied on for treatment.

Complications are associated with high parasitaemia and are therefore more common in non-immunes, children, travellers and areas of unstable transmission.

Infection with *P. vivax, P. ovale* or *P. malariae* is usually benign; fatal infections are rare in the immunologically competent. Treatment with chloroquine is effective. *P. vivax* and *P. ovale* will relapse unless treatment is given to eradicate the liver hypnozoite stage.

Patients should be reviewed 28 days after treatment to confirm parasitological and clinical cure. Patients who have splenic enlargement should avoid body contact sports and strenuous exercise due to a risk of splenic rupture.

Laboratory confirmation

Diagnosis is by demonstrating parasites in the peripheral blood. A minimum of three specimens should be taken at the height of fever. Thick films are of particular value when the parasitaemia is low; the technique requires experience. A thin film enables a parasite count (number of parasites per 100 RBC) to be per-

formed and the morphology of the parasites to be more clearly seen.

Slides should be reviewed by an expert so that a species diagnosis, essential to guide chemotherapy, can be made. Serology has no part to play in diagnosis of acute malaria. Antigen detection methods for malaria antigen are under development, but none yet compare with the sensitivity and specificity of microscopy.

Transmission

Malaria is transmitted by the bite of the female anopheline mosquito.

Increased ease, speed and availability of air travel has meant that many more people travel to infected areas; the failure of malaria eradication in Africa has resulted in an increase in the number of cases of imported *P. falciparum* infection.

Absence of the insect vector in the UK and Europe means that there is no risk of secondary cases. Rare cases of 'airport malaria' happen when an infected mosquito introduced to Europe bites a host before dying. There are also rare transmissions through blood donation or needlestick.

Pathogenesis

Incubation periods—time from infection to appearance of parasites in blood	
P. falciparum	5–7 days
P. vivax	6–8 days
P. malariae	12–16 days
P. ovale	8–9 days

Prevention

Good advice to those travelling is essential. The risk of those visiting relatives is often underestimated by travellers and those providing advice. Existing immunity will probably have waned.

Prevention of mosquito bites (the mosquitoes bite mainly at night).

- Sleep under bed nets; impregnation with pyrethrum enhances the efficacy of nets.
- Wear long-sleeved garments and long trousers between dusk and dawn.
- Use mosquito repellents.

Suppression of the malaria parasite with chemoprophylaxis. Regular antimalarial prophylaxis should be taken for one week before travel to an endemic area and six weeks after return. Changing patterns of resistance mean that specialist advice should be consulted.

Control of malaria in populations depends on diminishing or eradication of the vector, the anopheles mosquito. Methods include spraying of houses with insecticides and the destruction of larval sites by removing standing water.

Surveillance

Malaria is notifiable in many countries, including the UK. Cases should be reported to national authorities so that advice on prophylaxis can be based upon observed patterns of risk.

Response to a case

A travel history should be taken.

If there is no travel history, information about transfusions or injections (including drug misuse), airport vicinity should be sought.

Investigation of a cluster and control of an outbreak

If clusters arise from areas where malaria has not previously been recognized, the national authorities should be informed. Travel advice should be reviewed. If cases occur in people who have not been abroad, consider blood, nosocomial and airport exposures.

Case-definitions

Clinical: fever and/or compatible illness in person who has travelled to an area in which malaria is endemic.

Cases can also are classified according to the following World Health Organization categories.

- Autochthonous:
    indigenous: malaria acquired by mosquito transmission in an area where malaria is a regular occurrence;
    introduced: malaria acquired by mosquito transmission from an imported case in an area where malaria is not a regular occurrence.
- Imported: malaria acquired outside a specific area.
- Induced: malaria acquired through artificial means (e.g. blood transfusion, common syringes, or malariotherapy).
- Relapsing: renewed manifestation (i.e. of clinical symptoms and/or parasitaemia) of malarial infection that is separated from previous manifestations of the same infection by an interval greater than any interval resulting from the normal periodicity of the paroxysms.
- Cryptic: an isolated case of malaria that cannot be epidemiologically linked to additional cases.

3.47 Measles

Measles is a systemic viral infection caused by a paramyxovirus. Its main features are fever, rash and respiratory disease. The public health significance of measles is that it is highly infectious and can be prevented by vaccination.

Suggested on-call action

None usually necessary.

Epidemiology

In the prevaccination era, most people were infected in childhood; the average age at infection was four years. Large epidemics occurred every two years in the UK until 1968, the year that routine childhood immunization was introduced. Vaccine coverage was initially low (about 50%) and epidemics continued every 2–3 years, although the number of cases dropped by 80%. In epidemic years the peak incidence was in spring and early summer.

Vaccine coverage started to improve during the 1980s and reached 93% by 1997. This has broken the epidemic cycle: the last measles epidemic was in 1988. Measles is now rare: although 2000–4000 cases are notified each year, less than 5% are laboratory-confirmed. Most confirmed cases are in older unvaccinated children and in many there is a history of contact with an imported case. The case fatality rate has fallen from 1 per 100 in 1940 to 0.02 per 100 in 1999.

The epidemiology of measles varies considerably across Europe, depending on when vaccination was introduced, vaccine schedules and coverage. The disease has been virtually eliminated in Scandinavia, Holland and parts of eastern Europe where coverage has been high for many years. In Germany, France and Italy, coverage is below 90% and outbreaks are still common. The World Health Organization has set a target of measles elimination in Europe by 2007.

Clinical features

In an unvaccinated child, there is a prodromal illness with a high fever and a coryzal respiratory infection. There is cough, conjunctivitis and runny nose. Koplik's spots appear during the early part of the illness—these look like grains of salt on a red inflamed background and are found on the mucosa of the cheek next to the upper premolars and molars. The rash of measles starts on day three or four, initially in the hairline, but spreads rapidly to cover the face, trunk and limbs. It is maculopapular but not itchy. Koplik's spots fade as the rash appears. The rash fades over a week to 10 days.

In a vaccinated child, the illness is usually mild with a low-grade fever, transient rash and absent respiratory features.

Complications of measles include pneumonitis, secondary bacterial infection, especially acute otitis media and pneumonia, and encephalitis. Complication rates are higher in malnourished or immunosuppressed children. Subacute sclerosing panencephalitis is a late, slow-onset, progressive complication which occurs in about 1 per million cases. It is always fatal.

Laboratory confirmation

The diagnosis can be confirmed by culture (in blood, nasopharyngeal and conjunctival secretions and urine) or serology (single raised IgM or rise in IgG). Measles IgM can now reliably be detected in saliva if the specimen is collected between 1 and 6 weeks after the onset of symptoms.

Transmission

Man is the only reservoir. Carriers are unknown. Spread is from person to person by direct contact with nose and throat secretions or respiratory droplets; less commonly indirectly by articles freshly soiled with nose and throat secretions.

Pathogenesis

The incubation period (to onset of fever) is 8–13 days, usually about 10 days. The period of communicability starts just before the onset of the prodrome and lasts until four days after the rash appears. Measles is highly infectious, with a reproduction rate of 15–17, i.e. between 15 and 17 secondary cases in a susceptible population for every index case. Natural infection provides lifelong immunity. Vaccine-induced immunity is lower, but is also usually lifelong and can be boosted by exposure to circulating wild virus. In developed countries, maternal antibody persists for up to 12 months; this period may be shorter when the maternal immunity is vaccine-induced.

Prevention

Measles vaccine is highly effective (>90%) and is given as a combined measles/mumps/-rubella (MMR) vaccine at 12–15 months of age. A second dose of MMR is given at 4–5 years. The main purpose of this second dose is to protect children who failed to respond to the first dose; it also boosts waning vaccine-induced immunity in children who did respond to the first dose. The only contraindications to measles vaccine are immunosuppression, life-threatening egg allergy and a severe reaction to a previous dose.

Surveillance

Measles is notifiable in nearly all countries in Europe, including the UK. The clinical diagnosis is unreliable in a highly vaccinated population, so laboratory confirmation should be sought in all notified suspected cases.

Response to a case

• Obtain laboratory confirmation (e.g. saliva test).
• Check vaccination status of contacts.
• Immunize previously unimmunized contacts.
• Determine source of infection (including travel history).
• Exclude from school until five days from the onset of rash.
• Give HNIG to immunosuppressed close contacts and those under 12 months of age.

Response to a cluster and investigation of an outbreak

As per case investigation, but also check vaccination coverage in the population where the cluster is occurring, and arrange for vaccination of all children in that population without a documented history of vaccination. In a larger outbreak it may be necessary to conduct a mass campaign to interrupt transmission.

> **Suggested case-definition for an outbreak**
>
> *Suspected case:*
>   fever (>38°C if measured);
>   plus rash
>   plus one of: conjunctivitis, cough, coryza.
> *Confirmed case:*
>   measles virus in blood, urine, conjunctival or nasopharyngeal secretions;
>   *or*
>   measles IgM in blood or saliva; *or*
>   fourfold or greater rise in measles IgG in blood

3.48 Meningococcal infection

Meningococcal infection is the spectrum of disease caused by the bacterium *Neisseria meningitidis*. The infection may present as meningitis, septicaemia, or a combination of both. The public health significance of meningococcal infection lies in the severity of the disease, the absence of effective vaccines, the ability of the infection to cause unpredictable clusters, and the intense public anxiety that inevitably accompanies a case or cluster.

Epidemiology

The incidence of meningococcal infection in western Europe varies from 1 to 10 per 100000 population. In most countries the incidence is relatively stable, although the UK has seen an increase since the mid 1990s from 4 to 6 per 100000. Much of this increase is due to a rise in serogroup C cases among older children. Spain, Ireland, Holland and the Czech Republic have also experienced outbreaks of serogroup C disease during the 1990s.

There are 13 serogroups of *Neisseria meningitidis*. In Europe, serogroups B and C account for over 95% of cases. Serogroup B is commoner than C.

Children under the age of five are most frequently affected, with a peak incidence at about 6 months of age, which coincides with the loss of maternally derived immunity. There is a second, smaller peak in teenagers.

Most cases arise sporadically, although clusters occur from time to time. These are unpredictable, although they often occur in educational establishments or in the military. Serogroup C disease tends to cause clusters more than serogroup B.

The infection is seasonal, with a higher incidence in the winter months. There are geographical variations in the disease, although these are not consistent over time. Local increases are often associated with the arrival of a strain not previously seen in that community.

There are a number of factors that predispose to meningococcal infection. These include passive smoking, crowding, recent influenza type A infection, absence of a spleen and complement deficiency. Travellers to the meningitis belt of Africa (where outbreaks of serogroup A disease are common) may be at risk of disease. Cases (serogroup A, but more recently serogroup W135) among pilgrims to the Hadj in Mecca have prompted the government of Saudi Arabia to require a certificate of meningococcal vaccination from visitors.

Clinical features

The early symptoms are non-specific and are often mistaken for a viral infection. In infants there is fever, floppiness, high-pitched crying and sometimes vomiting. Older children and adults have a fever, malaise, increasing headache, nausea and often vomiting. The illness usually progresses rapidly, with the clinical picture changing hourly, although sometimes there is a slower onset, which causes diagnostic difficulty. In infants there is progressive irritability, altered consciousness and sometimes convulsions. Older children and adults develop photophobia and neck stiffness with a positive Kernig's sign, although these features are sometimes absent.

An important feature is the appearance of a petechial rash, which indicates that there is septicaemia. The rash is not always present, or there may be only a few petechiae, so a careful search for petechiae is important in suspected cases. The 'glass test' can be used to distinguish a haemorrhagic rash from other types of rash (Plate 1).

Patients with rapidly advancing disease may develop hypotension, circulatory collapse, pulmonary oedema, confusion and coma. The overall case fatality rate is about 10%, although for patients without septicaemia the outlook is better. Approximately 15% of survivors have permanent sequelae, including deafness, convulsions, mental impairment and limb loss.

Laboratory confirmation

Obtaining laboratory confirmation in suspected cases is essential for public health management. This requires close co-operation between clinicians, microbiologists and public health doctors. Specimens should be taken as soon as a suspected case is seen in hospital (see Box 3.48.1). The single most important specimen is blood for culture and PCR diagnosis (a 2.5-mL EDTA or citrated specimen is needed for PCR). There is often reluctance to do a lumbar puncture because of the risk of coning; however, where CSF sample has been obtained, this should be submitted for microscopy, culture and PCR. A throat swab should also be obtained for culture (the yield from cases is about 50% and is unaffected by prior administration of antibiotic). A rash aspirate for microscopy is a further useful specimen. A throat swab from family members before chemoprophylaxis may also help to identify the causative organism, although counselling is advised before swabbing to prevent feelings of guilt should a household member be found to be the source of infection. Acute and convalescent serology can also provide a diagnosis, although the result is often obtained too late to affect either clinical or public health management.

It is important determine the serogroup of the infecting organism, to inform decisions about vaccination. PCR diagnosis is

---

Box 3.48.1 Suggested laboratory specimens in suspected meningococcal infection

- Blood for PCR and culture.
- Throat swab for culture.
- CSF for microscopy, antigen detection, culture and PCR.
- Paired serum samples for serology.

---

serogroup-specific and a result is available within a few hours. Latex agglutination tests are also available as a rapid screening method when there is a positive culture, although the result should ideally be confirmed by the national reference laboratory. Genotyping methods such as multilocus sequence typing (MLST) are becoming increasingly available and provide a much more precise typing than phenotype-based methods.

Transmission

The infection is spread from person to person through respiratory droplets and direct contact with nose and throat secretions. Infectivity is relatively low, and transmission usually requires prolonged close contact such as occurs in the household setting or through 'wet' mouth kissing.

Man is the only reservoir, and the organism dies quickly outside the host. Approximately 10% of the population carry the organism harmlessly in the nasopharynx. Carriage confers natural immunity. Carriage rates are lowest in children under five, then rise to peak at 20–25% in teenagers and young adults. During outbreaks, carriage rates of the outbreak strain may rise sharply, to high as high as 50%. There is however, no consistent relationship between carriage rates and disease, and some outbreaks occur in the absence of normal carriage. This was the case during an outbreak at Southampton University, where there were six cases due to a C2aP1.5 strain: no carriers of this strain were identified among several hundred students who were swabbed before receiving chemoprophylaxis. Increased rates of carriage

have been observed in smokers, in crowded conditions, and among military recruits.

The most common setting for transmission to occur is within households, where a member of the household (usually an adult) has recently become a carrier and infects a susceptible household member (usually a child). The risk of a further case in the same household in the week following the index case is then increased by about 1000-fold. In comparison, transmission in other settings is uncommon; a recent study in England and Wales found that the relative risk of a second case in the week following an index case was approximately 60 in primary schools, 170 in secondary schools and two in universities (no secondary cases occurred within one week in nurseries during the study period). Transmission from patients to healthcare workers has been documented, but is rare, occurring where there has been direct exposure to nasopharyngeal secretions.

Pathogenesis

The incubation period is usually 2–5 days, although it may occasionally be up to 10 days. For public health purposes, an upper limit of 7 days is generally accepted. Patients are usually no longer infectious within 24 h of starting antibiotic treatment, although it should be noted that some antibiotics used in treatment (e.g. penicillin) will only temporarily suppress carriage. For this reason a chemoprophylactic antibiotic should be given before hospital discharge.

Maternal immunity to meningococcal infection is passed across the placenta to the neonate, but only lasts for a few months. Subsequent carriage of pathogenic and nonpathogenic meningococci (especially *Neisseria lactamica*) confers serogroup-specific natural immunity. Carriage of pathogenic meningococci is unusual in infancy and early childhood, rises progressively to peak at 25% in 15 to 19-year-olds and then slowly declines through adult life. Conversely, carriage of *N. lactamica* (which induces some cross-immunity to *N. meningitidis*) is predominantly in infants and young children, with carriage rates low in teenagers and young adults. It has been speculated that a variety of factors may affect susceptibility. This could for example account for the increased risk of invasive disease that follows influenza type A infection.

Prevention

Vaccines offer the only prospect for prevention. Polysaccharide vaccines against serogroups A, C, W135 and Y are available; however, they offer only short-lived (2–3 years) protection and are ineffective in young children, in whom the disease incidence is greatest. They are only of value where short-term protection is required, for example during outbreaks or for travellers to the meningitis belt or the Hadj.

Serogroup B vaccines have to date performed poorly in clinical trials (particularly in children) and are not yet generally available (with the exception of some Latin American countries). Genetically engineered serogroup B vaccines are now undergoing clinical trials and appear promising.

Improved polysaccharide-protein conjugate vaccines against serogroup A and C strains have recently become available. They are effective in young children and induce immunological memory, which is likely to be lifelong. A conjugate serogroup C vaccine has recently been introduced into the UK childhood immunization schedule. The UK is the first country in which this has been done. Three doses of the vaccines are given to infants at 2, 3 and 4 months; children over 12 months require only a single dose.

Surveillance

Both meningococcal infection and meningococcal disease are notifiable in most European countries, including the UK. Laboratory reports are another important source of data in most countries, although increasing use of preadmission antibiotics means that there is now greater reliance on non-culture diagnoses for surveillance.

Response to a case

There are four key actions for the CCDC:
1 Ensure rapid admission to hospital and that preadmission benzyl penicillin has been given (see Box 3.48.2). Prompt action may reduce the case fatality rate by up to 50%.
2 Ensure that appropriate laboratory investigations are undertaken (see Box 3.48.1).
3 Arrange for chemoprophylaxis for close contacts, and vaccine if the infection is due to a vaccine-preventable strain. (See Box 3.48.3.)

The aim of chemoprophylaxis is to eradicate the infecting strain from the network of close contacts, and thus prevent further cases among susceptible close contacts. Chemoprophylaxis should be given as soon as possible. Close contacts are defined as people who have had close prolonged contact with the case in the week before onset. This usually includes household members, girlfriends/boyfriends, regular childminders and sometimes students in a hall of residence. Classroom, nursery and other social contacts do not need chemoprophylaxis.

Box 3.48.2 Immediate dose of benzyl penicillin for suspected meningococcal infection

Adults and children aged 10 years or over	1200 mg
Children aged 1–9 years	600 mg
Children aged 1 year	300 mg

The dose should be given intravenously (or intramuscularly if there is peripheral shutdown). If there is a history of penicillin anaphylaxis (which is very rare), chloramphenicol by injection (1.2 g for adults, 25 mg/kg for children under 12 years) is a suitable alternative.

Box 3.48.3 Doses for chemoprophylaxis

Rifampicin: 600 mg twice daily for 2 days (adults and children over 12 years); 10 mg/kg twice daily for 2 days (children aged 1–12 years); 5 mg/kg twice daily for 2 days (infants under 12 months).
or
Ciprofloxacin (unlicensed for this use): 500 mg single oral dose (adults only)
or
Ceftriaxone: 250 mg single i.m. dose (adults); 125 mg in children under 12 years.

The aim of vaccination is to prevent late secondary cases. There is less urgency for vaccination, as chemoprophylaxis aims to prevent the early secondary cases. Vaccine should be offered to all close contacts as defined above; contacts under 2 years of age of serogroup C disease should be given conjugate and not polysaccharide vaccine.

4 Provide information about meningococcal disease to parents, GPs and educational establishments. The aim here is to improve the outcome of any secondary cases that may occur and to prevent rumours and anxiety.

Response to a cluster and control of an outbreak

In addition to the actions described above for single cases, links between cases should be sought. Expert advice should be obtained and an outbreak control team established. Information dissemination is essential. Where clusters occur in an educational establishment, the following action is recommended:

1 Two or more possible cases (see case definition): prophylaxis to household or institutional contacts is not recommended.

2 Two confirmed cases caused by different serogroups: only give prophylaxis to household contacts.

3 Two or more confirmed or probable cases within a four-week period: prophylaxis to household contacts and to a defined close contact group within the establishment. This may include, for example, classroom contacts, children who share a common social activity or a group of close friends.

4 Two or more confirmed or probable cases separated by an interval of more than four weeks: consider wider prophylaxis, but seek expert advice.

Where clusters occur in the wider community, age-specific attack rates should be calculated: the numerator is the number of confirmed cases and the denominator is the population within which all the cases reside. This may be difficult to define. Vaccination and chemoprophylaxis for the community may be indicated for clusters of serogroup C disease where attack rates are high (e.g. above 40 per 100 000). Establish an outbreak control team and seek expert advice.

Suggested case-definitions for public health action

Confirmed case: invasive disease (meningitis, septicaemia, or infection of other normally sterile tissue) confirmed as caused by *Neisseria meningitidis*.

Probable case: clinical diagnosis of invasive meningococcal disease without laboratory confirmation, in which the CCDC, in consultation with the clinician managing the case, considers that meningococcal disease is the likeliest diagnosis. In the absence of an alternative diagnosis a feverish, ill patient with a petechial/purpuric rash should be regarded as a probable case of meningococcal septicaemia.

Possible case: as probable case, but the CCDC, in consultation with the clinician managing the case, considers that diagnoses other than meningococcal disease are at least as likely. This includes cases treated with antibiotics whose probable diagnosis is viral meningitis.

3.49 Molluscum contagiosum

Molluscum contagiosum is a skin infection caused by a member of the Poxviridae family. It produces characteristic smooth-surfaced white or translucent papules 2–5 millimetres in diameter, which are seen on the face and body. Lesions vary in number; they may be extensive in HIV infection and sometimes coalesce to form giant lesions. Molluscum contagiosum resolves spontaneously after 6–24 months. The lifespan of individual lesions is 2–3 months. If necessary, diagnosis can be confirmed by the typical appearance of the contents of the lesions on light microscopy or by histology.

The infection has a worldwide distribution and is most frequently seen in children. Spread is by direct contact, both sexual and non-sexual, from human cases. Autoinoculation can occur as a result of scratching. The incubation period is variable and a person will remain infectious as long as the lesions persist. There is, however, no need to stay away from work or school. A child with molluscum contagiosum can take part in most school activities, including swimming, but it may be prudent to avoid close contact sports such as wrestling.

3.50 MRSA (methicillin-resistant *Staphylococcus aureus*)

Staphylococci are Gram-positive cocci which are classified as coagulase-positive (*Staphylococcus aureus*) or coagulase-negative (all other staphylococci).

Staphylococcus aureus is a common cause of acute pyogenic infection in man, ranging from minor skin sepsis to life-threatening septicaemia. There are numerous subtypes of *S. aureus*, which may be distinguished by phage typing.

Staphylococcal food poisoning is an intoxication rather than an infection and is dealt with separately (Chapter 3.71).

Over 80% of *S. aureus* produce penicillinases and are resistant to benzyl penicillin. Cloxacillin and flucloxacillin are not inactivated and were generally the antibiotics of choice before staphylococci resistant to these antibiotics became a common cause of infection, particularly in hospitals.

Laboratory identification of these resistant strains uses methicillin, an antibiotic no longer used therapeutically, and they are referred to as methicillin-resistant *Staphylococcus aureus* (MRSA). Some MRSA are sensitive only to vancomycin, but *S. aureus* with intermediate-level resistance to vancomycin (VISA) have been reported in Japan, the USA, France and Scotland.

The mechanism of methicillin resistance is usually the production of a low-affinity penicillin-binding protein rather than the production of a beta-lactamase.

On-call action

The public health doctor should be prepared to assist the infection control doctor to investigate and control nosocomial outbreaks of MRSA. The public health team may be asked to advise on the management of a cluster of cases of methicillin-sensitive *S. aureus* (MSSA) or MRSA infection in the community.

Epidemiology

Nasal carriage of *Staphylococcus aureus* can be detected in about 30% of the population at any given time and will occur at some time in about 80%.

The risk of staphylococcal infection is increased in vulnerable groups including newborn infants, the elderly, problem drug users and those who are admitted to hospital, particularly if undergoing surgery or other invasive procedures.

MRSA were first identified in the 1960s soon after the introduction of methicillin. MRSA re-emerged as a problem in the UK in the early 1980s following the introduction of newer penicillins and cephalosporins.

MRSA is now endemic in many hospitals worldwide and is an important cause of hospital-acquired infections, particularly in vulnerable patients, in whom they are often difficult and expensive to treat, delay discharge and are associated with increased morbidity and mortality.

In a typical general hospital with 500 beds there may be 300–400 first isolates of MRSA each year, with 10–25 patients affected at any one time.

MRSA is said to be uncommon in countries that have strict infection control policies, including the Netherlands and Scandinavia.

In England and Wales, the Communicable Disease Surveillance Centre collates laboratory reports of *S. aureus*-positive blood cultures and cerebrospinal fluid. The proportion of bacteraemias due to MRSA has risen in recent years to over 30%. The number of hospitals reporting MRSA and the number of MRSA hospital incidents (three or more patient isolates of the same MRSA strain in a month) have also increased.

Clinical features

The clinical syndromes associated with *S. aureus* infection are summarized in Table 3.50.1. MRSA causes infection or colonization in the same way as methicillin-sensitive *S. aureus*.

Table 3.50.1

Infection	Comments
Acute osteomyelitis	Infection is usually haematogenous but may spread from adjacent structures or arise in association with peripheral vascular disease.
Bacteraemia and septicaemia	Often associated with infection in other sites such as pneumonia, cellulitis or wound infection.
Skin infection	Folliculitis, carbuncle, furunculosis (boils), impetigo.
Cellulitis	May follow trauma.
Conjunctivitis	
Septic arthritis	May be due to spread of organisms from a distant site by the haematogenous route or direct inoculation from a penetrating wound or bite, from adjacent osteomyelitis, prosthetic joint surgery or when intra-articular injections are given. Risk factors include trauma, joint diseases such as rheumatoid arthritis or osteoarthritis, debility, immunosuppressive therapy and intravenous drug abuse.
Staphylococcal pneumonia	Staphylococcal pneumonia is rare unless the lungs have been affected by influenza, measles, chronic bronchitis or surgery. It may occur in children in the first eight weeks of life. It may be complicated by pleural effusion, empyema or lung abscess.
Staphylococcal scalded skin syndrome (SSSS)	Fever, tender erythematous rash, large bullae and exfoliation of sheets of skin due to certain *S. aureus* phage groups which produce an exotoxin.
Toxic shock syndrome (TSS)	Due to exotoxins produced by *S. aureus* and comprises fever, hypotension, thrombocytopenia, vomiting and diarrhoea, skin rash with later desquamation, renal, hepatic and CNS dysfunction. It occurs in menstruating females using tampons but can occur with infection at other sites and in males or children.

Laboratory confirmation

The laboratory diagnosis of *S. aureus* infection requires microbiological examination of appropriate clinical specimens. As a minimum a Gram stain, culture and antibiotic sensitivities should be requested. Biochemical tests, phage typing and genome analysis are available.

Using these techniques up to 16 different strains of MRSA have been characterized in the UK. These differ in their ability to spread in hospital and to colonize and cause infection. Currently EMRSA-15 and EMRSA-16 are the two dominant strains in the UK.

Transmission

The reservoir of *S. aureus* is colonized or infected humans and rarely animals. The main sites of colonization are the anterior nares and skin whilst purulent discharges from wounds and other lesions are the main source in infected persons.

Transmission is by direct contact. Some carriers are more efficient at spreading infection than others. Infection is spread mainly on hands but indirect spread via fomites, equipment and the environment may occur. It is estimated that in about a third of cases infection is endogenous.

Use of cephalosporins is associated with rapid acquisition of MRSA by hospital patients previously carrying methicillin-sensitive strains. Once selected in one patient MRSA may spread to others, particularly in modern hospitals where high bed turnover, frequent transfers between wards, hospitals and nursing homes, overcrowding and limited numbers of medical and nursing staff challenge basic infection control measures.

MRSA rarely invades intact skin but can invade pressure sores, surgical wounds, intravascular catheter sites and may then lead to severe infections.

Pathogenesis

The incubation period is 4–10 days and a person will remain infectious to others as long as the infection or carrier state persists.

Prevention

Prevention of staphylococcal infection depends on good personal hygiene, especially handwashing and prompt identification and treatment of cases.

Surveillance

In the community appropriate clinical specimens should be collected for microbiological examination from cases of suspected staphylococcal infection and clusters of cases should be reported to the local public health department.

In hospitals the infection control team should agree testing protocols. As a minimum all patients with clinical lesions should be sampled. In many hospitals nasal and skin swabs are collected routinely on patients who are admitted to high-risk areas of the

Table 3.50.2 Prevention of MRSA

Prevention of MRSA in hospitals depends on:
• Requesting appropriate specimens for microbiological testing when infection is suspected
• Sound antibiotic policies and practices
• Effective surveillance systems
• Infection control policies, co-ordinated and monitored by an infection control team
• Compliance with basic control measures such as handwashing, aseptic techniques, ward cleaning, dust control, handling of waste, use of disposable gloves and aprons

Prevention of MRSA in the community
• Basic infection control measures of handwashing, cleaning of equipment and handling of potentially contaminated dressings, catheters and linen should be applied routinely
• Wounds and pressure sores on residents, and skin lesions on staff or residents should be protected by an impermeable dressing

---

hospital such as ITU. Cases of MRSA will then be readily detected by alert organism surveillance.

Response to a case or carrier

Treatment

Localized infection may respond to warm soaks and topical antiseptics (e.g. triclosan and benzalkonium chloride) or antibiotics. Surgical drainage may be required. Until the results of diagnostic cultures are available a penicillinase-resistant penicillin should be given (e.g. flucloxacillin 0.5–1.0 g orally every 6 h). In severe cases parenteral therapy may be needed. In recurrent infection, the application of antibiotic ointment to the nares and oral rifampicin may be used to eradicate carriage.

MRSA may remain susceptible to fusidic acid, ciprofloxacin or trimethoprim, but in practice any severe suspected MRSA infection requires urgent parenteral treatment with a glycopeptide such as vancomycin or teicoplanin. Appropriate samples for culture and antibiotic sensitivity testing must be obtained. For small superficial MRSA infections, topical antiseptics or mupirocin ointment may be used.

MRSA nasal carriers are treated with mupirocin ointment. Skin carriage can be treated with daily antiseptic baths and shampoos with hexachlorophane powder for axillary or groin carriage. The importance of throat carriage in relation to spread is unclear. A 5-day course of oral treatment with an appropriate combination of antibiotics may be considered.

Control of infection

It is not usually necessary to report individual cases of MRSA in the community. Cases should be started on appropriate treatment and discharging lesions should be covered with impermeable dressings if practicable. Contact with infants and other susceptible groups should be avoided. School-age children and cases in high-risk occupations should stay at home until no longer infectious.

Guidelines have been published on infection control for MRSA in hospitals and other inpatient settings including high-risk areas such as ITU, special care baby units and orthopaedic units and lower-risk areas such as care of the elderly wards and nursing homes.

Hospitals

Every effort should be made to keep MRSA out of high-risk hospital areas where it can cause problems. Patients should be placed under source isolation in a side room. If several patients are affected they may be cohort nursed in a separate area of the ward. Efforts should be made to clear the MRSA with antiseptic baths, shampoos and skin powders and antibiotic ointments.

Nursing homes

Colonization with MRSA should not prevent a patient being discharged to their own home or to a nursing home in the community if their general clinical condition allows it. Although in the UK 4–7% of elderly nursing home residents are colonized with MRSA, clinical infections in such settings are uncommon. Routinely high standards of infection control should be observed. There should be good communication between the hospital infection control team and the nursing home staff. In nursing homes with high-dependency patients or early postoperative patients, control measures should resemble those in hospitals (see above).

Investigation of a cluster and control of an outbreak

Despite the implementation of infection control measures, outbreaks of MRSA (and less commonly of MSSA) are reported from hospitals, community nursing homes, day-care settings and amongst groups of people participating in contact sports such as rugby and wrestling.

An MRSA outbreak may be defined as either an increase in the rate of MRSA cases (defined statistically or experientially) or a clustering of new cases due to the transmission of a single strain in a particular setting and includes both infected and colonized patients.

In hospitals, infected or colonized patients form the main source of MRSA and transmission is usually via the transiently colonized hands of healthcare staff. However staff who are nasal carriers and environmental sources have been implicated in some outbreaks.

Outbreaks are investigated in a systematic fashion.

• Search for infected cases and carriers.

• Request appropriate laboratory tests including antibiotic sensitivity patterns, phage typing and pulsed-field gel electrophoresis (PFGE) to confirm that cases are caused by the same strain and to rule out a pseudo-outbreak.

• Screen staff to detect carriers who may be the source of infection.

• Carry out an environmental investigation and microbiological sampling.

• Review clinical practice such as wound closure, antibiotic use, etc.

• Review infection control practice, including handwashing, cleaning of equipment, care of catheter sites, etc.

In an MRSA outbreak, in addition to the standard control measures detailed above the following measures may be required:

• Restrict or suspend admissions.

• Restrict movement of staff and patients.

• Limit use of temporary agency staff.

• Ward closure.

Definitions for MRSA surveillance

New isolates

A patient or staff member who has MRSA isolated for the first time from a clinical sample or screening swab.

or

A patient or staff member who is positive for a second or subsequent time having been successfully treated and shown to be microbiologically clear of MRSA.

New isolates are classified as infected if any of these signs and symptoms are present, otherwise new isolates will be classified as colonized.

• The cardinal signs and symptoms of infection are present at the time the laboratory specimens are obtained. These include fever >37.7 °C and inflammation as indicated by redness, swelling, pain, heat, pus.

• A clinician has diagnosed infection.

• In the case of a positive urine culture there is fever and urgency, frequency or dysuria (if a catheter is in place fever alone is sufficient).

• A medical diagnosis of pneumonia or chest infection has been made.

• There are chest signs, X-ray changes or increased sputum and fever.

• In the case of a positive blood culture there is fever or chills or rigors or hypotension.

• In the case of a wound culture there is a purulent discharge in or exuding from the wound.

• In the case of skin infection there are signs of inflammation with or without pus.

• In the case of a burn infection or eye infection there is a purulent discharge.

• There is a clinical diagnosis of septic arthritis or osteomyelitis.

• In the case of a faecal isolate there is diarrhoea and vomiting.

• There is a clinical diagnosis of abscess or peritonitis.

• In the case of a genital isolate there is a purulent discharge.

Continued

Continued.

Hospital in-patients

Patients in NHS accommodation including long-stay hospitals, mental health units, etc.

Patients in the community
- Patients in private nursing homes and private and social services residential accommodation, usually cared for by GPs.
- Patients in their own homes.

3.51 Mumps

Mumps is a systemic viral infection characterized by parotitis. It is caused by a paramyxovirus. The public health significance of mumps is that complications are common and it is preventable by vaccination.

Suggested on-call action

None usually required.

Epidemiology

Before vaccination was introduced in 1988, mumps caused epidemics every three years, with highest attack rates in children aged 5–9. It is now uncommon; between 1500 and 2000 cases are notified every year, although only about 30% of these are confirmed on laboratory testing. Most cases are in unvaccinated older children. Deaths are rare, although meningitis is a relatively common complication: in the prevaccine era, mumps was the commonest viral cause of meningitis.

Clinical features

Tenderness and swelling of the parotid occur in about 70% of cases. It can be confused with swelling of the cervical lymph nodes. Other common features of mumps include meningitis (which is mild), orchitis (in adult males) and pancreatitis. Rare features are oophoritis, arthritis, mastitis and myocarditis.

Laboratory confirmation

Saliva, CSF or urine may be collected for viral culture. Serological diagnosis is best achieved either by demonstrating S antibody by complement fixation or IgM antibody by ELISA.

Transmission

Man is the only reservoir. Carriage does not occur. Mumps is moderately infectious, with transmission occurring through droplet spread and direct contact with saliva of a case.

Pathogenesis

The incubation period is 2–3 weeks (average 18 days). Cases are infectious for up to a week (normally two days) before parotid swelling until nine days after.

Prevention

Mumps vaccine is a live attenuated vaccine. In the UK schedule, two doses are given (in combination with measles and rubella) at 12–15 months and 3–5 years of age.

Surveillance

The disease is notifiable in the UK. Laboratory confirmation should be sought in all cases.

Response to a case

- Consider exclusion from school for 10 days from onset of parotid swelling, if many school contacts are unvaccinated.

- Check vaccination status.
- Arrange for laboratory confirmation (e.g. saliva test).

Response to a cluster and control of an outbreak

As for a case, but also consider community-wide vaccination if coverage is low.

Suggested case-definition for an outbreak

Clinical: acute onset of parotid swelling, in the absence of other obvious cause.
Confirmed: positive by culture, IgM or four-fold rise in IgG. Does not need to meet clinical case-definition.

3.52 *Mycoplasma*

Mycoplasma pneumoniae causes acute respiratory infection and is an important cause of community-acquired pneumonia during its four-yearly epidemics.

Suggested on-call action

None, unless outbreak suspected in institution containing frail individuals (treat symptomatic contacts if so).

Epidemiology

Most *M. pneumoniae* infection is never diagnosed. During the epidemics which occur approximately every 3–4 years in the UK and last 12–18 months, peaking in winter(s), *M. pneumoniae* may be responsible for up to a third of community-acquired pneumonia. The most recent epidemic in the UK was late 1997 to early 1999. Outside of epidemic periods, as little as 1% of pneumonias may be due to this organism. Incidence rates are highest in school-aged children, with a secondary peak in adults aged 30–39. Outbreaks occur in institutions and military barracks.

Clinical diagnosis

Mycoplasma classically presents with fever, malaise and headache with upper respiratory tract symptoms such as coryza, sore throat or unproductive cough. Up to 10% then progress to tracheobronchitis or 'atypical' pneumonia with a more severe cough, although muco-purulent sputum, obvious dyspnoea and true pleuritic pain are rare. Onset is usually insidious, with presentation often delayed 10–14 days. Asymptomatic infection may also occur. Those with sickle-cell anaemia may be more severely affected.

Laboratory confirmation

The mainstay of diagnosis is demonstration of a fourfold rise in serum-specific IgG antibodies. However, it may take several weeks for such a rise to become apparent. Quicker but less sensitive alternatives may be available, including culture on special media, detection of serum-specific IgA or IgM (positive after 8–14 days of illness), and antigen detection or PCR testing of sputum or nasopharyngeal aspirates (or less optimally throat swabs).

Transmission

Humans are the sole reservoir. Transmission requires relatively close contact: although school-age children appear to be the main vectors of transmission, they usually only infect family members and close playmates and rarely start classroom epidemics. Airborne spread by inhalation of droplets produced by coughing, direct contact with an infected person (perhaps including asymptomatics) and indirect contact with items contaminated by nasal or throat discharges from cases probably all contribute to transmission.

Pathogenesis

The *incubation period* is reported as ranging from 6 to 32 days. Two weeks is a reasonable estimate of the median.

The *infectious period* probably does not start until coryza or cough is evident. The length of infectiousness is unclear: three weeks from onset of illness can be used as a rule of thumb if coughing has ceased, although excretion may be prolonged despite antibiotics.

Immunity does occur postinfection, but later re-infection is recognized.

Prevention

- Avoid overcrowding in closed communities.
- Safe disposal of items likely to be contaminated by respiratory secretions.

Surveillance

Not statutorily notifiable in the UK. Report to local public health authorities if associated with institution. Report laboratory-confirmed cases to national surveillance systems.

Response to case

- Hygiene advice. Care with respiratory secretions.
- Not to attend work or school whilst unwell.
- Treat cases with lower respiratory tract infection with erythromycin or tetracycline (i.e. drugs which are not usually first choice for pneumonia).

Investigation of a cluster

- Look for links to institutions: however, more likely to be links between families via school-age children.
- If increase in community, warn local clinicians and remind them of appropriate antibiotics.

Control of an outbreak

- Reinforce hygiene and infection control practices, especially relating to respiratory secretions and handwashing.
- Avoid introduction of new susceptibles into institutions with frail individuals (e.g. nursing home).
- Offer antibiotic treatment to those with respiratory symptoms.
- Consider feasibility of separating coughing residents from asymptomatic ones.

Suggested case-definition for use in outbreak

Confirmed: serological confirmation of illness (IgM, IgA or fourfold rise in IgG) or demonstration of antigen or PCR in respiratory secretions.

Clinical: pneumonia, bronchitis or pharyngitis without other identified cause in member of affected institution.

3.53 Ophthalmia neonatorum

Ophthalmia neonatorum (ON) is acute infection of the eye or conjunctiva occurring in the first three weeks of life, caused by a variety of bacteria present in the birth canal. Infection due to *Neisseria gonorrhoea* is the most serious and that due to *Chlamydia trachomatis* the most common. ON may also be caused by staphylococci.

On-call action

None.

Epidemiology

The incidence of ON depends on the prevalence of maternal infection in any given population. Gonorrhoea is now uncommon in pregnant women, but the prevalence of genital chlamydial infection in some studies is around 5%. Up to 30% of neonates exposed to maternal infection will develop ON, giving an estimated incidence of 1–2% of births.

ON is a legally notifiable infection in the UK. Historically this was because of the serious nature of gonococcal ON and the need for prompt treatment. Recently in England and Wales there have only been 200–400 reports per year, but this almost certainly underestimates the true incidence.

Diagnosis

In gonococcal ON there is swelling and redness of the eye, with purulent discharge, within 1–5 days of birth. Without prompt treatment the cornea may be damaged. Chlamydial ON starts between 5 and 12 days after birth. There is an acute purulent phase, which may be followed by chronic inflammation with corneal scarring. Diagnosis may be confirmed by microscopy using appropriate staining or culture.

Transmission

Spread is by direct contact with an infected birth passage. Secondary spread may take place by direct or indirect contact with eye discharges. The infant will remain infectious until treated.

Prevention

Infection may be prevented by identification and treatment of infection in pregnancy. Routine use of appropriate prophylactic eye-drops for newborn infants prevents gonococcal but not chlamydial ON.

Surveillance

ON is notifiable in many countries, including England and Wales.

Response to a case

Treat with appropriate antibiotics and obtain microbiological diagnosis. Contact precau-

tions should be observed. If the infection is chlamydial or gonococcal, the mother and her sexual partners should be investigated and treated for genital infection, even if they are symptom-free.

Case-definition
Purulent conjunctivitis within three weeks of birth.

3.54 Paratyphoid fever

Paratyphoid fever is caused by *S. paratyphi* A, B or occasionally C. It produces an illness similar to typhoid (see Chapter 3.80), though usually less severe.

Suggested on-call action
• Exclude cases and contacts who are food-handlers. • Exclude cases and symptomatic contacts in other risk groups (see below).

Epidemiology

Infection results from the ingestion of water or food contaminated by human faeces. Infection occurs worldwide and is associated with poor sanitation. About 170 laboratory confirmed cases of paratyphoid are reported annually in England and Wales. 80–90% are imported, most commonly from the Indian subcontinent.

Clinical features

S. paratyphi may cause gastroenteritis or enteric fever (EF). EF begins with fever, and rigors may occur. Patients complain of headache, cough, malaise, myalgia and may be constipated. Later in the course, diarrhoea, abdominal tenderness, vomiting, delirium and confusion may occur. In paratyphoid fever cases, spots are more frequent and brighter red than in typhoid. Complications are less common than for typhoid and typically arise in the third week. Up to 5% cases may relapse.

Laboratory confirmation

Blood, urine, faeces and bone marrow aspirate can be cultured. Definitive diagnosis is by culture of the organism from a normally sterile site (e.g. blood). Over 80% of UK cases are serogroup A, with the remainder group B.

Transmission

Transmission is predominantly food-borne from the consumption of foods contaminated by a human case or occasionally by an asymptomatic carrier, including fruit or vegetables washed in water contaminated by sewage. Water-borne outbreaks and milk-borne infection are recorded. Person-to-person spread is possible in poor hygienic conditions. Serogroup B is occasionally associated with cattle.

Pathogenesis

The incubation period for enteric fever is usually between 1 and 2 weeks, and for paratyphoid gastroenteritis 1–10 days.

Commonly bacteria are excreted up to two weeks after convalescence. A small number of persons infected with *S. paratyphi* become chronic carriers.

Partial immunity results from infection.

Prevention

Control depends on sanitation, clean water and personal hygiene. There is no effective vaccine against paratyphoid.

Surveillance

Paratyphoid is a notifiable disease in most countries, including the UK, and should be reported to local public health departments on clinical suspicion.

Response to a case

- Check antibiotic resistance of isolate.
- Enteric precautions and hygiene advice for cases; isolation if hospitalized.
- Obtain food and travel history for the 3 weeks prior to onset of illness.
- Cases who have not visited an endemic country in the 3 weeks before onset should be investigated to determine the source of infection.
- Exclude cases who are food handlers (Box 2.2.1: risk group 1) until 6 consecutive negative stool specimens taken at 2-week intervals and commencing 2 weeks after completion of antibiotic therapy.
- Exclude cases who are children aged under 5 years and cases with poor personal hygiene (risk groups 3 and 4) until 3 consecutive negative faecal samples taken at weekly intervals.
- Exclude cases who are health workers (risk group 2) until clinically well with formed stools and hygiene advice given. Tell hospital infection control team.
- Exclude all other cases until clinically well with formed stools.
- Investigate household and other close contacts with a faecal specimen for culture. If positive, treat as case.
- Do not treat contacts in groups at risk for further transmission (Box 2.2.1) as negative until three consecutive negatives taken at weekly intervals commencing 3 weeks after last exposure to case. Exclude contacts who are food handlers until these results are known. Exclude others only until formed stools for 48 h and hygiene advice given.
- Quinolones may reduce the period of carriage in those for whom exclusion is producing social difficulties.

Investigation of a cluster

Clusters should be investigated to ensure that secondary transmission has not occurred. Check each case (and their household contacts) for travel abroad. Obtain and compare food histories. Explore family and social links between cases.

Control of an outbreak

Outbreaks of paratyphoid should be investigated as a matter of urgency. All cases and contacts should be investigated to identify the source of the outbreak. This could be due to contact with a chronic carrier, with faecal material, or with contaminated food, milk, water or shellfish.

Contacts should be observed and investigated if they develop symptoms suggestive of paratyphoid after appropriate specimens are taken.

Suggested case-definition

Clinical illness compatible with paratyphoid and isolate from blood or stool.

3.55 Parvovirus B19 (fifth disease)

Parvovirus B19 is the cause of a common childhood infection, erythema infectiosum, also known as fifth disease or slapped cheek syndrome. It is important because of the risk of complications in pregnancy, in those with haemoglobinopathies and the immunocompromised.

Suggested on-call action

If case is a HCW in contact with high-risk patients, consider either exclusion from work or avoiding contact with high-risk patients.

Epidemiology

Infection occurs at all ages, although children aged 5–14 years are at greatest risk. School outbreaks usually occur in early spring. Fifth disease is now more common than rubella in children in the UK.

Clinical features

The first symptom is fever, which lasts for two or three days until the rash appears. The rash is maculopapular and is found on the limbs, less commonly the trunk. The cheeks often have a bright red ('slapped cheek') appearance. In a healthy person, the illness is usually mild and short-lived, although persistent joint pain, with or without swelling sometimes occurs, especially in young women, most commonly in knees, fingers, ankles, wrists and elbows.

Parvovirus infection in the first 20 weeks of pregnancy can cause fetal loss (9%) and hydrops fetalis (3%); it is however, not teratogenic. In patients with haemoglobinopathies it can cause transient aplastic crises, and in immunodeficient patients red cell aplasia and chronic anaemia can occur.

Laboratory confirmation

This is important to distinguish from rubella, especially in pregnant women or their contacts. The diagnosis can be confirmed by testing serum for B19 IgM or by electron microscopy.

Transmission

Man is the only reservoir; cat and dog parvoviruses do not infect humans. Transmission is from person to person by droplet infection from the respiratory tract; rarely by contaminated blood products. Long-term carriage does not occur.

Pathogenesis

Parvovirus is highly infectious. The incubation period is often quoted as 4–20 days, but is usually between 13 and 18 days. The infectious period is from 7 days before the rash appears until the onset of the rash. In aplastic crises infectivity lasts for up to a week after the rash appears, and immunosuppressed people with severe anaemia may be infectious for several months or even years.

Prevention

Only patients likely to develop complications (see above) need consider specific preventive measures. These individuals may choose to avoid exposure to potential cases in outbreak situations.

Surveillance

The disease is not notifiable in the UK or most other European countries, and may only come to the attention of the public health department as a result of investigation of a case of suspected rubella, or when there is an outbreak of a rash illness in a school.

Diagnosis confirmed in HCW
Was the HCW in contact with any patient from the following groups : in the same room for a significant period of time (15 minutes or more); or face to face contact during the period from seven days before the appearance of a rash to the date of appearance of the rash; in the absence of respiratory isolation precautions?
- Pregnant women <21 weeks gestation
- Immunocompromised
- Haemoglobinopathies

Consider need for action in light of risk assessment

HCW in contact with pregnant women <21 weeks	HCW in contact with patients with haemoglobinopathies	HCW in contact with immunocompromised patients

If the decision is made to investigate **Check antenatal/ booking serum** to identify seronegative susceptible women (40%)

Check serology to identify IgG-negative patients at risk and monitor IgG-negative patients for development of aplastic crisis

Contact reference laboratory for DNA testing as antibody testing may be unreliable. If infected, consider human normal intravenous immunoglobulin 400 mg/kg per day for 5–10 days

Contact exposed susceptible women or those for whom no previous serum available Inform them of low risk of infection but need to follow up their serology 21 days after exposure or if a rash develops

Take serum if rash appears or at 21 days after contact. Test for IgG and IgM

IgG positive IgM negative REASSURE – NO RISK	**IgG negative IgM negative** SUSCEPTIBLE BUT NOT INFECTED – need to follow up future rash contacts	**IgM positive** INFECTED – refer for specialist follow-up by ultrasound to detect fetal hydrops and intrauterine transfusion if necessary

Fig. 3.55.1 Response to parvovirus B19 infection in a healthcare worker (HCW): protection for those at risk (to be incorporated into advice for acute potentially infectious illness in HCW including rash with fever). With permission from N.S. Crowcroft *et al.* (1999). Guidance for the control of parvovirus B19 in healthcare. *Journal of Public Health Medicine*, **21** (Suppl. 4), 439–446.

Response to a case

Arrange for laboratory confirmation. Isolation or school exclusion of cases is of no value as any transmission occurs before the onset of symptoms.

Where a healthcare worker (HCW) has been exposed to a case, and is found to be susceptible, it may be necessary to exclude the HCW if a fever develops, until either the rash appears or for 15 days from the last contact with the case. Alternatively the HCW may be advised to avoid contact with high-risk patients (women in the first 20 weeks of pregnancy, those with haemoglobinopathies and the immunocompromised), or to take respiratory precautions until a rash appears or for 15 days. Screening of HCWs may be justified for those who have frequent contact with high-risk patients, or for laboratory workers who work with infectious material known to contain B19 virus.

Where infection is confirmed in a HCW, high-risk contacts (as above) should be tested for immunity and monitored for evidence of infection, as they need specialist care if infected. Human normal immunoglobulin 400 mg/kg intravenously for 5–10 days should be considered for immunosuppressed contacts (efficacy uncertain).

Investigation and control of an outbreak

In addition to measures described above for a case, it may be worth excluding susceptible teachers who are in the first 20 weeks of pregnancy from a school in which an outbreak is occurring, until they are more than 20 weeks pregnant.

Suggested case-definition

IgM or em positive in presence of clinically compatible illness.

3.56 Plague

Plague is a serious and potentially highly infectious disease caused by *Yersinia pestis*.

On-call action

- Ensure that cases are isolated.
- Ensure staff monitoring is instituted.
- Ensure samples are handled appropriately.
- Identify contacts and others at risk.
- Liaise with rodent and flea control experts if possibility of local acquisition.

Epidemiology

Yersinia pestis is a pathogen of rodents in many parts of the New and Old World. Man comes into contact with infected fleas by disturbing the natural hosts (ground squirrels, gerbils, etc.) or if domestic rats acquire them. Northern Europe is free of plague, but cases occur in the former Soviet Union.

Clinical features

Bubonic plague: high fever, malaise and delirium develop rapidly. Regional adenopathy and tender buboes draining the site of infection develop. Petechial or purpuric haemorrhages are common. The disease progresses to septic shock, with an untreated mortality of 60–90%.

Pneumonic plague is acquired by respiratory spread. The patient becomes severely ill with a high fever, tachypnoea, restlessness and shortness of breath. Respiratory signs are often absent. Frothy blood-tinged sputum is usually produced as a preterminal event. The untreated mortality is 100%.

Laboratory confirmation

The organism can be isolated from the blood, sputum and buboes. Organisms in smears can be Gram-stained. Serology and antigen detection may also be available.

Transmission

Bubonic plague is transmitted by the bite of infected rat fleas. Spread is from the bite site to lymph nodes, rapidly followed by septicaemia and pneumonia. Pneumonic plague is acquired directly by the respiratory route from another case of pneumonic plague.

Pathogenesis

Incubation period as follows:
- Bubonic plague: one to six days.
- Pneumonic plague: 10–15 h.

Prevention

Control of rats and fleas is essential. Laboratory staff likely to come into contact with the organism should be vaccinated. The organism should be handled only in Class 4 laboratory facilities.

Surveillance

Notifiable: cases should be reported to national authorities and to WHO. Any suspected case should be reported to local public health departments as a matter of urgency.

Response to a case

Streptomycin and tetracyclines or chloramphenicol are the drugs of choice. Patients are highly infectious. All care should be taken with specimens. Patients and possessions must be disinfected of fleas. Patients should be strictly isolated. Staff should be monitored carefully for fever and treated promptly. Household contacts should be offered tetracycline prophylaxis. Treatment after 15 h probably does not influence the course of pneumonic plague.

Investigation of a cluster and control of an outbreak

The source should be identified as a matter of urgency and rodent and flea control instituted as necessary. Contacts should be offered prophylaxis.

Suggested case-definitions

Suspected: clinically compatible case.
Probable: clinically compatible case with single high antibody titre or detection of antigen.
Confirmed: clinically compatible case with isolate or fourfold rise in titres.

3.57 Pneumococcal infection

Streptococcus pneumoniae ('pneumococcus') is the commonest cause of community-acquired pneumonia and a common cause of bacteraemia and meningitis.

Suggested on-call action

- If case of meningitis, reassure contacts that no prophylaxis is needed.
- If outbreak in institution suspected, consult local outbreak control plan.

Epidemiology

Pneumococcal pneumonia is estimated to affect 0.1% of the population per annum. 4000 isolates of pneumococcus from blood or CSF were reported in the UK in 1999. All ages are affected but the distribution is bimodal: half of cases occur in the over-65s, but the highest rates are in infants. Both pneumonia and meningitis are more common in the winter. Pneumococcal infection is more common in smokers, heavy drinkers and those who live in overcrowded sleeping quarters. Incidence increases during influenza epidemics.

Although the incidence of pneumococcal meningitis is highest in young children, its relative importance is highest in middle-aged and elderly adults, in which it is the most common cause of bacterial meningitis.

Resistance to antibiotics such as erythromycin and penicillin has been increasing in most European countries and is particularly high in Spain.

Clinical features

Approximately a third of pneumococcal infections affect the respiratory tract, a third are focal infections (mostly otitis media) and a third are fever or bacteraemia without obvious focus. The most common symptoms of pneumococcal pneumonia are cough, sputum and fever. Factors that suggest pneumococcal rather than 'atypical' pneumonia in an outbreak include mucopurulent or bloodstained sputum, pleuritic chest pain and prominent physical signs. Respiratory symptoms may be less obvious in the elderly. Many cases have predisposing illnesses such as chronic respiratory, cardiac, renal or liver disease, immunosuppression or diabetes. Bacteraemia may occasionally lead to meningitis. Case fatality for bacteraemia or meningitis is 20%.

Asymptomatic carriage of pneumococci in the nasopharynx is common, affecting approximately 25% of healthy people, although not all are serotypes commonly associated with illness.

Laboratory confirmation

Gram staining and culture of good-quality sputum specimens are the mainstay of diagnosis of pneumococcal pneumonia, although they are only 60% sensitive and 90% specific. 25% of cases of pneumonia will also have a positive blood culture, which can be useful confirmation that the pneumococcus is a pathogen rather than a coincidental commensal. Antigen detection in sputum or urine may be available in some laboratories. Gram-positive diplococci in CSF suggest pneumococcal meningitis.

Transmission

Pneumococci are spread by extensive close contact with human cases or carriers. Transmission is usually by droplet spread but may also be via direct oral contact or articles soiled by respiratory discharges. Pneumococci remain viable in dried secretions for many months and may be cultured from the air or dust in hospitals, although the importance of this for transmission is unclear. In hospitals, spread is usually to patients in the next one or two beds. Staff may also become colonized.

Cases of pneumococcal meningitis are viewed as sporadic; indeed, many cases are autoinfections.

Prevention

• A polysaccharide vaccine with approximately 65% efficacy for pneumonia in those over 2 years of age is available and conjugate vaccines are under development. Current UK recommendations are that the vaccine should be given to all those in whom pneumococcal infection is likely to be more common and/or dangerous. This includes those with chronic renal, heart, lung or liver disease, splenic dysfunction, immunosuppression or diabetes. The present vaccine covers all common antibiotic-resistant strains.
• There is some evidence that pneumococcal vaccination of all over-65s would be beneficial; this is not currently recommended in the UK.
• Avoid overcrowding in institutions such as hospitals, day-care centres, military camps, prisons and homeless shelters.
• Safe disposal of discharges from nose and throat.

Surveillance

Possible outbreaks of pneumococcal infection should be reported to local public health authorities, e.g. CCDC in England and Wales. Isolates from blood, CSF or other normally sterile sites should be reported to national surveillance systems (e.g. CDR report via CoSurv in England and Wales). Isolates from sputum are not reported in England and Wales because of their uncertain clinical significance. Antibiotic sensitivity (especially penicillin) should be given for all recorded cases.

Response to a case

• Safe disposal of discharges from nose and throat.
• Antibiotic therapy as appropriate to clinical condition and sensitivity. Penicillin eliminates infectivity in susceptible strains within 48 h.
• There may be some value in separating patients from others with an increased risk of serious disease until 48 h of appropriate antibiotics received.

Investigation of a cluster

• Organize serotyping of strains.
• Check for links via institutions. Otherwise no action necessary.

Control of an outbreak

• Immunize all contacts that are at higher risk of serious infection.
• Check antibiotic sensitivity and serotype of isolates.
• If outbreak in institution/ward, vaccinate all residents (unless known to be strain not in vaccine). Institute case-finding and early treatment of symptomatics for at least 7–10 days.
• Ensure adequate environmental decontamination.

Suggested case-definition for an outbreak

Confirmed: clinically compatible illness with isolate from normally sterile site (e.g. blood or CSF).
Probable: clinically compatible illness with either:
  (i) isolate of outbreak serotype from non-sterile site (e.g. sputum), *or*
  (ii) antigen positive from normally sterile site (e.g. urine).

3.58 Poliomyelitis

Poliomyelitis is an acute viral infection of the nervous system caused by poliovirus types 1, 2 and 3. Its public health importance lies in the ability of polioviruses to cause permanent paralysis and sometimes death. It is readily transmitted, causing both endemic and epidemic disease.

Suggested on-call action

• Arrange for urgent laboratory confirmation.
• Obtain vaccination and travel history.
• Notify national surveillance unit.

Epidemiology

Poliomyelitis has been eliminated from most developed countries by vaccination. The last indigenous case of polio in the UK (an unvaccinated gypsy boy) was in 1983, and the WHO declared the UK polio-free in 1997. Imported cases occur occasionally, mainly from the Indian subcontinent. Vaccine-associated polio, a complication of live oral polio vaccine (OPV), occurs at a rate of two cases per million doses. There are on average two cases of vaccine-associated polio a year in the UK, half of which are in vaccine recipients (usually an infant following the first dose of OPV) and half are in unvaccinated contacts of recently vaccinated individuals (usually a parent of a recently vaccinated infant).

The epidemiology in other countries of western Europe is similar, although there was an outbreak in the Netherlands during the 1990s among unvaccinated members of a religious community. Many countries have switched to using inactivated polio vaccine (IPV), which carries no risk of vaccine-associated polio.

The WHO aims to eradicate polio globally by the end of 2000. At time of going to press, polio has been eradicated in two of the six WHO regions (the Americas and the Western Pacific) and no cases have been reported in Europe since 1998. More than half the world's cases occur in the Indian subcontinent.

Clinical features

Most cases of polio are asymptomatic or present with a sore throat or diarrhoea. A few cases develop meningitis that is indistinguishable from other causes of viral meningitis. Paralysis is relatively rare: the proportion of paralytic cases increases with age from about 1 in 1000 in infants to 1 in 10 in adults.

Poliomyelitis should be considered in any patient with acute flaccid paralysis with a history of recent travel to an endemic area. Vaccine-associated polio should be considered in a recently vaccinated individual with acute flaccid paralysis (particularly after the first dose) or in a close contact of a recently vaccinated individual. The main differential diagnosis is Guillain–Barré syndrome. The paralysis in polio is usually asymmetric, whereas in Guillain–Barré syndrome it is usually symmetrical. There is always residual paralysis in polio, whereas patients with Guillain–Barré syndrome usually recover completely.

Laboratory confirmation

The most important diagnostic specimen is a stool sample, which should be sent for viral culture. Poliovirus can be recovered from faeces for up to six weeks and in nasopharyngeal secretions for up to one week from onset of paralysis. At least two stool samples, 24 h apart, should be obtained within seven days of the onset of paralysis. All cases of acute flaccid paralysis should be investigated to exclude polio. The diagnosis can also be made serologically or by CSF examination.

Transmission

Polio is spread by the faecal–oral route. Man is the only reservoir. Long-term carriage does not occur. Poor hygiene favours spread.

Pathogenesis

The usual incubation period is 7–14 days for wild cases and vaccine-associated (recipient) cases, although it may be as long as 35 days. For vaccine-associated (contact) cases the incubation period may be up to 60 days.

Immunodeficiency is a risk factor for vaccine-associated paralysis, and immunodeficient patients with either vaccine-associated or wild polio may excrete virus for many months.

Prevention

OPV has been used in the UK since 1962 (IPV was used from 1956 to 1961). Three doses are given at 2, 3 and 4 months of age with boosters at 3–5 years and 15–19 years (see Box 4.7.1). IPV should be used for immunodeficient individuals and their household contacts. Further boosters are required at 10-yearly intervals for travel to endemic areas. No individual should remain unvaccinated against polio.

Surveillance

Notifiable in most countries, including the UK. Report on clinical suspicion.

Response to a case or cluster

A single case of indigenous wild polio would be a national public health emergency. The case should be notified **immediately**, by telephone, to the CCDC and to the regional and national epidemiologist. Urgent stool virology should be requested. If confirmed, mass vaccination with OPV would be required, possibly at the national or subnational level. In the event of an outbreak, international agencies such as WHO would be involved.

For vaccine-associated and imported cases, no specific action is required, although such incidents may provide an opportunity to review local immunization coverage.

3.59 Q fever

Q fever is a zoonotic disease caused by the rickettsia *Coxiella burnetii*. It causes an acute febrile illness or, more rarely, a serious chronic infection.

Suggested on-call action

None required unless outbreak suspected.

Epidemiology

Around 70 cases of Q fever are reported to CDSC per annum, but because much infection with *C. burnetii* is mild or asymptomatic, the true incidence of infection is not known. Reported cases in children are rare, probably because of an increased likelihood of infection being asymptomatic, and males are 2.6 times more likely to be reported with Q fever than females, mainly due to occupational exposure. In Europe, human infection increases in the spring (particularly April and May). Reported incidence has not increased over the last decade in the UK (although reports have trebled in Germany, mainly due to outbreak-associated cases). Most UK cases are sporadic or associated with occupational exposure to animals, but occasionally large outbreaks occur, including in urban areas. *C. burnetii*

infection occurs in most countries, although New Zealand is an exception.

Clinical features

Infection may be asymptomatic, an acute febrile or pneumonic illness, or chronic infection, particularly endocarditis or hepatitis. Almost all acute clinical cases have fever and fatigue, and most have chills, headaches, myalgia and sweats. Other features may be cough, weight loss and, particularly in the UK, neurological symptoms. Tiredness and malaise may persist for months after infection.

Laboratory confirmation

The diagnosis of Q fever is usually confirmed by the demonstration of a fourfold rise in complement-fixing antibodies: this usually takes 14–20 days to become apparent, although it may occur within 7 days or, take up to 6 weeks. IgM may be detected earlier than IgG (7–10 days) and usually persists for 6 months, although occasional persistence up to 2 years makes a single high titre non-diagnostic of an acute event. Phase II antibody generally occurs in acute infection and 'phase I' in chronic. Culture of this organism is potentially hazardous. Strain typing is not routinely available.

Transmission

The natural reservoir for *C. burnetii* is a number of animal species, particularly sheep, cattle, goats, cats, dogs, wild rodents, birds and ticks. Most infected animals are asymptomatic, although abortions may occur. In mammals such as sheep and cats, the infection localizes to the endometrium and mammary glands and is reactivated during pregnancy to be aerosolized during parturition. These aerosols may be inhaled directly or may contaminate the environment for many months, leading to the creation of secondary aerosols. Animal excreta or carcasses may also contaminate the environment with *C. burnetii*. Human infection is usually via inhalation from close exposure to animals, wind-borne aerosols (possibly over many miles) or contaminated fomites such as wool, straw and fertilizer. Person-to-person spread is rare. Infection via raw milk is described but its importance is unclear. Blood and marrow transfusion, necropsy and laboratory animals (especially pregnant sheep) have all been a source of infection.

Pathogenesis

The incubation period varies from 14 to 39 days (average 20 days) and is generally shorter the larger the infecting dose.

Although person-to-person spread has been reported, in practice human cases can be viewed as non-infectious to others under normal circumstances.

The infective dose is low, perhaps only 1–5 organisms. One gram of placenta from an infected sheep may contain 10^9 infective doses.

Immunity to previous illness is probably lifelong. Children may be less susceptible to clinical disease than adults, females less susceptible than males, and the immunocompromised and cigarette smokers more susceptible than the general population.

Prevention

- Vaccination of high-risk occupations.
- Adequate disposal of animal products of conception.
- Pasteurization of milk.
- Good infection control in microbiology and animal research laboratories.

Surveillance

Q fever is statutorily notifiable in some countries (e.g. Germany, Netherlands and Switzerland), but not in others, including the UK. However, all laboratory-confirmed cases should be reported to the relevant surveillance centre (e.g. CDSC for England and Wales). Potential clusters or linked cases should be reported to local public health authorities (e.g. the CCDC in England and Wales).

Response to a case

- Check for exposure to animals.

- No exclusion/isolation necessary, although avoid blood/tissue donation.

Investigations of a cluster

Undertake a hypothesis-generating study to cover six weeks before onset, including:
- full occupational history;
- full travel history;
- exposure to sheep, cattle, goats and other farm animals (ask about recent parturition), or farm equipment, clothing, etc.;
- exposure to pets, especially cats, or pet owners/household after parturition;
- possible visit to pet shop;
- exposure to potentially contaminated fomites, including straw, hay, peat, manure and wool; or
- general outdoor exposure.

Check local veterinary and meteorological data for clues (e.g. sheep abortions, wind conditions).

Control of an outbreak

- Plot dates of onset as an epidemic curve: is there ongoing exposure?
- Remove any continuing source.
- Treat human cases. No need to isolate.

Suggested case-definition for an outbreak

1 Fourfold rise in serum antibodies to *C. burnetii*. No need to demonstrate symptoms.
or
2 Acute febrile or pneumatic illness with single high convalescent IgM and no other cause identified.

3.60 Rabies

Rabies is an infection of the central nervous system caused by a rhabdovirus. The public health significance of rabies is that there are many animal hosts, the disease is always fatal and both human and animal vaccines are available.

Suggested on-call action

Possible exposure:
- Advise cleaning of wound if recent.
- Assess need for postexposure prophylaxis. If in doubt, seek expert advice.

Possible case:
- Seek history of animal bite, travel and vaccination status.
- Contact virus reference laboratory to arrange lab confirmation.
- Arrange admission to specialist unit.
- Prepare list of close contacts.
- Inform CDSC (or equivalent).
- Inform state veterinary service (or equivalent).

Epidemiology

There is no animal rabies in the UK, and the last indigenous human case was in 1902. Since 1946 there have been 20 imported cases. Rabies exists in animal and bat populations in many countries of western Europe, although human cases are extremely rare.

Clinical features

The early features of human rabies are often mistaken for hysteria, with altered personality and agitation. Pain or numbness at the site of an animal bite is a useful early clue. Painful spasms of the face and induced by attempts to drink ('hydrophobia') are the classical feature. The case fatality is 100%.

Laboratory diagnosis

This is only possible after the onset of symptoms. The national virus reference laboratory must be involved. Serum antibodies appear after six days. Rabies virus can be isolated from saliva, brain, CSF and urine, or demonstrated by immunofluorescent antibody staining of impression smears of skin, cornea or other material.

Transmission

Animal reservoirs include dogs, cats, foxes, wolves, bats, squirrels, skunks and occasionally horses. Transmission is from the bite or scratch of an infected animal, or a lick on a mucosal surface such a conjunctiva. Airborne spread has been demonstrated in bat caves, but this is unusual. Rare cases have occurred in recipients of corneal grafts from patients who died of undiagnosed rabies.

Pathogenesis

The incubation period is usually 3–8 weeks, but may be as short as 9 days or as long as 7 years, depending on the amount of virus introduced, the severity of the wound, and its proximity to the brain.

Prevention

Historically, this has been by quarantine of animals. A new scheme has recently been introduced to allow domestic pets from EU countries to enter the UK without quarantine, provided there is evidence of successful vaccination against rabies and a microchip detection device has been implanted in the animal. In western Europe, the use of live oral vaccines in animal bait has greatly reduced the incidence of rabies in foxes, the principal reservoir in Europe.

An inactivated vaccine is available for travellers and those at occupational risk such as some laboratory workers and animal handlers. The primary course is three doses at days 0, 7 and 28, given in the deltoid (NB the response may be reduced if vaccine is given in the buttock) with a booster at 6–12 months.

Postexposure prophylaxis should be given following a bite in an endemic area. The wound should be thoroughly cleansed as soon after injury as possible. As a minimum, this should be with soap or detergent under running water; antiseptics such as iodine or 40–70% alcohol (gin, vodka or whisky will do if stuck) should also be used. Factors used in deciding need for vaccine and immunoglobulin are given in Box 3.60.1: each case should be assessed on its own merits using these factors. Countries are classified as *no-risk* (usually no postexposure prophylaxis needed), *low-risk* (usually vaccine sufficient) or *high-risk* (immunoglobulin and vaccine usually given). Human rabies specific immunoglobulin is given at 20 iu/kg body weight, half the dose infiltrated around the wound, and the rest by i.m. injection. Five doses of vaccine should be given, on days 0, 3, 7, 14 and 30.

Surveillance

Rabies is notifiable. The public health department should be notified immediately.

Response to a case

• Isolation in a specialist unit for the duration of the illness.
• Healthcare workers attending the case should wear masks, gloves and gowns.
• Vaccination and immunoglobulin for contacts who have open wound or mucous membrane exposure to the patient's saliva (according to the schedule above).
• Investigate source of infection.
• Disinfect articles soiled with patients' saliva.

Investigation of a cluster and control of an outbreak

A cluster of human cases from an indigenous source is unlikely in the UK. Local authorities should have plans to eradicate rabies in the animal population should it occur.

Suggested case-definitions

Clinical: acute encephalomyelitis in an exposed individual.
Confirmed: clinically compatible case confirmed by vial antigen, isolate or rabies neutralizing antibody (prevaccination).

Box 3.60.1 How to evaluate an animal bite

• Risk of rabies in country visited: no risk, low risk or high risk?
• Exposure to saliva of animal?
• Contact with broken skin, e.g. bite? (NB: cat-scratch will contain saliva).
• Site and severity of bite? (NB: bat bites may not be obvious).
• Is the animal a known rabies host?
• Behaviour of animal? Provoked or unprovoked bite?
• Animal wild, domestic or pet?
• Can the animal be followed up?
• Vaccination status of the animal?
• Did the animal become ill?
   Sources of advice (UK): JCVI Green Book, PHLS Virus Reference Laboratory, local public health laboratories, CDSC, SCIEH (Scotland).

3.61 Relapsing fever

Louse-borne relapsing fever is a systemic disease due to *Borrelia recurrentis*. Tick-borne disease may be caused by a number of different *Borrelia* species. The illness is characterized by periods of high fever lasting up to 9 days, which are interspersed with afebrile periods of 2–4 days. Laboratory diagnosis is by visualization of the spirochaete in dark field examination of blood.

Relapsing fever is vector-borne; there is no person-to-person spread. The disease is classically epidemic where spread by lice, and endemic when spread by ticks. Louse-borne fever is found in Africa, especially highland areas of E. Africa and S. America. Endemic disease is widespread, including foci in Spain. The incubation period is 5–11 days.

Prevention is by maintenance of personal hygiene and by impregnation of clothes with repellents and permethrin in endemic areas.

Relapsing fever is a notifiable disease in the UK, and should also be reported to WHO. The case does not need isolation once deloused. The immediate environment should also be deloused.

3.62 Respiratory syncytial virus (RSV)

Respiratory syncytial virus (RSV) causes bronchiolitis in infants and upper and lower respiratory tract infection at all ages. It may cause serious nosocomial outbreaks in children, the elderly and the immunocompromised.

***

Suggested on-call action

- Suggest case limits contact with infants, frail elderly and immunocompromised.
- If linked cases in an institution suspected, activate outbreak control plan.

***

Epidemiology

RSV epidemics occur every winter in December and January. Almost all children who have lived through two epidemics in urban areas will have become infected. However, reinfections occur throughout life. Most cases are not specifically diagnosed as RSV. 80% of cases of bronchiolitis and 20% of pneumonia in young children are caused by RSV. About 5% of elderly people suffer RSV infection each year, and it is a significant cause of infection and outbreaks in nursing homes, day units and hospitals, particularly neonatal units. Large families and passive smoking are recognized risk factors for infection.

Clinical diagnosis

The most common presentation is upper respiratory tract infection with rhinitis, cough and often fever. Children may also get otitis media or pharyngitis. Bronchiolitis (wheeze, dyspnoea, poor feeding), pneumonia or croup may develop after a few days. Infants with congenital heart disease or chronic lung disease risk severe disease. In adults, RSV infection is usually confined to the upper respiratory tract, but it may cause exacerbations of asthma or chronic bronchitis, or, particularly in the elderly, acute bronchitis or pneumonia. Few infections are asymptomatic.

Laboratory confirmation

Nasopharyngeal aspirates (NPAs) taken early in the illness may be positive for RSV by antigen detection, which can provide immediate results, or viral culture, which takes 3–7 days but is slightly more sensitive. NPAs may not be obtainable from elderly patients: nose or throat swabs are less sensitive, and as the elderly do not shed the organism for as long as infants and often present later in the illness, the diagnosis rate is low in this group. PCR is available from some specialist laboratories and is more sensitive for these patients. Serology is also available for retrospective diagnosis.

Transmission

Humans are the only known reservoir of RSV. Spread occurs from respiratory secretions either directly, through large-droplet spread, or indirectly via contaminated hands, handkerchiefs, eating utensils or other objects or surfaces. RSV may survive for 24 h on contaminated surfaces and 1 h on hospital gowns, paper towels and skin. Infection results from contact of the virus with mucous membranes of the eye, mouth or nose. Hospital staff and visitors are thought to be important vectors in hospital outbreaks.

Pathogenesis

The incubation period is 2–8 days, with an average of 5 days.

The infectious period starts shortly before to (usually) one week after commencement of symptoms. Some infants may shed RSV for many weeks.

Immunity is incomplete and short-lived.

Prevention

• Personal hygiene, particularly handwashing and sanitary disposal of nasal and oral discharges.
• Good infection control in hospitals, nursing homes and day units. Avoid overcrowding.
• Avoid young infants, frail elderly and immunocompromised coming into contact with individuals with respiratory infection.
• RSV vaccines are under development.

Surveillance

RSV infection is not notifiable in the UK, but cases associated with institutions should be reported to local public health authorities. Laboratory-confirmed cases should be reported to the relevant national surveillance system. Hospitals should include RSV in nosocomial surveillance programmes.

Response to a case

• Contact isolation for hospital patients.
• Avoid contact with infants, frail elderly and immunocompromised until well.
• Exclude from nursery, work, school or non-residential institution until well.
• Sanitary disposal of nasal and oral discharges.

Investigation of a cluster

• Rarely investigated unless link to institution thought likely. Undertake case-finding at any institution containing infants, elderly or immunosuppressed if linked to a case.
• Antigenic and genomic fingerprinting may be useful in investigating hospital clusters, but beware that more than one strain may be involved, i.e. there may be more than one source.

Control of an outbreak

• Contact isolation and cohorting of suspected cases in hospitals. Nearest feasible equivalent in nursing and residential homes.

• Reinforce hygiene and infection control measures, particularly handwashing and sanitary disposal of nasal and oral discharges.
• Exclude staff and day attenders at institutions with respiratory infection until well. Restrict visiting.
• Active surveillance of new and existing patients in hospital for respiratory infection with rapid testing for RSV.
• Cancel non-urgent admissions.
• Consider other measures to limit transfer of RSV by hospital staff (e.g. use of eye–nose goggles, gloves and perhaps gowns and masks).
• Maintaining adequate compliance with the above recommendations will require constant monitoring and reinforcement.

Suggested case-definition for use in an outbreak
Upper or lower respiratory tract infection and antigen or culture positive for RSV.

3.63 Ringworm

The dermatophytoses, tinea and ringworm are synonymous terms that refer to fungal infections of the skin and other keratinized tissues such as hair and nails. These infections affect millions of people throughout the world. They are caused by various species of the genera *Trichophyton*, *Epidermophyton* and *Microsporum*, and are classified according to the area of the body that is affected, namely corporis (body), faciei (face), cruris (groin), pedis (foot), manuum (hand), capitis (scalp), barbae (beard area) and unguium (nail) variants.

On-call action
Advise on laboratory diagnosis and treatment. Recommend immediate control measures. Enquire about linked cases and record details. Arrange environmental investigation.

Epidemiology

There has been a recent increase in the frequency of dermatophyte infections along with changes in the epidemiology and distribution of the fungal species responsible. The reasons for this are not known.

Scalp ringworm, mainly affecting children, is becoming more common in the UK, particularly in urban areas. Until recently, *Microsporum canis*, spread from infected animals, accounted for most cases, but now *Trichophyton tonsurans* spread from humans is more common. Infections that could previously be considered sporadic and associated with exposure to infected animals now risk being spread within families and in schools.

M. canis is still a prevalent agent of ringworm in many regions of the world, and this could be related to the close association of humans with their pets. *Trichophyton violaceum* is endemic in certain parts of eastern Europe, Africa, Asia, and South America, but not in North America. *Trichophyton rubrum* is the most common cause worldwide of tinea pedis, onychomycosis, tinea cruris and tinea corporis. The wearing of athletic shoes by men and women and communal bathing could be responsible for the increase in tinea pedis and onychomycosis.

Persons who are immunosuppressed, including those with HIV infection, are at increased risk of dermatophyte infection. Certain occupations, such as veterinary surgeons, face a risk of infections of animal origin.

Clinical features

Tinea capitis, ringworm of the scalp	Infection starts as a small red spot which spreads leaving a scaly bald patch. The hair becomes brittle and breaks easily. Variable degrees of inflammation are present
Zoophilic: *M. canis* (cat, dog), *T. verrucosum* (cattle)	Infection with *T. verrucosum* acquired from cattle may be very inflammatory and produce large pustular lesions called kerions. Infection with *T. schoenleinii* produces an inflammatory crust, a condition called favus
Anthrophilic: *T. tonsurans, T. violaceum, T. soudanense, M. audouinii, T. schoenleinii*	The clinical picture with *T. tonsurans* varies from light flaky areas, often indistinguishable from dandruff, to small patches of hair loss on the scalp. There may be affected areas on the face, neck and trunk in some children
Tinea corporis, ringworm of the body Tinea cruris, ringworm of the groin *M. canis* *T. tonsurans* *T. rubrum* *T. mentagrophytes* *E. floccosum*	Lesions are found on the trunk or legs and have a prominent red margin with a central scaly area
Tinea barbae, barber's itch	Infection of the beard area of the face and neck with both superficial lesions and deeper lesions involving the hair follicles
Tinea pedis, athlete's foot *T. rubrum* *E. floccosum*	Affects the feet particularly the toes, toe webs, and soles
Onychomycosis (tinea unguium) *T. rubrum*	Infection of the nails, usually associated with infection of the adjacent skin. There is thickening and discoloration of the nail

Laboratory confirmation

Hairs infected with *Microsporum* species fluoresce green under filtered ultraviolet (Wood's) light. Hairs infected with most *Trichophyton* species do not fluoresce. Fungus can sometimes be detected by microscopic examination of the hair after preparation in potassium hydroxide. Definitive diagnosis requires culture of the infecting fungus. Specimens for culture are collected by scraping the affected area with a scalpel or glass slide. Specimens can also be obtained using a scalp massage brush. The scalp is brushed 10 times, and the contaminated brush pressed into the surface of an agar-coated Petri dish, which is then incubated for up to three weeks. A culture taken from an infected child will usually produce a fungal colony from each of the 130 inoculation points, whereas one taken from a carrier often produces only 1–10 colonies. Identification of the fungus helps determine the source of infection (either an animal or another child) and allows appropriate treatment and control measures.

Transmission

The reservoir of some of the dermatophyte species such as *T. rubrum* and *T. tonsurans* are exclusively human. Others such as *M. canis* have animal reservoirs, including cats, dogs, cattle, horses and rodents. Soil species rarely cause infection in humans.

Transmission is by direct skin-to-skin contact with an infected person or animal or by indirect contact with objects (seat backs, combs and brushes) or environmental surfaces (showers, changing-rooms) contaminated with hair or skin scales. Viable fungus may persist on these items for long periods.

T. tonsurans in humans and some animal species can produce an asymptomatic carrier state. This atypical presentation of some infections may lead to misdiagnosis and allow further spread.

Pathogenesis

The incubation period varies with the site of infection, but it usually takes 3–5 days for infection to become established and a further two to three weeks for symptoms to appear. The infectious period lasts for as long as infection is present—it may be from months to years if untreated.

Prevention

• Early recognition of animal and human cases and carriers and prompt effective treatment.
• Maintain high levels of personal and environmental hygiene with attention to hand-washing, care of pets, regular cleaning and maintenance of floors and surfaces at home, in schools and in swimming pools and communal changing rooms.

Surveillance

Cases of scalp and body ringworm in school-age children should be reported to the school nurse. Clusters of cases should be discussed with the CCDC.

Response to a case

• Human-source fungi can be transmitted between children at school, but exclusion of an infected pupil from school is probably unnecessary once treatment has started. However, activities involving physical contact or undressing, which may lead to exposure of others, should be restricted. There is no evidence that shaving the head aids therapy or reduces the risk of transmission.
• Confirm diagnosis and identity of infecting fungus with skin, nail or hair samples for microscopy and culture.
• Start effective treatment. Most cases of dermatophyte infections respond readily to topical agents used for 2–4 weeks. Oral treatment is required for nail and scalp infection.
• Topical antifungals alone are ineffective in treating scalp ringworm, since infection of the hair shaft begins beneath the skin. Scalp ringworm and intractable cases of body ringworm are treated with oral griseofulvin. The optimal duration of treatment is 8–10 weeks, but with

T. tonsurans treatment may need to be given for 12 weeks. Referral to a specialist is needed only if the response to treatment is poor, if the diagnosis is uncertain or if infection recurs.

• Selenium sulphide lotion (used as a shampoo) has been shown to kill fungal spores on scalp hair when applied twice weekly for 2 weeks. It may therefore be used to limit the spread of infection in combination with oral griseofulvin. It is not recommended for use in children under the age of five, for whom an alternative antifungal lotion may be used.

• If cultures show that the infecting fungus is of human rather than animal or soil origin, a search should be made for other cases. Signs of infection in others may be minimal and so samples should be requested for culture. Those with mycological evidence of carriage should be offered topical treatment. Griseofulvin therapy should be used if positive cultures persist.

• If the source is an animal, family pets should be screened by a veterinary surgeon.

Investigation of a cluster

• Clusters of cases of scalp or body ringworm may be reported from schools or nurseries. Spread is well recognized amongst members of wrestling teams (tinea corporis gladiatorum). Nosocomial spread has also been documented from patients to nursing staff.

Control of an outbreak

• Confirmation of the diagnosis is important and all contacts should be examined to identify cases and carriers. Samples should be requested for culture.

• The Consultant for Communicable Disease Control and the Community Infection Control Nurse should be available to give advice and practical assistance.

• Prompt effective treatment should be offered to cases and carriers (see above).

• Exclusion from school is not normally necessary once treatment has started, but may be considered if control proves difficult.

• An environmental investigation should be carried out to ensure a high standard of hygiene, particularly in communal changing rooms. Additional cleaning may be recommended. Possible animal sources should be investigated.

• In hospitals and nursing homes, cases should be nursed with source isolation precautions, and gloves and aprons should be used.

Suggested case-definition for cluster investigation

Characteristic lesions reported amongst household or other close contacts, with or without laboratory confirmation by microscopy or culture.

3.64 Rotavirus

Rotaviruses are the commonest cause of childhood diarrhoea. The public health significance of rotavirus diarrhoea is the high level of morbidity and the imminent availability of vaccines.

Suggested on-call action

• Exclude cases in risk groups (Box 2.2.1) until 48 h after the diarrhoea and vomiting have settled.
• If linked to other cases in an institution, consult outbreak control plan.

Epidemiology

Over 10 000 laboratory-confirmed cases are reported in the UK every year, although this only represents a small fraction of the total. It has been estimated that a third of hospital admissions for childhood diarrhoea are due to rotavirus.

The peak incidence is between 6 months and two years of age; clinical infection is unusual above 5 years, although subclinical infection is probably common. Most cases occur in winter. Mortality is low in developed countries, although there are an estimated one million deaths each year in developing countries. Around 15 outbreaks are reported a year in England and Wales, mostly associated with residential institutions, nurseries or hospitals.

Clinical features

There is sudden onset of diarrhoea and vomiting, often with a mild fever. Occasionally there is blood in the stools. The illness usually lasts for a few days only.

Laboratory confirmation

This is needed to differentiate rotavirus infection from other viral infections of the gastrointestinal tract. Rotavirus particles can usually be demonstrated in diarrhoea stools by electron microscopy. Serology is also available. There are three serogroups, of which group A is by far the commonest.

Transmission

There are both animal and human rotaviruses, although animal-to-human transmission does not occur. Person-to-person transmission is mainly by the faecal–oral route, although there may also be spread from respiratory secretions and sometimes via contaminated water. Long-term carriage does not occur. Outbreaks may occur in nurseries, and nosocomial spread may occur in paediatric, and occasionally geriatric units, where the virus may contaminate the environment. It is resistant to many disinfectants, but is inactivated by chlorine.

Pathogenesis

The incubation period is one to three days. Cases are infectious during the acute stage of the illness and for a short time afterwards; this is usually for less than a week in a healthy child, but may be as long as a month in an immunocompromised patient. Re-infection may occur after some months.

Prevention

Until vaccines become available, there are no specific preventive measures. General enteric precautions may help limit spread in households, nurseries and hospitals. In nurseries, children should have clothing to cover their nappies.

A live human-rhesus reassortant rotavirus vaccine was recently licensed in the US, but has been withdrawn following reports of vaccine-associated intussusception. Other vaccines are in development.

Surveillance

The disease is indistinguishable from many other types of viral gastroenteritis, so surveillance must be based on laboratory reports to local public health departments and national surveillance. This significantly underestimates the true incidence, as only hospitalized cases are likely to be investigated. Gastroenteritis in children under 2 years of age is formally notifiable in Northern Ireland.

Response to a case

Cases should be isolated with enteric precautions in hospital. Give hygiene advice to the family in the community. Exclude from nursery or school (or risk occupation—see Table 2.2.1) until 48 h after the diarrhoea and vomiting have settled.

Investigation of a cluster and control of an outbreak

An outbreak of rotavirus diarrhoea provides the opportunity to remind the local population of the importance of good hygiene (although this will probably not play an important role in controlling the outbreak). Consider also the possibility of a common source, e.g. contaminated water supply. In institutions with cases, public health authorities must satisfy themselves of the adequacy of hygiene and toilet facilities.

3.65 Rubella

Rubella is a systemic virus infection characterized by a rash and fever. Rubella virus is a member of the Togaviridae. The public health importance of rubella is the consequences of infection in pregnancy and the availability of a vaccine.

Suggested on-call action

• Exclude from school until five days from onset of rash.
• Advise limiting contact with those known to be pregnant.

Epidemiology

Rubella is now rare in most countries in western Europe, including the UK, where vaccination programmes have been in place for many years. Before vaccination, epidemics occurred at six-yearly intervals, affecting mainly children in primary school but also adolescents and some adults. During epidemics, up to 5% of susceptible pregnant women caught the disease, leading to subsequent outbreaks of congenital rubella syndrome and rubella-associated terminations of pregnancy.

In the postvaccination era, rubella outbreaks still occur among susceptible young adult males who are too old to have been vaccinated. There are now fewer than 10 cases a year of congenital rubella syndrome in the UK.

Clinical features

The main differential diagnosis is parvovirus, which is now commoner than rubella. In rubella, there is sore throat, conjunctivitis and mild fever for two or three days before the macular rash appears. The lymph nodes of the neck are often swollen. Recovery is usually rapid and complete, although, as in parvovirus infection, persistent joint infection sometimes occurs, especially in adults.

The features of congenital rubella syndrome range from mild sensorineural deafness to multiple defects of several organ systems.

Laboratory confirmation

This is particularly important in pregnancy. The simplest method is by IgM detection in serum or saliva. Other methods are viral culture from serum or urine, or a rising IgG antibody titre.

Transmission

Man is the only reservoir. Transmission is by direct person-to-person contact by respiratory droplets. There are no carriers.

Pathogenesis

Rubella is moderately infectious, although not as infectious as parvovirus or measles. The incubation period is 2–3 weeks. Infectivity is from one week before the onset of rash to about four days after.

The risk of congenital rubella syndrome in a susceptible pregnant woman infected in the first trimester is greater than 90%. This risk declines to about 50% in the second trimester and is zero near term.

Prevention

Rubella vaccine is a live attenuated vaccine that provides long-term immunity in approximately 95% of recipients. It was introduced in the UK in 1970, initially for adolescent school-girls and older susceptible women. In 1988, universal immunization of children aged

12–15 months was introduced, as part of a combined measles/mumps/rubella (MMR) vaccine. A mass measles/rubella campaign was carried out in 1994 for children aged 5–16 years, and in 1998 a second dose of MMR, given at 3–5 years, was introduced into the UK schedule.

The only contraindications to rubella vaccine are immunosuppression and pregnancy, although women accidentally vaccinated in pregnancy can be reassured that the risk of fetal damage is minimal. All women should be screened in early pregnancy and vaccinated postpartum if found to be susceptible. It is particularly important that all healthcare workers who are likely to be in contact with pregnant women are vaccinated.

Surveillance

Rubella is notifiable in the UK, although the diagnosis is unreliable and surveillance should be based on laboratory-confirmed cases.

Response to a case

Laboratory confirmation should be sought (saliva test in the UK), especially in pregnancy or if the case has been in contact with a pregnant woman. Check vaccination status of the case and arrange for vaccination if unvaccinated. Exclude children from school for five days from the onset of rash.

Pregnant women who have been in contact with a case, particularly during the first trimester, should be tested serologically for susceptibility or evidence of early infection (IgM antibody) (Fig. 2.4.2). Susceptible women should be vaccinated postpartum; infected women should be offered termination. In later pregnancy there is balance between the risk of fetal damage and the desirability of termination.

Investigation of a cluster and control of an outbreak

Laboratory confirmation is essential. In addition to the measures described above for all cases, there may be need to conduct a community-wide vaccination programme if coverage is low.

Suggested case-definitions

Confirmed:
- presence of IgM in blood, urine or saliva; or
- fourfold or greater rise in haemagglutination inhibition antibody in serum; or
- positive viral culture in blood, urine or nasopharyngeal secretions.

Suspected (for investigation):
- generalized maculopapular rash, fever and one of cervical lymphadenopathy or arthralgia or conjunctivitis.

3.66 Salmonellosis

Salmonella infection is a common cause of gastro-enteritis resulting in substantial social/economic costs; large outbreaks, particularly due to food-borne transmission; and severe infection in the elderly, immunosuppressed and pregnant women. One outbreak of salmonellosis in a hospital in England in 1984 led to 19 deaths.

For *S. paratyphi* and *S. typhi*, see Chapters 3.54 and 3.80, respectively.

Suggested on-call action

- Exclude cases in risk groups for onward transmission (Box 2.2.1) until formed stools for 48 h.
- If you or reporting laboratory/clinician aware of other potentially linked cases, consult local outbreak plan.

Epidemiology

Salmonellae are the second most commonly reported cause of infectious intestinal disease in the UK: approximately 30 000 laboratory confirmed cases per year were reported in England and Wales in 1989–97. However, salmonellae were only responsible for about 3% of community cases of gastro-enteritis with an identified pathogen; this discrepancy is due to the relative severity of salmonellosis.

Laboratory reports of *Salmonella* doubled during the late 1980s, in common with many countries in western Europe, almost entirely due to *S. enteridis* PT4, the strain associated with poultry and eggs. More recently there has been an increase in *S. typhimurium* DT104 resistant to a number of antibiotics. The reported incidence of salmonellosis remained stable throughout the 1990s, although a substantial decrease occurred in 1998–2000 particularly affecting *S. enteridis* PT4. *Salmonella* is recorded as the cause of death in an average of 40 people per year in England and Wales.

Salmonellosis occurs at all ages, although incidence rates of confirmed infection are highest in young children, partially due to testing bias. Laboratory isolates of *Salmonella* show a consistent seasonal pattern, peaking in late summer (Fig. 2.2.1); this is thought to be related to more rapid multiplication at higher ambient temperatures and perhaps seasonal variation in raw food consumption.

Although most cases are sporadic or part of family outbreaks, outbreaks associated with institutions or social functions are not uncommon. In recent years, there have been more than 100 *Salmonella* outbreaks in England and Wales reported to CDSC each year—approximately one per district.

Salmonella infection occurs worldwide. In Europe, variations include a decrease in cases in the Netherlands in the late 1980s, when other countries were experiencing increases, and the predominance of *S. enteritidis* PT1 in eastern Europe.

Clinical features

It is difficult to differentiate salmonellosis from other causes of gastro-enteritis on clinical grounds for individual cases. The severity of the illness is variable, but in most cases stools are loose, of moderate volume, and do not contain blood or mucus. Diarrhoea usually lasts 3–7 days and may be accompanied by fever, abdominal pain, myalgia and headache. Other symptoms, particularly nausea, may precede diarrhoea, and malaise and weakness may continue after resolution of the gastro-enteritis. Rare complications include septicaemia and abscess formation. Factors that may suggest salmonellosis as the cause of a cluster of cases of gastro-enteritis include fever in most cases, headache and myalgia in a significant minority, and severe disease in a few. With some serotypes, e.g. *S. dublin*, *S. cholerae-suis* and, to a lesser extent *S. virchow*, septicaemia and extraintestinal infection are more common.

Laboratory confirmation

Diagnosis is usually confirmed by culture of a stool specimen, rectal swab or blood culture. Using a stool sample rather than a rectal swab, collecting at least 5 g of faecal material and, especially when looking for asymptomatic excretors, collecting two or more specimens over several days all increase sensitivity. Excretion usually persists for several days or weeks beyond the acute phase of the illness. Refrigeration and/or a suitable transport medium may be necessary if there will be a delay in processing specimens, especially in warm weather.

The laboratory may be able to issue a provisional report within 48 h of receiving the specimen (further confirmatory tests will be necessary), although a further day is often required. Both serotyping (e.g. 'typhimurium') and phage typing ('PT' or 'DT') are routinely available, usually via national reference laboratories. These tests are often useful in detecting and controlling outbreaks of rarer salmonellae (e.g. *S. goldcoast* from cheddar cheese in the UK in 1997). However, as approximately 70% of UK isolates are *S. enteritidis* PT4 or *S. typhimurium* DT104, further more discriminatory tests are urgently required: pulsed field gel electrophoresis (PFGE) 'fingerprinting' has already been shown to be useful in subdividing *S. enteritidis* PT4. Antibiograms were found to be a useful marker for case finding in an outbreak of *S. typhimurium* DT104 in Birmingham.

Transmission

Salmonella infection is acquired by ingestion of the organisms. In most cases this is through the consumption of a contaminated food.

Salmonella infection or carriage affects many animals (Box 3.66.1), leading to contamination of foodstuffs before their arrival in the kitchen. If such foods are eaten raw or undercooked then illness can result. Such food sources include undercooked poultry or meat, raw or undercooked eggs (often used in mayonnaise, sweets such as mousse or tiramisu, and 'egg nog' drinks) and raw or inadequately pasteurized milk. Such foodstuffs, particularly raw poultry or meat, may be the source of cross-contamination to other foods that may not be cooked before eating (e.g. salad). This cross-contamination may also occur via food surfaces or utensils. Contamination of food by an infected food handler may occur but is thought to be uncommon in the absence of diarrhoea. Salmonellae can multiply at temperatures ranging from 7 to 46 °C: thus inadequate temperature control will allow a small number of contaminating organisms to develop into an infective dose. Heating to at least 70 °C for at least two minutes is required to kill the organism.

Person-to-person spread via the faeco–oral route may occur without food as an intermediary. The risk is highest during the acute diarrhoeal phase of the illness. Person-to-person spread due to inadequate infection control practices may prolong food-borne outbreaks in institutions. Children and faecally incontinent adults pose a particular risk of person-to-person spread.

Other, rarer, causes of salmonellosis include direct contact with animals, including exotic pets; contamination of non-chlorinated water; nosocomially via endoscopes, breast milk and blood transfusion; and contamination of bedding, toys and clothing by excreta.

Pathogenesis

The incubation period may range from six hours to three days or occasionally longer and is affected by the number of organisms ingested. Most cases occur within 12–36 h of ingestion.

The infectious period varies enormously: most cases excrete the organism for a few days to a few months, with a median duration of five weeks. Approximately 1% of adults and 5% of children under five years of age will excrete the organism for at least a year.

Box 3.66.1 Frequency and some possible animal sources of common *Salmonella* serotypes

	Number of human cases 1998*	Animal reservoirs
S. enteritidis	16196	Chickens, other poultry
S. typhimurium	2994	Cattle, pigs, poultry, sheep
S. virchow	604	Chickens
S. hadar	476	Chickens, other poultry
S. heidelberg	254	Chickens
S. newport	205	Turkeys, chickens
S. infantis	156	Calves
S. agona	135	Turkeys, chickens
S. braenderup	127	–
S. java	100	Tropical fish, terrapins
S. montevideo	94	Sheep, chickens

Rarer serotypes associated with particular animals include *S. arizonae* (sheep), *S. binza* (gamebirds), *S. derby* (pigs, sheep), *S. dublin* (cattle) and *S. mbandaka* (chicken).

*England and Wales. Source: PHLS.

In most cases the infective dose for salmonellae is 10^3–10^5 organisms, but certain food vehicles are thought to protect the organism against gastric acid, reducing the infective dose to only a few organisms. High fat foods such as chocolate and cheese may be examples.

Immunity to *Salmonella* infections is partial, with reinfection possible if milder. Those at increased risk include patients with low gastric acidity (including antacid therapy), immunosuppression, debilitation or on broad-spectrum antibiotics.

Prevention

Prevention of food-borne salmonellosis is a classic case of the need for a 'farm to fork' strategy:
• At the farm, action is required to reduce infection and carriage in food animals, particularly poultry to reduce contaminated meat and eggs. Vaccination of poultry flocks is now possible. Slaughter and processing practices for poultry also require attention to reduce cross-contamination. The Scandinavian experience suggests that *Salmonella*-free poultry can be achieved.
• Commercial food processing should be subject to the HACCP (Hazard Analysis Critical Control Point) system to identify, control and monitor potential hazards to food safety. Specific measures for *Salmonella* include use of only pasteurized eggs and milk; adequate cooking of meat and poultry; practices to avoid cross-contamination; exclusion of food handlers with diarrhoea; and adequate temperature control.
• In the home, routine food and personal hygiene measures need to be supplemented by particular care with raw poultry and eggs. The public need to be made aware that all poultry should be viewed as contaminated and how to prevent cross-contamination from it. Consumption of raw or undercooked eggs should be avoided.

Surveillance

Salmonellosis is notifiable in the UK as suspected 'food poisoning'. Laboratory isolates of *Salmonella* should be reported to local and the national surveillance systems. Isolates should be sent for further typing to aid epidemiological investigation. On a European level, salmonellosis is monitored via the EnterNet System (Chapter 5.1).

Response to a case

• Hygiene advice, particularly on handwashing, should be given to all cases: ideally, the case should not attend work or school until he/she has normal stools.
• Occupational details should be sought: cases in risk groups 1–4 (Box 2.2.1) should be excluded until 48 h after the first normal stool.
• Enquiry for symptoms in household contacts (or others exposed to the same putative source) should be made: those with symptoms, particularly diarrhoea, should be treated as cases.
• Enteric precautions for those admitted to hospital (especially for handling faeces or soiled bedding or clothing) should be followed.
• Asymptomatic excretors rarely require exclusion, provided adequate personal hygiene precautions are followed. This requires adequate knowledge and co-operation of the individual (or a responsible adult) and adequate facilities.
• Antibiotics should not routinely be given in uncomplicated gastroenteritis or to eliminate carriage. Those at risk of severe disease (e.g. immunosuppressed, newborn infants, elderly/debilitated, sickle cell, inflammatory bowel disease, cardiovascular abnormalities, chronic arthritis, prostheses) may be exceptions, as are patients with signs of systemic disease.

Investigation of a cluster

• If an increase in reports of *Salmonella* isolates is noted, arrange with local and reference laboratories for serotyping and phage typing of strains to check if similar organisms.
• Although some clues may be obtained by analysis of person/place/time variables, administration of a hypothesis-generating questionnaire is usually necessary (see Chap-

ter 4.3). A general semistructured question-naire for investigating clusters of food-borne illness should be available in each district; this can be modified in light of the epidemiology of the specific pathogen (e.g. known animal reservoirs or vehicles associated with previous outbreaks) and outbreak-specific factors (e.g. most cases in children).

Control of an outbreak

In food-borne outbreaks, microbiological ex-amination of faeces from infected patients and food can reveal the organism responsible and a cohort or case–control study may reveal the vehicle of infection. However, in order to pre-vent recurrence the question 'how did the food consumed come to contain an infec-tive dose of the organism?' needs to be an-swered. Particular factors to bear in mind in a food-borne outbreak of salmonellosis are as follows.

• Were any potentially contaminated foods consumed raw or inadequately cooked? In the case of *S. enteritidis* PT4, was poultry inade-quately cooked or were raw eggs used in any recipes? Can the raw food be checked for the organisms?

• Are food preparation procedures and hy-giene practices adequate to prevent cross-contamination, particularly from raw meat or poultry?

• Did any food handlers have symptoms of gastrointestinal infection? All relevant food handlers should provide faecal samples for analysis, but remember that they may also have eaten the vehicle of infection and so be victims of the outbreak rather than the cause.

• What happened to the food after cooking? Was there scope for contamination? Was it refrigerated until just before eating? Was it adequately reheated?

Many outbreaks require more than one thing to be done incorrectly. An example is a sandwich tea made for a cricket match that used raw egg mayonnaise and then was stored in the boot of a car on a hot summer day until consumed.

Secondary spread is common in outbreaks

of *Salmonella* infection: outbreak cases should receive intervention as outlined earlier for sporadic cases. Plotting of an epidemic curve may help identify the contribution of per-son to person spread (see Box 2.2.3 for other clues).

Case-definition for analytical study of a *Salmonella* outbreak

Clinical: diarrhoea or any two from abdom-inal pain/fever/nausea with onset 6–72 h after exposure.
Confirmed: clinical case with isolate of out-break strain.

3.67 Scabies

Scabies is an inflammatory disease of the skin caused by the mite *Sarcoptes scabiei* var. *hominis*.

On-call action

Advise on treatment and recommend im-mediate control measures. Enquire about linked cases and record details. Arrange environmental investigation.

Epidemiology

The prevalence is unknown, but in England and Wales consultation rates in general prac-tice are about 23 per 1000 population per year. This probably underestimates the true incidence.

In the past, scabies was associated with over-crowding and poor personal hygiene. The prevalence of scabies infection shows a cycli-cal pattern with a periodicity of 10–30 years. Various sources indicate that a major increase has been underway since 1991and there have been reports of outbreaks in hospitals, particularly on geriatric, psychiatric and long-stay wards, in AIDS units, and in residential homes for the elderly, where patients and staff may be affected.

Clinical features

Scabies is diagnosed by its typical appearance, the presence of itching, particularly at night, and the clustering of cases. A high level of diagnostic suspicion should be observed.

There may be no sign of infection for 2–4 weeks after exposure, when an allergy develops to the mites and an itchy symmetrical rash may appear anywhere on the body. If the person has had scabies before, the rash may appear within a few days of re-exposure. The itching is intense, particularly at night.

The appearance of the rash is variable but pimples, vesicles and nodules are characteristic. With scratching, reddening and secondary infection can occur. Burrows are the only lesions caused directly by the mite and may be seen in the webs of the fingers.

If there is impaired immunity or altered skin sensation, large numbers of mites may be present and the skin thickens and becomes scaly. This condition is known as atypical scabies, which is also called crusted or Norwegian scabies.

Laboratory confirmation

Skin scrapings can be examined under the microscope for mites, eggs or faeces.

Transmission and pathogenesis

Biology and life cycle

The pregnant female mites burrow in the epidermis and lay about 2–3 eggs per day before dying after four or five weeks. They burrow at a rate of 0.5–5 mm per day and feed on cells and tissue fluid. The eggs hatch after 3–4 days into larvae that move to hair follicles before developing into adults after a further 7–10 days. Mating takes place and the female embeds in a new burrow within one hour. The pregnant female is about a third of a millimetre long, slightly larger than the male.

The scabies mites are attracted to folded skin such as the webs of the fingers, but other areas can be affected, including wrists, elbows, feet, genitalia, buttocks, axillae, and nipples. In infants and those with impaired immunity, the face and scalp can be affected.

Spread

Adult scabies mites are passed from person to person by prolonged skin-to-skin contact. This is often non-sexual contact such as hand holding.

Scabies remains infectious until treated. Infectiousness depends on the number of mites on the affected person. Usually there are only 10–20 mites, but in atypical scabies there are many more and this form of scabies is particularly infectious.

Scabies is not usually spread by clothing or bedding. However, in atypical scabies skin scales with mites attached may spread into the environment.

Animal scabies is called mange or scab. It can be passed to humans but only causes a temporary problem since the mites cannot multiply and soon die out.

Prevention

Prevention of scabies depends on early recognition of cases and prompt effective treatment. This in turn depends on public and professional education and a high level of awareness and diagnostic suspicion.

Surveillance

Scabies is not notifiable. In England and Wales, newly diagnosed cases of scabies in general practice are reported to the Birmingham Research Unit of the Royal College of General Practitioners by participating practices.

Clusters of cases of scabies in residential and day care settings should be reported to the CCDC or community infection control nurse.

Response to a case

Specific scabicides in the form of aqueous malathion lotion or permethrin dermal cream are recommended. A single topical application to all areas of the body below the neck should be sufficient. A second application after 5–7 days will kill any larvae that hatch from eggs that survived the first application.

A single oral dose of ivermectin has been shown to be effective in difficult cases and in those with HIV infection.

In children, in those with impaired immunity or if an atypical form is suspected, the scabicide should also be applied to the face, neck and scalp but avoiding mouth, nose or eyes. In children permethrin should be used. Extra care is needed when treating pregnant and breast-feeding women.

Generally scabicides should be left on for 24 h and washing should be avoided during this time. This is easier if the scabicide is applied at bedtime. After 24 h the patient should have a bath or shower, dress in clean clothes and change bed sheets.

Itching may continue for 2–3 weeks after successful treatment, which may sometimes actually make the rash worse due to an allergic reaction to the killed mites. It is important not to interpret this as a treatment failure or mistaken diagnosis.

Cases can return to school or work after the scabicide has been applied.

All contacts in the same house are treated even if they do not have any symptoms. Everyone should be treated at the same time to ensure that they do not re-infect each other. Boyfriends and girlfriends should also be treated.

Clothing and bedding should be laundered on a hot washing machine cycle. Any items that cannot be washed in this way should be set aside and not used for seven days. Under these conditions mites will quickly become dehydrated and die.

In crusted or Norwegian scabies more intensive treatment is necessary, which may be continued for some time. Normal hygiene and vacuuming of chairs, beds and soft furnishings will minimize environmental contamination with skin scales. Atypical scabies can spread from patients to nurses and others who provide close care. Use of gloves, aprons and handwashing afterwards will minimize this.

Investigation of a cluster

Clusters of cases of scabies are usually reported from hospitals, nursing homes or other residential health or social care settings.

Confirmation of the diagnosis is important in these settings. All patients and residents may need to be examined in an attempt to identify the index case, or someone with an unrecognized case of atypical or crusted scabies. The GP of the patient, client or service user should be asked to advise. He/she may ask for a second opinion from a consultant dermatologist. A high level of diagnostic suspicion should be maintained.

Control of an outbreak

The Consultant for Communicable Disease Control and the Community Infection Control Nurse should be available to give advice and practical assistance.

The cases, whether members of staff or residents, should be promptly treated (see above). Staff can return to work once treatment has been completed. If practicable, while affected residents are undergoing treatment they should be separated from other residents. If the case is a member of staff, treatment is recommended for his/her close household contacts. If the case is a client it may not be practicable to treat everyone else in the residential setting but if there are several cases and the situation appears to be out of control then treatment of all residents and staff may be necessary. It is recommended that a scabies monitoring record sheet is used for each person with scabies following treatment so that apparent treatment failures and recurrences can be assessed.

Table 3.67.1 Responsibilities in control of scabies

Consultant for Communicable Disease Control and Community Infection Control Nurses	To receive reports of scabies within institutions and day care settings and to advise on management
	To involve other carers, such as District Nurses, Health Visitors or School Health Nurses and GPs and managers and owners of residential and nursing homes as appropriate
	To make available information on scabies for the public and professionals
General practitioners	To maintain a high level of diagnostic suspicion, to diagnose, treat and follow up cases of scabies amongst their patients and contacts. To make referrals and request second opinions as appropriate
	To discuss with the Consultant for Communicable Disease Control (CCDC) or Community Infection Control Nurse (CICN) whenever an outbreak of scabies is suspected in a residential or nursing home
	To co-operate with the CCDC/CICN in dealing with such an outbreak
Residential and nursing home managers and owners	To remain vigilant to the possible diagnosis of scabies in their residents
	To involve the GP in diagnosing, treating, referral if necessary and follow-up of the resident
	To recognize outbreaks and to alert the CCDC/CICN if an outbreak is suspected
	To co-operate with the CCDC/CICN in dealing with such an outbreak
Families of those with scabies	To ensure that treatment is carried out properly
	Inform all close contacts, particularly those in a day care or nursing setting if scabies is suspected
	Follow advice from their General Practitioner or the CCDC/CICN, particularly relating to treatment and exclusion from work or school

---

Suggested case-definition for outbreak

A rash of typical appearance and itching particularly at night. Often with other similar cases reported amongst household and other close contacts.

3.68 *Shigella*

Shigellae are a genus of bacteria that cause intestinal infection, including 'bacillary dysentery'. *S. sonnei* is the most common species in the UK and causes relatively mild illness. Most *S. flexneri* and all *S. boydii* and *S. dysenteriae* are imported and are more severe. *S. dysenteriae* type 1 may cause very severe illness due to production of an exotoxin.

Suggested on-call action

• If case in risk group for further transmission, advise exclusion as suggested in Table 3.68.1.
• If you or reporting clinician/microbiologist aware of other linked cases, activate local Outbreak Plan.
• If infection with *S. dysenteriae*, obtain details of household and ensure symptomatic contacts excluded as suggested in Table 3.68.1.
• If *S. dysenteriae*, ensure symptomatic contacts receive medical assessment.

Epidemiology

Shigella infection has decreased dramatically since the peak incidence period of 1950–69, when 20–40 000 cases per annum were reported in the UK. Most years since 1980 have

Table 3.68.1 Suggested criteria for return to work, nursery, school and other institutions for groups at risk of transmission of shigellosis

Risk group (see Box 2.2.1)	S. sonnei	S. flexneri* S. boydii* S. dysenteriae (non-1)*	S. dysenteriae 1 (toxin producer)
Food handlers	48 hours symptom-free	Assess individually (minimum 48 hours symptom-free and hygiene advice is likely to be implemented)	Two consecutive negative faecal specimens
Healthcare and nursery staff	Symptom-free	48 hours symptom-free and hygiene advice given	Two consecutive negative faecal specimens
Children aged under 5 years	Symptom-free	48 hours symptom-free and adequate toilet facilities and supervision available	Two consecutive negative faecal specimens
Others with poor personal hygiene (including infant school pupils)	Assess individually (minimum until symptom-free)	Assess individually (minimum until 48 hours symptom-free)	Two consecutive negative faecal specimens

* Current PHLS guidelines (1995) for England and Wales suggest that groups with these organisms should be excluded as for the *S. sonnei* column. We have given slightly more rigorous criteria because of the risk of more severe illness in the few secondary cases that would occur from this group.

seen less than 5000 reports, with the exception of a small epidemic in the mid-1980s and a larger one in the early 1990s, both due primarily to *Shigella sonnei*. There were only 1264 laboratory-reported cases in England and Wales in 1999; in recent years, around 70% of reports were *S. sonnei*, 20% *S. flexneri*, 6% *S. boydii* and 3% *S. dysenteriae*.

Shigellosis is primarily a disease of children, with the highest rates reported in those under five years of age, followed by those aged 5–14. Boys have higher rates than girls, but the reverse is seen in those aged 15–44. There is no longer a winter excess of cases in the UK. The most common settings for *S. sonnei* outbreaks are schools and nurseries. Large outbreaks of non-*sonnei* infection are uncommon in the UK, but family outbreaks appear to be more frequent in those of south Asian ethnicity.

Clinical diagnosis

S. sonnei infection often causes only mild and transient diarrhoea and rarely causes dysentery. Other species are more likely to follow the classic picture of an initial illness of abdominal pain and diarrhoea (often watery) which may be accompanied by malaise, fever, nausea, vomiting, tenesmus and toxaemia. Approximately 40–50% then develop mucus and/or frank blood in the stool (dysentery). In developed countries illness is usually self-limiting, lasting an average of seven days. *S. dysenteriae* 1 may cause toxic megacolon and haemolytic uraemic disease, and has a case-fatality rate of 10–20%.

Asymptomatic infection and excretion may also occur.

Laboratory confirmation

Diagnosis is usually confirmed by isolation (and subsequent biochemical testing) of the organism from faeces; testing is routine in most laboratories. Provisional results are usually available within 48 h. Speciation should always be carried out as control measures vary between species. Serotyping based on 'O'antigens is also available if epidemiologically indicated, e.g. any case of *S. dysenteriae* or possible clusters of *S. boydii* (18 serotypes) or *S. flexneri* (six serotypes, and two variants, e.g. 'type 2a'). *S. sonnei* is antigenically homogeneous: colicin typing or phage typing may be available if necessary from some specialist laboratories.

Transmission

Man is the only significant reservoir of infection. Transmission to other humans is via the faeco–oral route either directly or by contamination of food, water or the environment.

Direct person-to-person spread is extremely common in households and institutions, particularly those containing young children. Studies in the UK have found that 30–50% of contacts of cases became infected. Cases with diarrhoea are a much greater risk than asymptomatic excretors, with inadequate handwashing after defaecation the main cause. Such individuals may also contaminate food. Young children may act as a transmission link between households.

Shigellae, particularly *S. sonnei*, may also survive for up to 20 days in favourable environmental conditions (i.e. cool, damp and dark). This may lead to transmission via lavatory seats, towels and any other vehicle that could become contaminated by faeces, either directly or via unclean hands. Flies may also transfer the organism from faeces to food.

Food-borne outbreaks are relatively uncommon but do occur: *Shigella* transmitted from imported iceberg lettuce affected several European countries in 1994.

Pathogenesis

The incubation period is between 12 and 96 h, but may be up to one week for *S. dysenteriae* 1.

The infectious period is primarily during the diarrhoeal illness. However, cases maintain a low level of infectivity for as long as the organism is excreted in the stool, which is 2–4 weeks on average.

The infective dose is very low: infection may follow ingestion of as few as 10 organisms of *S. dysenteriae* 1. The average infective dose for *S. sonnei* is about 500 organisms.

Immunity post infection does occur and lasts for several years, at least for the same type. Longer-term immunity does not appear to be important.

Prevention

- Adequate personal hygiene, particularly handwashing after defaecation.
- Adequate toilet facilities in schools. Supervised handwashing in nursery and infant schools.
- Regular and frequent cleaning of nurseries and schools, particularly for toilet areas.
- Safe disposal of faeces and treatment of drinking and swimming water.
- Care with food and water for travellers to developing countries.
- Routine cooking kills shigellae.

Surveillance

All clinical cases of diarrhoea or dysentery should be reported to local public health authorities: dysentery is formally notifiable in the UK. Laboratory isolates of *Shigella* species from symptomatic patients should be reported to the relevant national surveillance system.

Response to a case

- Report to local public health authority, e.g. CCDC in England and Wales.
- Hygiene advice to case and contacts.
- Enteric precautions for case and symptomatic contacts. In institutions, isolate if possible.
- If case or symptomatic contact, exclude

from work or school until well. For particular risk groups, consult Table 3.68.1.

• Obtain details of any nursery or infant school attended. Check to see if other cases and reinforce hygiene measures.

• For species other than *S. sonnei*, check that case has been abroad in the four days before onset (seven for *S. dysenteriae* 1) or has been in contact with another case who was ill abroad or on return. If no link abroad, obtain details of contacts and full food history for four days before onset.

• Mild cases will recover without antibiotics and multiple drug resistance is increasing. Antimotility drugs should be avoided.

Investigation of a cluster

• Liaise with microbiologist to organize typing of isolates.

• Does epidemic curve suggest point source (plus secondary cases) or continuing exposure? Does age/sex/ethnic/geographical analysis of cases suggest common factor?

• Look for links via institutions such as nurseries, schools, social clubs, care facilities and links between affected families via child networks. Administer hypothesis generating food questionnaire for 12–96 h before onset. Ask about water consumption, hobbies, swimming, social functions and occupation. For non-*sonnei* species, look for social networks that include travellers to developing countries.

Control of an outbreak

• Reinforce hygiene measures, particularly handwashing. Supervised handwashing for children aged under eight.

• Check toilet and handwashing facilities are adequate. Increase cleaning of risk areas in toilets (e.g. seats and 'touch points') to at least twice a day.

• Ensure regular and frequent cleaning of all other areas and objects which could become contaminated, including facilities for disinfection after faecal accidents.

• Exclusion of cases as per Table 3.68.1.

• Provide hygiene advice to families of those in affected institutions.

Suggested case-definition for outbreak

Confirmed: Diarrhoea and/or abdominal pain with *Shigella* species of outbreak strain identified in faeces.
Clinical: Diarrhoea in member of population of affected institution, without alternative explanation

---

3.69 Smallpox

The World Health Organization confirmed the global eradication of smallpox in 1980. There is therefore no need for any individual to be vaccinated, with the exception of a very small number of laboratory workers. Individuals such as archaeologists who have direct contact with corpses that may have died from smallpox are not at risk.

Any suspected case must be reported to and investigated by WHO. A number are investigated every year; these usually turn out to be another poxvirus infection such as monkey pox. However, smallpox is a potential bioterrorism weapon.

3.70 Small round structured viruses (SRSV)

This section covers gastro-enteritis caused by caliciviruses, particularly Norwalk-like agents. Although generally causing mild illness, spread, particularly in institutions, may be rapid. Other causes of viral gastroenteritis include rotavirus (Section 3.64), adenovirus and astrovirus.

Suggested on-call action

• If in group at risk for further transmission (Box 2.2.1), exclude from work or nursery.
• If you or reporting clinician/microbiologist are aware of related cases, consult local outbreak plan.

Epidemiology

Approximately 2000 laboratory-confirmed cases of SRSV infection are now reported annually in England and Wales. However, true incidence of disease is likely to be at least 1% of the population per year. All age groups are affected. Infection occurs throughout the year, but reported cases in the UK are more common during the cooler months. Recorded outbreaks in the UK occur mainly in hospitals or residential institutions (e.g. nursing homes) but are occasionally reported from hotels and schools. SRSV has a worldwide distribution.

Clinical features

SRSV infection is relatively mild, lasting 12–60 h. Abdominal cramps and nausea are usually the first symptoms, followed by vomiting and/or diarrhoea. Forceful vomiting is particularly characteristic. Diarrhoea is usually mild, with no blood, mucus or white blood cells in the stool. Other symptoms may include anorexia, lethargy, myalgia, headache and fever. Illness may be debilitating in elderly patients.

Laboratory confirmation

The mainstay of confirmation in the UK is electron microscopy (EM) of faecal specimens, which should be collected within the first day or two of illness and preferably be unformed. Many laboratories do not routinely test all stools, due to the limited availability of EM. Samples of vomit may also be examined by EM. PCR tests, which are more sensitive than EM, are also available from some national reference centres and may be available for suspected SRSV outbreaks where EM is negative. Serology (paired samples 3–4 weeks apart) may also be available.

If laboratory confirmation is lacking or awaited, epidemiological criteria can be used to assess the likelihood of an outbreak being due to SRSV (Box 3.70.1).

Transmission

Humans are the only known reservoir of SRSV. Spread between humans may occur via:
• Infected food handlers: may contaminate food during the preparation of foods to be

---

Box 3.70.1 Epidemiological criteria for suspecting that an outbreak is due to SRSV

• Stool cultures negative for bacterial pathogens*.
(NB, check that all relevant pathogens have actually been tested for).
• Incubation period, if known, of 15–50 h*.
• Vomiting in over 50% of cases*.
• Diarrhoea generally mild without blood or mucus.
• Over half have nausea and abdominal cramps, and over a third have malaise, low-grade fever, myalgia and headache.
• Mean duration of illness is 12–60 h*.
• High secondary attack rate. Even if originally food-borne, likely to be signs of ongoing person-to-person spread (see Box 2.2.3).
• Staff are also affected.

* 'Kaplan criteria.'

eaten raw (e.g. salads) or food postcooking, via hands contaminated by faeces. Vomiting nearby may also contaminate food.

• Contaminated foods: the most commonly contaminated food is shellfish that have concentrated the virus from sewage-contaminated waters. If eaten raw (e.g. oysters) or insufficiently cooked, such shellfish can cause disease. Outbreaks have also been linked to imported fruits such as raspberries and strawberries.

• Person to person: SRSV is easily spread via the faeco–oral route, either directly or indirectly due to contamination of environmental surfaces and other items. SRSV may remain viable for many days on carpets or curtains. Airborne transmission may occur due to suspended viral particles. This may explain spread in some outbreaks in hospitals and residential institutions.

• Water-borne: drinking water which is inadequately chlorinated or contaminated post treatment may transmit SRSV, as may swimming in contaminated water.

Pathogenesis

The incubation period is usually 15–50h but ranges of 4–77h have been reported from outbreaks.

The infectious period lasts until 48h after the resolution of symptoms.

The infective dose is extremely low.

Immunity occurs postinfection, but may only last a few months (sufficient to remove recovered cases from the pool of susceptibles in an outbreak). This, plus the existence of several antigenic types, means later reinfection is possible.

Prevention

• Good standards of personal and food hygiene.

• Good standards of infection control in hospitals and residential homes, including adequate cleaning arrangements.

• Cook raw shellfish before consumption and wash fruit if to be eaten raw.

Surveillance

Cases should be reported to local public health authorities. Not formally notifiable in the UK except as 'suspected food poisoning' (although gastro-enteritis in children under two years is notifiable in Northern Ireland). Only an estimated six in every 10000 community cases are reported to national surveillance in England.

Response to case

• Report to local public health authority, e.g. CCDC in England and Wales.

• Exclude cases in groups with risk of further transmission (Box 2.2.1) until 48h after resolution of diarrhoea and vomiting.

• Enteric precautions with particular attention to environmental contamination related to vomitus.

• Cases in institutions should be isolated where practicable.

• Treat symptomatic contacts in high-risk groups (Box 2.2.1) as cases.

• Hygiene advice to cases and contacts.

• Collect risk factor data including food history in 10–50h before onset. Ask specifically about seafood, fruit, salad and sandwiches.

Investigation of a cluster

Most recognized clusters are associated with an institution or a social function.

• If an institution, use Box 2.2.3 to help assess likelihood of person-to-person or food-borne source.

• If a social function, consider infected food handler, contaminated premises and contaminated food, especially shellfish.

• If a community outbreak, describe by person, place and time and obtain full food, occupational, family and social histories 10–50h before onset as a hypothesis generating exercise. Organize further case-finding, e.g. requesting faecal samples from cases of gastroenteritis presenting to GPs for EM.

Control of an outbreak

• For outbreaks in institutions, form an outbreak team, which includes a senior manager who has authority to commit the institution to agreed action.
• Reinforce good infection control (especially handwashing) and food hygiene practices. Ensure toilet facilities are adequate.
• Increase cleaning, particularly of toilet areas and 'contact points' (e.g. taps and door-handles). Wear disposable gloves and aprons for cleaning potentially contaminated areas.
• Disinfect contaminated areas with 1000 p.p.m. hypochlorite. Immediate cleaning of areas contaminated by vomiting.
• Isolate cases where practicable in residential institutions. Cohorting of cases otherwise.
• Exclude cases in non-residential institutions until symptom-free for 48 h.
• Staff to wear gloves and aprons and to observe enteric precautions when dealing with infected patients.
• Exclude staff with gastrointestinal symptoms until 48 h after resolution. Nausea and cramps may precede vomiting and diarrhoea; do not wait until they vomit on the premises!
• Do not admit more susceptible individuals into an outbreak area, preferably until 72 h since last episode of diarrhoea or vomiting.
• Do not discharge potentially incubating patients into another institution.
• Restrict unnecessary patient and staff movements between wards.
• Give advice on SRSV to adult visitors. Restrict visiting by children if possible.
• Thoroughly clean before re-opening to admissions. Change curtains in hospital.
• The Infection Control Nurse or Environmental Health Officer will need to maintain constant supervision to ensure that the agreed actions are fully implemented and maintained.

3.71 Staphylococcal food poisoning

Staphylococcal food poisoning is a relatively rare food intoxication (rather than an infection), caused by heat-stable enterotoxins produced when certain phage types of *Staphylococcus aureus* multiply in food. It is the main form of food-borne disease that arises from human rather than animal or environmental contamination of food.

Suggested on-call action

If you or reporting clinician/microbiologist know of associated cases, consult outbreak control plan.

Epidemiology

Staphylococcal food poisoning occurs worldwide but is now rare in the UK. A handful of outbreaks are reported each year, compared with around 150 each year in the 1950s.

Clinical features

There is abrupt, sometimes violent, onset with nausea, cramps, vomiting, diarrhoea, hypotension and prostration. The illness lasts 1–2 days; serious sequelae are uncommon, but admission to hospital may occur because of the intensity of symptoms.

Laboratory confirmation

Gram-positive cocci may be seen on Gram staining of food vehicles. *S. aureus* may be cultured from unheated food at levels of 10^5–10^6 organisms per gram or from the vomit or faeces of cases. Enterotoxin may be detected in food samples. *S. aureus* of the same phage type may be found in the implicated food vehicle and on the skin or lesions of food handlers.

Transmission

Food handlers colonized with *S. aureus* or with infected skin lesions contaminate foods such as cooked meats, sandwiches and pastries. These are stored with inadequate refrigeration, allowing the organism to multiply and produce toxin before being eaten—2 h at room temperature is often quoted as sufficient to create a large enough dose. Even with further cooking or heating the toxin may not be destroyed. Some outbreaks have followed contamination of dairy products as a result of staphylococcal mastitis in cattle.

Pathogenesis

The incubation period is 1–7 h (usually 2–4 h). Staphylococcal food poisoning is not communicable from person to person.

Prevention

- Ensure strict food hygiene including kitchen cleaning, temperature control, food storage and handwashing.
- Reduce food-handling time to a minimum.
- Store cooked foods at above 60 °C or below 10 °C before re-heating or consumption.
- Exclude food handlers with purulent lesions until successfully treated. Nasal carriers do not need to be excluded.

Surveillance

- Staphylococcal food poisoning should be reported to local public health departments; in the UK, notify as 'food poisoning'.
- Outbreaks should be reported to national surveillance centres.

Response to a case

- Report to local public health department.
- Enquire about food consumed in the 24 h before onset of symptoms.
- Exclude risk groups (Box 2.2.1) with diarrhoea or vomiting.

Investigation of a cluster

- Discuss further microbiological investigation (e.g. phage typing) with microbiologist.
- Undertake hypothesis generating study covering food histories particularly restaurants, social functions and other mass catering arrangements.
- Investigate the origin and preparation methods of any food items implicated in the outbreak. Submit any leftover food for laboratory analysis.
- Search for food handlers with purulent lesions.

Control of an outbreak

- Identify and rectify faults with temperature control in food preparation processes.

Suggested case-definition for an outbreak
Vomiting occurring 1–7 h after exposure to potential source with appropriate laboratory confirmation.

3.72 Streptococcal infections

Streptococci are part of the normal flora and colonize the respiratory, gastrointestinal, and genitourinary tracts. Several species cause disease, including:
- Group A streptococci (beta-haemolytic streptococci, BHS, *Streptococcus pyogenes*) cause sore throat and skin infection (impetigo, cellulitis, pyoderma), scarlet fever, necrotizing fasciitis, streptococcal toxic shock syndrome, wound infections, pneumonia and puerperal fever.
- Group A organisms may also cause postinfectious syndromes, such as rheumatic

fever, glomerulonephritis; and Sydenham's chorea.

• Group B streptococci cause neonatal meningitis and septicaemia.

• Group C and G streptococci can cause upper respiratory infections such as tonsillitis.

• Viridans streptococci are a common cause of bacterial endocarditis.

Suggested on-call action

Not usually necessary unless outbreak suspected.

Epidemiology

Streptococcal sore throat and scarlet fever are found worldwide, though less commonly in the tropics. Up to 20% of individuals may have asymptomatic pharyngeal colonization with group A streptococci. Particular 'M types' are associated with various sequelae (for example 1, 3, 4, 12 with glomerulonephritis). The incidence of sequelae depends upon the circulating M types. Acute rheumatic fever has become rare in most developed countries, though occasional cases and outbreaks are seen. It is associated with poor living conditions and is most common in the 3–15 age group.

Impetigo is most commonly seen in younger children. The M types associated with nephritis following skin infection are different from those associated with nephritis following upper respiratory infection.

Asymptomatic carriage of group B streptococci (GBS) is common in pregnant women.

Clinical features

Sore throat: it can be difficult to differentiate streptococcal from viral sore throat; various scoring systems have been proposed but they lack predictive power. The presence of an exudate suggests a bacterial sore throat.

Skin infection: streptococcal skin infection commonly presents as acute cellulitis or impetigo.

Scarlet fever: may accompany pharyngeal or

skin infection and is characterized by a skin rash, classically a fine punctate erythema, sparing the face, but with facial flushing and circumoral pallor. During convalescence, desquamation of the finger and toe tips may occur.

Puerperal infection: puerperal fever occurs in the postpartum or postabortion patient and is usually accompanied by signs of septicaemia.

Necrotizing fasciitis: involves the superficial and/or deep fascia; group A streptococci are implicated in about 60% of cases.

Laboratory confirmation

Streptococci are classified by a number of systems including haemolytic type, Lancefield group and species name.

Group A streptococcal antigen can be identified in pharyngeal secretions using rapid antigen detection; negative tests require confirmation. Detection of antibody to streptococcal extracellular toxins may be useful in the diagnosis of necrotizing fasciitis.

Confirmation is by culture on blood agar, the production of a zone of haemolysis and showing inhibition with bacitracin.

A rise in antistreptolysin O, anti-DNA-ase or antihyaluronidase antibodies between acute and convalescent sera may be helpful in retrospective diagnosis.

Transmission

Streptococcal infection is commonly acquired by contact with patients or carriers, particularly nasal carriers. Transmission via contaminated foodstuffs, particularly unpasteurized milk and milk products is recognized.

Group B disease is acquired by the newborn as (s)he passes through the genital tract of the mother.

Pathogenesis

Group A streptococcal pharyngitis

The incubation period is 1–4 days for acute infection.

> Mean time for appearance of immunological sequelae:
> Acute glomerulonephritis: 10 days
> Acute rheumatic fever: 19 days
>   (1–5 weeks)
> Sydenham's chorea: Several
>   months

The infectious period is commonly 2–3 weeks for untreated sore throat. Purulent discharges are infectious. Penicillin treatment usually terminates transmissibility within 48 h.

Group B infection in infants

Early-onset infection: mean age of 20 h.
Late-onset infection: occurs in infants with a mean age of 3–4 weeks, range 1 week to 3 months.

Immunity develops to specific M types and appears to be long-lasting. Repeated episodes due to other M types occur.

Prevention

Primary:
- Personal hygiene.
- Avoid unpasteurized milk.
- Reduce need for illegal abortions.
  Secondary: prevention   of   immune-mediated sequelae.
- Prompt recognition, confirmation and treatment of streptococcal infection.
- Those with a history of rheumatic fever should be offered antibiotic prophylaxis to prevent cumulative heart valve damage.

Prevention of group B streptococcal infection: GBS is a significant cause of neonatal morbidity and mortality. Intrapartum antibiotic treatment of women colonized with group B streptococcus appears to reduce neonatal infection. Screening strategies to detect maternal colonization are under development and should be considered.

Surveillance

Scarlet fever and/or puerperal fever are notifi-able in some countries including England, Wales and Northern Ireland (SF), and Scotland (PF).

Response to a case

- Report acute cases of scarlet fever, puerperal fever and post-streptococcal syndromes to local health authorities.
- Careful handling of secretions and drainage fluids until after 24 h penicillin treatment.
- Personal hygiene advice to case and contacts.

Investigation of a cluster

- Does epidemic curve suggest point source, ongoing transmission (or both) or continuing source?
- Determine mode of transmission, exclude food-borne source particularly milk urgently.
- Search for and treat carriers if considered a potential source of infection.

Control of an outbreak

- Activate outbreak plan.
- Identify and treat carriers.
- Identify and remove contaminated food sources.

3.73 Tetanus

Tetanus is an acute illness caused by the toxin of the tetanus bacillus, *Clostridium tetani*. Its public health significance is the severity of the disease and its preventability by vaccination.

Suggested on-call action
None required for public health team.

Epidemiology

There are 10–15 cases notified a year in the UK, although there is probably significant under-ascertainment of mild cases. Most cases are in unvaccinated people over 65 years of age. The case fatality is about 10%. The epidemiology is similar in other western European countries.

Clinical features

In classical tetanus there are painful muscular contractions, especially of the neck and jaw muscles (hence the name 'lockjaw'), muscular rigidity and painful spasms. The symptoms can be mild in a vaccinated person. There is often a history of a tetanus-prone wound, although not always.

Laboratory confirmation

This is infrequently obtained and unnecessary in typical cases. It is sometimes possible to culture the organism from the site of the original wound.

Transmission

The reservoir is the intestine of horses and other animals, including humans. Tetanus spores are found in soil contaminated with animal faeces. Transmission occurs when spores are introduced into the body through a dirty wound, through injecting drug use, and occasionally during abdominal surgery. The illness is caused by a toxin. Person-to-person spread does not occur.

Pathogenesis

- The incubation period is 3–21 days, depending on the site of the wound and the extent of contamination; occasionally it may be up to several months.
- Natural immunity may not follow an attack of tetanus.

Prevention

Tetanus vaccine is a toxoid preparation. The UK schedule is three doses in infancy (in combination with pertussis, diphtheria and Hib) at 2, 3 and 4 months, with boosters at 3–5 years and 13–18 years. Further boosters may be re-

quired at the time of injury. Tetanus vaccine and tetanus immunoglobulin should be given at the time of injury in tetanus-prone wounds where more than 10 years have elapsed since the last dose of vaccine. The dose of tetanus immunoglobulin is 250 iu by i.m. injection; 500 iu if more than 24 h have elapsed since the time of injury.

Surveillance

Tetanus is notifiable in most European countries, including the UK.

Response to case

Seek injury history, ascertain vaccination status and arrange for primary course or booster, depending on history.

Response to a cluster or outbreak

Outbreaks of tetanus are rare. Look for a common source, e.g. surgery, i.v. drug abuse.

Suggested case-definition
Physician diagnosis of tetanus.

3.74 Threadworms

On-call action
None.

Threadworm (pinworm) infection is an intestinal infection with *Enterobius vermicularis,* a nematode of the family Oxiuridae. It is ubiquitous in temperate regions, particularly amongst children.

In symptomatic infections there is perianal itching and sleep disturbance. Appendicitis and chronic salpingitis are rare complications of worm migration.

The diagnosis can be confirmed by the presence of eggs on a strip of transparent adhesive tape that has been pressed on to the anal region and then examined under a microscope. Adult worms may be seen in faeces or on perianal skin.

Adult worms live in the small intestine. Females are 8–12 mm long but males, which die soon after mating and are rarely seen, are between 2 and 2.5 mm long.

Mature female worms migrate through the anus and lay thousands of eggs on the perianal skin. Infective embryos develop within 5–6 h and these are transferred to the mouth on fingers as a result of scratching. Larvae emerge from the eggs in the small intestine and develop into sexually mature worms. Re-infection is common and infectious eggs are also spread to others directly on fingers or indirectly on bedding, clothing and in environmental dust. Adult worms do not live for longer than six weeks. Direct multiplication of worms does not take place and eggs must be swallowed for new worms to develop, although retro-infection may occur as a result of hatched larvae migrating back through the anus from the perianal region.

Prevention is by prompt recognition and treatment of cases and their household contacts, health education and attention to personal and environmental hygiene, particularly handwashing. The perianal area may be washed each morning to remove eggs and bedding and nightclothes should be changed regularly.

Response to a case

Anti-helminthics such as mebendazole or piperazine are effective against adult worms but must be combined with hygienic measures to break the cycle of auto-infection. All household members should be treated.

An initial course of treatment should be followed by a second course two weeks later to kill worms which have matured in that time.

3.75 Tick-borne encephalitis

Tick-borne encephalitis (TBE) is a flavivirus infection of the CNS, characterized by a biphasic meningo-encephalitis. It has a focal distribution throughout central and eastern Europe and parts of Scandinavia. Related infections occur in Russia and North America. The disease is commonest in early summer and autumn. Cases have not been reported in the UK, although louping ill, a related tick-borne flavivirus infection, occurs occasionally in Scotland and Ireland.

Ixodes ricinus, the woodland tick, is the principal reservoir in Europe; sheep and deer are also hosts for louping ill. The incubation period is 7–14 days. Person-to-person transmission does not occur.

The diagnosis should be considered in a patient with neurological symptoms with a history of a tick bite in an endemic area. Laboratory confirmation is by serology or virus isolation from blood (only in specialist laboratory).

Prevention is by wearing of protective clothing against tick bites in endemic areas. A killed vaccine is available; postexposure prophylaxis with a specific immunoglobulin is also available in some countries.

3.76 *Toxocara*

Toxocara canis is an ascarid parasite of dogs. It occasionally causes ocular infection in man.

On-call action
None required.

Epidemiology

Toxocara canis infection is found worldwide. Infection is more common in young children.

Clinical features

Infection may be asymptomatic, produce the visceral larva migrans syndrome or ocular disease. Visceral larva migrans mostly occurs in younger children in association with pica. The features include fever, eosinophilia and bronchospasm and an urticarial skin rash. Hepatosplenomegaly may be present. Ocular disease is found in older children; vision may be compromised.

Laboratory confirmation

Diagnosis is based on detecting antibodies to *T. canis* larvae using an ELISA test.

Transmission

The larvae can remain dormant in dogs for long periods, migrate transplacentally and through bitches milk to infect the pups. Most pups are infected at the time of whelping; the adult worms produce eggs until the majority are expelled when the pups are six months old. The eggs, which are the source of human infection, survive in the environment for many years.

Prevention and control

Toxocariasis may be controlled by regular worming of dogs and disposal of dog faeces hygienically. Contact between animal faeces and children should be minimized. No public health response is usually needed in response to cases.

3.77 Toxoplasmosis

Toxoplasma gondii is a protozoan parasite that causes a spectrum of disease from asymptomatic lymphadenopathy to congenital mental retardation, chorioretinitis, and encephalitis in the immunocompromised.

> **On-call action**
>
> None required unless outbreak suspected.

Epidemiology

Human exposure to toxoplasmosis is worldwide and common. 20–40% of healthy adults in developed countries are seropositive. It is more common in Mediterranean countries than in Northern Europe.

Clinical features

There are a number of clinical presentations. Acute infection is usually asymptomatic, but may produce a mononucleosis-like illness. Congenital infection may occur following acute infection during pregnancy. Congenital toxoplasmosis is characterized by fetal hepatosplenomegaly, chorioretinitis, and mental retardation. In the immunocompromised, cerebral reactivation of toxoplasmosis may occur, with presentation as an encephalitis.

Laboratory confirmation

Acute toxoplasmosis may be diagnosed serologically. Specific IgM antibodies appear during the first 2 weeks, peak within 4–8 weeks, and then typically become undetectable within several months. IgG antibodies rise more slowly, peak in 1–2 months, and may remain high for years.

Congenital infection requires the demonstration of IgM in neonatal blood; evidence of acute infection during pregnancy indicates the need for fetal blood sampling at 18 weeks and cord blood at delivery.

Serology is not useful for diagnosis of toxoplasmosis in patients with AIDS. Cerebral toxoplasmosis is usually diagnosed on the basis of clinical features, a positive agglutination test and CT/MRI scan appearance. Specific diagnosis in patients with AIDS and CNS symptoms requires a brain biopsy.

Transmission

The cat is the definitive host and transmits the

infection through faecal shedding of oocysts. Children may come into contact with oocysts from pets, soil or sandpits. Adults are usually infected by ingestion of undercooked meat. Congenital infection usually occurs following primary infection in a pregnant woman.

Pathogenesis

• Incubation period: 10–25 days.
• Transmissibility: No person-to-person spread.

Prevention

• Pregnant women in particular should avoid raw or undercooked meat. Contact with soil or food possibly contaminated with cat faeces should be avoided.
• Chemoprophylaxis has been recommended for AIDS patients with positive IgG serology once CD4 cells are low.
• Protect sandpits and play areas from cats.

Surveillance

Report to local public health authorities. Some countries have surveillance of congenital cases.

Response to a case

Investigate likely exposure to cat faeces and raw/undercooked meat.

Investigation/control of a cluster/outbreak

As for response to case.

Suggested case-definition for an outbreak

Confirmed: Isolate or IgM antibody confirmed.
Clinical: Acute fever and lymphadenopathy in person linked epidemiologically to confirmed case.

3.78 Tuberculosis

Tuberculosis (TB) is an infection of the lungs and/or other organs, usually by *Mycobacterium tuberculosis* but occasionally by *M. bovis* or *M. africanum*. TB has a long incubation period, produces chronic disease with risk of reactivation, and without treatment may be fatal.

Suggested on-call action

If the case is a healthcare worker, teacher or another individual in contact with particularly susceptible individuals, consult the outbreak control plan. However, action can usually wait until the next working day.

Epidemiology

The incidence of tuberculosis has fallen in western European countries throughout this century. In the UK the rate of decline slowed in the 1960s due to increased immigration from higher-prevalence countries, and has plateaued since 1987. Current annual notification rates in the UK are 1.1 per 10000 population, similar to much of western Europe except Scandinavia (lower rates) and Iberia (higher). High rates of drug-resistant TB are reported from countries of the former Soviet Union.

Within the UK, TB rates are highest in Black Africans (48 times higher than for the indigenous population in the 1998 national survey), South Asians (28 times higher) and Afro-Caribbeans (six times higher). Sixty-two percent of cases are now in non-white groups. Rates also increase with age and, at least in whites, are higher in deprived communities. Other risk factors for TB include HIV infection, other causes of immunosuppression, chronic alcohol misuse and homelessness. In the 1993 UK TB survey only 2% of TB patients tested were HIV-infected. The overall TB mortality rate is around 8 per million population per year.

Clinical features

TB is a biphasic disease. Only about 5% of whose who contract primary infection go on to develop clinically apparent primary disease, either as a result of local progression in the lungs, or haematogenous or lymphatic spread to other sites. Such spread may lead to serious forms of the disease such as meningitis or milary TB occurring within a few months of the initial infection.

In the remaining 95%, the primary TB lesion heals without intervention, although in at least half of patients, bacilli survive in a latent form which may then reactivate in later life. Five percent of those originally infected will develop postprimary disease. The risk of reactivation increases with age, chronic disease and immunosuppression (e.g. HIV/AIDS). Reactivated TB is often pulmonary and, without treatment, carries a high mortality.

Two thirds of TB in the UK is pulmonary disease, which is initially asymptomatic, although it may be detected on chest X-ray. Early symptoms may be constitutional, such as fatigue, fever, night sweats and weight loss, and often insidious in onset. Chest symptoms often occur in later disease, including cough (usually productive), haemoptysis and chest pain. Hoarseness and difficulty swallowing may occur in laryngeal TB. Symptomatic screening for cases is highly sensitive (most cases have symptoms on enquiry) but not very specific (many other diseases also cause similar symptoms). Chest X-ray has high sensitivity and medium specificity. Specificity is high for sputum smear and very high for sputum culture but both are of only moderate sensitivity.

Non-pulmonary TB is more common in children, ethnic minorities and those with impaired immunity. The most commonly affected sites are lymph nodes, pleura, genitourinary system and bones and joints. Constitutional or local symptoms may be reported. Diagnosis may be supported by tuberculin test and biopsy results. Almost all non-AIDS cases are tuberculin test–positive.

Laboratory confirmation

Rapid presumptive diagnosis of infectious cases can be achieved by microscopy of sputum (preferably early morning) samples: *M. tuberculosis*, *M. bovis* and *M. africanum* all stain poorly with Gram stain, but staining with Ziehl–Neelson (ZN) stain reveals acid-fast (and alcohol-fast) bacilli (AFB). As a general rule, sufficient bacilli in the sputum to be detectable by standard methods are sufficient to be infectious and three consecutive negative sputum smears are usually assumed to represent non-infectiousness. Although this test is usually sufficient to begin treatment and contact tracing, follow-up culture is essential as AFBs may occasionally be other species of *Mycobacteria* (see Box 3.78.1), culture increases the sensitivity of diagnosis for cases of lower infectivity, and antibiotic sensitivities need to be checked.

Table 3.78.1 Typical action in response to tuberculin testing

Test result		Interpretation and action	
Heaft grade	*Mantoux* (100 units/mL)*	*Scar from previous BCG*	*No BCG scar*
0/1	0–4 mm	Negative No action†	Negative Give BCG†
2	5–14 mm	Positive No action‡	Positive Investigate?‡
3/4	15 mm plus	Strongly positive Investigate	Strongly positive Investigate

* Source: JCVI, 1996.
† Unless contact of case (repeat test in 6 weeks).
‡ Will vary with age and reason for doing test.

Box 3.78.1 Mycobacteria other than tuberculosis (MOTT)

• Also known as atypical, environmental, anonymous, non-tuberculous, tuberculoid or opportunistic.
• Includes *M. avium, M. intracellulare,* and *M. scrofulaceum* (collectively known as *M. avium* complex). Also includes *M. kansasii, M. malmoense, M. marinum, M. xenopi, M. fortuitum, M. chelonei, M. abscessus, M. haemophilum* and others.
• Common environmental contaminants. Occasionally found in water supplies, swimming pools or milk. May cause nosocomial infection. Person-to-person spread rare.
• Rarely cause disease in immunocompetent individuals. *M. avium* complex and some others may cause disseminated disease in those with AIDS.

In 1998, 6.6% of isolates of *M. tuberculosis* in the UK were resistant to at least one first-line drug and 1.3% were multidrug-resistant ('MDR'). Culture and sensitivity testing has routinely taken around 6–12 weeks, but rapid culturing at a reference laboratory may reduce this to 30 days. New molecular techniques may reduce this wait to 3–4 days when results are urgent. Genotyping may also be useful in investigating clusters of cases.

Transmission

Almost all TB in Europe is contracted by inhalation of *M. tuberculosis* bacilli in droplet nuclei. These nuclei derive from humans with pulmonary or laryngeal TB, predominantly by coughing, although sneezing, singing, and prolonged talking may contribute. Such nuclei may remain suspended in air for long periods. The risk of transmission depends upon the amount of bacilli in the sputum, the nature of the cough, the closeness and duration of the interaction and the susceptibility of the contact (Box 3.78.2).

Bovine TB may be contracted by ingestion of raw milk from infected cows and occasionally via the airborne route. Although *M. bovis* has increased in cattle in the UK in recent years, most human cases probably represent reactivation of infection acquired before routine treatment of milk supplies and testing of cattle.

Direct transmission either through cuts in the skin or traumatic inoculation (e.g. prosector's wart) is now rare. Aerosols may be gener- ated from surgical dressing of skin lesions or autopsy.

Pathogenesis

The incubation period, as defined by reaction to a tuberculin test, is usually 3–8 weeks (occasionally up to 12 weeks). The latent period may be many decades.

The infectious period is for as long as there are viable organisms in the sputum (usually considered infectious if organisms demonstrable on sputum smear). Appropriate chemotherapy renders most patients non-infectious in two weeks.

Acquisition of an infective dose usually requires prolonged exposure and/or multiple aerosol inocula, although some strains appear to be more infectious.

Immunity usually occurs after primary infection and involves several responses, including delayed-type hypersensitivity, the basis of the tuberculin test. Conditions such as AIDS, which affect cellular immunity, increase the risk of disease. Other risks are given in Box 3.78.2.

Prevention

Control of TB in the UK has a number of components.
• Limitation of infectiousness by targeted case-finding and early treatment.
• Limitation of antimicrobial resistance by multidrug therapy (e.g. British Thoracic Society guidelines) and measures to maxi-

mize compliance, such as directly observed therapy (DOTS).

• Identification and treatment of further cases by contact tracing in response to notifications of TB (see Chapter 4.15). Up to 10% of clinical cases in the UK are found by this method. In addition, potentially latently infected individuals can be offered chemoprophylaxis and non-immune contacts offered BCG immunization.

• BCG vaccine has an efficacy against TB of about 75%, lasting at least 15 years in British schoolchildren. It should also offer similar protection against drug resistant strains. In the UK vaccination is recommended (provided the individual has no BCG scar and is tuberculin test—negative) for the following groups.

Schoolchildren between the ages of 10–14 years.

Higher-risk occupations, e.g. those working in healthcare premises, prisons or certain hostels.

Immigrants, students and refugees from high-prevalence countries.

Children born in the UK to ethnic minorities with links to high-prevalence countries (e.g. Indian subcontinent or Africa, but not the West Indies) should be vaccinated within a few days of birth.

Children born to families with a history of TB.

Travellers to higher-prevalence countries planning to stay over one month.

Contacts of cases of active pulmonary disease.

• Screening of immigrants and refugees from high-prevalence countries for active disease, latent infection and lack of immunity should be offered as part of a total health package in their new district of residence. Such individuals can be identified from a combination of port health forms, GP registers, school registers, refugee hostels and community groups.

• Infection control in hospitals, with particular care in units dealing with immunocompromised patients and units likely to admit patients with TB.

• Those contacts with evidence of infection (tuberculin test) but not disease can be protected by isoniazid prophylaxis to prevent later disease. Prophylaxis is also recommended for young children who are contacts of an infectious case of TB, even if tuberculin-negative.

Surveillance

• The two main sources of cases are notifications of clinical cases from clinicians (such as respiratory physicians) and positive reports from microbiology laboratories. Other potential sources are pathologists (histology and autopsy), surgeons and pharmacists. Reliance on only one source will lead to incomplete ascertainment.

• District TB registers are useful and may include data on:

age, sex, ethnicity, country of birth, place of residence;

type of disease, sputum status, antibiotic sensitivities;

treatment outcome.

• Enhanced surveillance of TB was introduced into the UK in 1999. District co-ordinators collect a standardized dataset on all new cases which is forwarded to CDSC for collation.

• The 'EuroTB' programme collects data on TB from national centres throughout Europe. However, reporting systems differ substantially between contributing countries, making comparisons difficult.

Response to a case

• All TB cases should be notified to local public health departments.

• Investigate whether infectious by three early morning sputum samples for microscopy and culture.

• Ensure isolate tested for drug resistance.

• Early treatment with standard multidrug therapy. Take appropriate measures to maximize compliance.

• Most cases can be treated at home: there is no need to segregate cases from other household members, unless they are neonates or immunocompromised.

• Those treated in hospital who are smear-positive (or pulmonary or laryngeal disease with results pending) should be segregated in a single room, preferably with measures

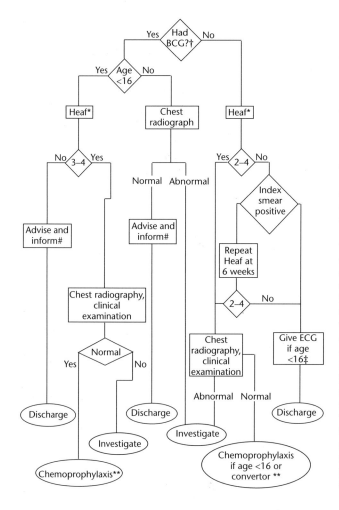

Figure 3.78.1 Recommendations for the investigation and management of TB contacts. Contact tracing: examination of close contacts of patients with pulmonary tuberculosis. Contacts of patients with non-pulmonary tuberculosis need not usually be examined. Note: children under two years who have not had a BCG vaccination and who are close contacts of a smear-positive index patient should receive chemoprophylaxis irrespective of tuberculin status. †Previous BCG vaccination cannot be accepted as evidence of immunity in HIV-infected subjects. *A negative test in immunocompromised subjects does not exclude tuberculosis infection. #Advise patient of tuberculosis symptoms and inform GP of contact. **Persons eligible for, but not given, chemoprophylaxis should have follow-up chest radiographs at 3 and 12 months. ‡See text. With permission from The Joint Tuberculosis Committee of the British Thoracic Society (1994). Control and prevention of tuberculosis in the UK: code of practice. *Thorax*, 2000; **55**: 887–901.

to reduce airflow to other patient areas. Particular care is needed in units containing immunocompromised patients or if the case is suspected to have drug-resistant TB.

• Adults with smear-negative disease, non-pulmonary disease or those who have been on appropriate treatment for 2 weeks do not require isolation. Persons visiting children with TB in hospital (one of whom may be the source case) should be segregated from other hospital patients until they have been screened.

• Screen household contacts of cases of pulmonary disease. Contacts of non-pulmonary cases need only be screened if the case is thought to have been recently infected (e.g. a young child).

• Casual contacts need only be screened if the case is smear positive and either: the contact is unusually susceptible to TB (e.g. young child or immunocompromised adult), or the case appears to be highly infectious (e.g. more than 10% of contacts infected).

• The recommendations of the British Thoracic Society for investigation and management of contacts are shown in Fig. 3.78.1.

• Check that the index case and any secondary cases are not healthcare workers,

---

Box 3.78.2 How to assess the likelihood of transmission of TB

1 How infectious is the source case?
- Sputum smear positive: infectious to any close contact.
- Smear negative, culture positive: possibly infectious to highly susceptible contacts.
- Sputum negative, bronchial washings positive: possibly infectious to highly susceptible contacts.
- Three consecutive sputum negatives: not infectious.
- Two weeks *appropriate* treatment: not infectious.
- Non-pulmonary/laryngeal disease: not infectious.
- Children, even if smear positive, less infectious than adults.

2 How great is the exposure?
- Exposure to coughing is the most important risk, but sneezing, singing and long (more than five minutes) conversation can also produce many infectious droplets.
- Prolonged multiple indoor exposure usually needed to infect most contacts.
- Risk highest in household and close associates of case (*c*.10% risk if smear positive).
- Brief contact: low risk.
- Outdoor contact: very low risk.
- Aerosols may persist after case leaves room.
- Dishes, laundry, etc. not infectious.

3 How susceptible is the contact to infection and disease?
- Susceptibility by age.
  Neonates: Very high
  Age under three years: High
- BCG reduces risk by 50–80% in developed countries.
- Immunosuppressed at very high risk: includes AIDS, lymphoma, leukaemia, cancer chemotherapy and oral corticosteroids (equivalent to 15 mg prednisolone per day).
- Severe malnutrition leads to increased risk. Post-gastrectomy or jejunal—ileal bypass patients   at risk if underweight.
- Silicosis or drug abuse increases risk.
- Diabetics and those with chronic renal failure have increased risk of reactivation of latent disease.

---

teachers or others who work with susceptible people.

Investigation of a cluster

- Aim is to discover whether there is an unrecognized infectious source.
- Check diagnosis of cases. Are they confirmed microbiologically? Beware the occasional 'pseudo-outbreak' caused by laboratory false positives.
- Any clinical or epidemiological clues as to whether cases have recent or old infection?
  Age and previous residence abroad.
  Clinical and radiological signs.
  Risk factors for new infection (e.g. contact with case or travel to high prevalence country)?
  Risk factors for reactivation (e.g. diabetes, renal failure)?
- Obtain microbiological samples on all non-confirmed cases. Liaise with reference laboratory for genotyping of all isolates (e.g. RFLP) to look for linked cases.
- Undertake hypothesis-generating study. Include family links, social networks, leisure and hobbies, links to institutions, especially those containing highly susceptible individuals and/or overcrowding (hospitals, nursing homes, schools, jail, homeless hostels) and

---

Box 3.78.3 How to manage specific TB scenarios

1 If the case is a healthcare worker with patient contact (or a patient found to have TB after admission):
- Decide how infectious the case is:
  Respiratory or laryngeal TB?
  Cough or cavities on chest X-ray?
  Sputum smear and/or culture positive?
  Results of screening of close contacts?
- Decide how long case has been infectious, in particular duration of cough.
- If case thought to be infectious, convene incident management team including hospital control of infection staff:
  senior hospital manager;
  public health physician (CCDC);
  physician with expertise in TB contact tracing services (and/or TB Health Visitor);
  medical records manager;
  manager of affected ward/unit;
  occupational health;
  press officer.
- Draw up list of contacts. Consider:
  inpatients, outpatients, referrals from other consultants;
  other members of staff;
  classifying contacts by level of exposure (e.g. patients for which case was 'named nurse' could be classified higher exposure and other patients on ward as lower exposure).
- Decide whether any of these contacts are particularly susceptible to TB (see Box 3.78.2): ask medical and nursing staff who treated them.
- Review case-notes.
- Organize screening of highly susceptible contacts (remember incubation period of up to two months since last contact with case).
- Write to GPs of other contacts so that exposure is noted.
- Consider need for helpline and press release for worried patients.
- Reconsider actions when results of screening and culture results are known.

2 If case is a teacher or pupil at a school:
- Consider teacher potentially infectious even if only sputum culture positive (smear negative). Screen children in relevant teaching groups (including games) if they have not had BCG or are under 11 years of age and close staff or other contacts.
- Although children rarely infectious, if child case is sputum smear positive, screen close contacts and other children in same class. Screen casual contacts (e.g. same year if not had BCG).
- If more than one child infected, screen staff. Also consider potential staff source if no further cases found in screening household of child.

3 If the case has recently travelled on an aircraft:
- Check if patient sputum smear and culture positive.
- Was flight within last three months and over eight hours in duration?
- Did the passenger have a cough at time of flight?
- If criteria above are satisfied, ask airline to identify passengers in the same compartment of the aircraft and contact them by letter.
- Letter to recommend passengers contact their own doctor and to give central telephone number for advice.
- Inform health authorities for areas with affected passengers.

travel to (or visitor from) a high prevalence country.
• Check drug sensitivities and compliance with treatment for known respiratory cases associated with cluster.

Control of an outbreak

Undertake contact tracing for known cases to identify and treat undiscovered infectious cases (and others with infection or disease who would benefit from treatment).
   In outbreaks linked to hospitals:
• Look for an unsuspected infectious source, e.g.:
   patient with MDR TB remaining infectious despite prolonged therapy (check sensitivity results);
   smear-negative cases infecting highly susceptible contacts (check culture results);
   delayed diagnosis in AIDS cases (don't rely on classic clinical picture);
   healthcare worker, patient or visitor with undiagnosed TB (chronic cough unresponsive to antibiotics?).
• Consider breakdown in infection control procedures, e.g.:
   procedures such as bronchoscopy, sputum induction and pentamidine inhalation may generate aerosols;
   inadequate isolation of sputum-positive patients;
   inadequate decontamination of multiuse equipment.

Suggested case-definition for use in an outbreak

Confirmed: culture or PCR positive with clinically compatible illness.
Probable: demonstration of acid-fast bacilli with clinically compatible illness.
Clinical: clinical diagnosis leading to initiation of antituberculous therapy.

3.79 Tularaemia

Tularaemia (rabbit fever; deer-fly fever; Ohara disease; Francis disease) is a zoonotic disease caused by an infection with the bacteria *Francisella tularensis* normally transmitted to humans from animal hosts.

Suggested on-call action

None usually required.

Epidemiology

Tularaemia is endemic in many parts of the world, including eastern Europe, Scandinavia, North America, China and Japan. Large outbreaks in Europe were recently reported from the Balkans (e.g. Kosovo in 2000).

Clinical features

A variety of clinical manifestations are common. They depend on the portal of entry into the human body. Symptoms include high fever, body aches, swollen lymph glands and difficulty swallowing. Fatal outcomes are rare in Europe. Fatalities occur mainly from typhoidal or pulmonary disease. With appropriate antibiotic treatment, the case-fatality rate is negligible.

Laboratory confirmation

Diagnosis is mostly made clinically and confirmed by a rise in specific serum antibodies. These are usually detectable after two weeks of the illness. Cross-reactions with *Brucella* species occur. Two biovars can cause human disease. Type A is more virulent than type B (case-fatality rate 5–15% vs. < 1%).

Transmission

Tularaemia is a zoonosis; reservoirs include wild rabbits, hares and musk-rats as well as some domestic animals and ticks. The most prevalent modes of transmission include arthropod bites, drinking water or food contaminated by rodents, handling of undercooked infected meat, or inhalation of dust from contaminated hay.

Pathogenesis

The incubation period varies depending on virulence of infecting strain and size of inoculum. It is usually 3–5 days, but may be as long as 2 weeks. Person-to-person transmission has not been reported.

Prevention

Health education to avoid tick bites and untreated potentially contaminated water, and to ensure meat from rodents is cooked thoroughly.

Surveillance

Tularaemia is notifiable in many countries (not UK). Cases should be reported to the public health authorities so that assessments of risk can be made.

Response to a case

No public health action usually necessary.

Investigation of a cluster/control of an outbreak

Search for a common source of infection related to arthropods, animal hosts, water or food.

Case-definition

Compatible clinical illness with laboratory confirmation of tularaemia.

3.80 Typhoid fever

Typhoid fever is caused by *Salmonella typhi*. A clinically similar, though usually less severe, illness may be caused by *S. paratyphi* (see Chapter 3.54). The collective name for these conditions is enteric fever.

Suggested on-call action

- Exclude cases and contacts who are food-handlers.
- Exclude cases and symptomatic contacts in other risk groups (see below).

Epidemiology

Infection occurs worldwide and is associated with poor sanitation. In underdeveloped countries the incidence of infection is around 50/100 000/year and is more common in summer. This compares with around 150 cases a year in England and Wales, with most of these cases being imported, often from the Indian subcontinent.

Clinical diagnosis

The illness begins with fever; rigors may occur. Patients complain of headache, cough, malaise, myalgia and may be constipated. Later in the course diarrhoea, abdominal tenderness, vomiting, delirium and confusion may occur. A few inconspicuous pale red spots (rose spots), scattered over the trunk, are seen in less than 20% of cases and are undetectable in pigmented skin. The spleen may be enlarged and abdominal tenderness is common but not severe.

Complications typically arise in the third week. In the abdomen, ulceration of Peyer's patches may result in haemorrhage (1.7%) or intestinal perforation (1–4%). DIC and renal failure occur in severe cases. Osteomyelitis may develop, especially in those predisposed by sickle cell disease. Other rare complications include cholecystitis, meningitis and typhoid pneumonia. Relapses occur in 5–10% of cases, and may be more common following antibiotic treatment.

Laboratory diagnosis

Definitive diagnosis of typhoid is by culture of the organism from a normally sterile site (e.g. blood). Blood, urine and faeces should be cultured: faeces are usually positive after the first week of illness and results should be available in 72 h. Culture of a bone marrow aspirate may be positive when there is no growth from other sites. The Widal agglutination test detects antibody to the somatic 'O', flagellar 'H' and Vi antigens of typhoid bacilli. Acute and convalescent sera may provide a retrospective diagnosis when a fourfold rise in titre occurs. Interpretation of a single high positive (for rapid diagnosis) is difficult. Phage typing may be available for unexplained clusters.

Transmission

Infection results from the ingestion of water or food contaminated by faeces from a human case or occasionally by an asymptomatic carrier. This may include fruit or vegetables washed in water contaminated by sewage, and shellfish. Water-borne outbreaks may occur. Person to person spread is possible in poor hygienic conditions and, rarely, between homosexual men. Urinary carriers are very rare in developed countries.

Pathogenesis

The incubation period ranges from 1 to 3 weeks.

The infectious period lasts as long as bacilli are present in the stool. This usually begins in the first week of illness. Approximately 10% of patients will be excreting bacilli 3 months after the onset. Approximately 3% of persons infected with *S. typhi* become chronic carriers; this carrier state may last many years and is more common in females and those with gallbladder disease.

S. typhi is extremely infectious; infection may occur with ingestion of fewer than 100 000

organisms. Achlorhydria and disturbance of bowel flora (e.g. by antibiotics) decrease the minimum infective dose. Splenectomy (e.g. in sickle cell disease, or immune defects) makes it more difficult to eradicate *S. typhi*.

Prevention

The control of the enteric fevers depends on sanitation, clean water and personal hygiene. Vaccination has had a limited effect as a control measure, although it provides useful protection in individuals. Vaccination is recommended for travellers to endemic countries, including ethnic minorities visiting their country of origin.

Surveillance

Typhoid is notifiable in most countries, including the UK. It should be reported on clinical suspicion to local public health authorities.

Response to a case

- Check antibiotic resistance of isolate.
- Enteric precautions and hygiene advice for cases; isolation if hospitalized.
- Obtain food and travel history for the 3 weeks prior to onset of illness.
- Cases who have not visited an endemic country in the 3 weeks before onset should be investigated to determine the source of infection.
- Exclude cases who are food handlers (Box 2.2.1: risk group 1) until 6 consecutive negative stool specimens taken at 2 week intervals and commencing 2 weeks after completion of antibiotic therapy.
- Exclude cases who are children aged under 5 years and cases with poor personal hygiene (risk groups 3 and 4) until 3 consecutive negative faecal samples taken at weekly intervals.
- Exclude cases who are health workers (risk group 2) until clinically well with formed stools and hygiene advice given. Tell hospital infection control team.
- Exclude all other cases until clinically well with formed stools.

• Investigate household and other close contacts with a faecal specimen for culture. If positive, treat as case.

• Do not treat contacts in groups at risk for further transmission (Box 2.2.1) as negative until three consecutive negatives taken at weekly intervals commencing 3 weeks after last exposure to case. Exclude contacts who are food handlers until these results are known. Exclude others only until formed stools for 48 h and hygiene advice given.

• Quinolones may reduce the period of carriage in those for whom exclusion is producing social difficulties.

Investigation of a cluster

Clusters should be investigated to ensure that secondary transmission has not occurred. Most clusters in developed countries will result from exposure to a common source abroad, or transmission within close family groups. Chains of transmission can be investigated through phage typing.

Control of an outbreak

Outbreaks of typhoid should be investigated as a matter of urgency. All cases and contacts should be investigated to identify the source of the outbreak. This could be due to contact with a chronic carrier, with faecal material, or with contaminated food, milk, water or shellfish.

Contacts should be observed and investigated if they develop symptoms suggestive of typhoid after appropriate specimens are taken.

Suggested case-definition

Probable: a clinically compatible case epidemiologically linked to a confirmed case in an outbreak.
Confirmed: a clinically compatible case that is laboratory-confirmed.

3.81 Typhus and other rickettsial infections

(Tables 3.81.1 and 3.81.2)

Rickettsia are small bacteria which only replicate within another cell. Transmission is by means of an arthropod vector. The natural mammalian host is typically a rodent; man acquires the infection as a zoonosis. Only epidemic typhus is primarily a disease of man.

Following an infected arthropod bite, replication of the organism at the site may give rise to a characteristic skin lesion, a small painless ulcer with a black centre, called an eschar. The infection then becomes generalized, and there is a fever, which in more severe infections is high and unremitting. If there is a rash, it appears around the fourth or fifth day of illness and may have either a dusky macular appearance or be petechial. In the most serious infections multiple organ damage may develop, usually towards the end of the second week.

Rickettsial infection should be considered if there is fever with either the typical rash or an eschar and an appropriate travel history. Confirmation by specific serology is now available for many of the rickettsia.

Prevention

Tick-borne disease can be prevented by reducing the incidence of tick bite through wearing long trousers and using repellents. For louse-borne disease, in an epidemic delousing measures with changing of clothes and impregnation with insecticide may be necessary.

There is no person-to-person spread. Typhus is formally notifiable in the UK.

Investigation

Diagnosis is usually clinical. To confirm serologically, use assays that detect antibodies to rickettsial antigens such as the indirect fluorescence antibody test or latex agglutination rather than the non-specific, insensitive Weil–Felix test.

Table 3.81.1 Rickettsial infections

Disease and organism	Incubation period	Mode of transmission & epidemiology	Clinical
Epidemic typhus (louse-borne typhus) *R. prowazeki*	1–2 weeks	The natural reservoir is amongst rodents. The illness reaches humans via infected dogs and their ticks. It is transmitted directly between humans by the human body louse, which feeds on the body but lays its eggs in clothing. It is now principally a disease of tropical highlands such as Ethiopia and the Andes. Infestation tends to occur where poverty and a cold climate coincide	The illness is relatively mild in children but mortality increases with age; untreated, about 50% of 50-year-olds will die. There is no eschar, but there is usually a rash, which is often petechial. The high fever may be associated with severe headache, vomiting and epistaxis. Complications include diminished consciousness, pneumonia and renal failure
Trench fever *R. quintana*	1–2 weeks	Louse-borne	The illness resembles epidemic typhus, but is milder. The rash may be macular or maculopapular
Murine typhus *R. typhi*	1–2 weeks	Transmitted from rats to man by fleas. It occurs worldwide, but particularly in tropical Asia	Resembles epidemic typhus, but milder
Rocky Mountain spotted fever *R. rickettsii*	3–14 days	Various reservoir hosts are described; rodents are most significant. The principal vector is the dog tick, thus bringing the risk of infection close to humans. This North American disease occurs widely in the eastern U.S. as well as in the Rocky Mountains	It is a severe illness. The rash is typically petechial and complications, including pneumonia and myocarditis, are common. Untreated, the mortality is around 20%
Boutonneuse fever *R. conorii*	5–8 days	Similar tick typhus syndromes, caused by *Rickettsia conorii* or its close relatives, occur in the Mediterranean, Asia, Australia and Brazil	An eschar is usual, sometimes with regional lymphadenopathy, and a macular rash may occur. Fatality is rare
Rickettsial pox *R. akari*	1–2 weeks	Transmitted naturally between rodents by mites. Humans are usually infected in recently cleared ground where the mites abound in South and East Asia and in parts of Queensland, Australia. Also reported from Russia, eastern USA and South Africa	Disseminated vesicular rash which may be confused with chickenpox. Fatality is low
Scrub typhus *R. tsutsugamushi*	6–21 days	Mite-borne scrub typhus occurs widely, including Japan, China, the Philippines, New Guinea, Indonesia, other islands of the southwest Pacific Ocean, southeastern Asia, northern Australia, India, Sri Lanka, Pakistan, Russia, and Korea	Only fever, headache, and swollen lymph nodes and in some cases myalgia, gastrointestinal complaints, or cough. Mortality about 5% untreated

Table 3.81.2 Infection due to *Ehrlichia*

Disease and organism	Incubation period	Mode of transmission and epidemiology	Clinical
E. chaffeensis	? 3–4 weeks	Transmission follows when the deer ticks bite human skin and inoculate organisms. Found in the USA	Illness similar to Rocky Mountain spotted fever
E. sennetsu	14 days	Found in USA, Japan and Malaysia	Illness similar to Rocky Mountain spotted fever

Ehrlichiosis

Ehrlichiosis is a recently recognized pathogen that causes an illness similar to the spotted rickettsioses. *Ehrlichia sennetsu, E. chaffeensis*, and the human granulocytic ehrlichiosis have been described. About 1200 cases of human ehrlichiosis have been recognized in the USA. Diagnosis is made on the clinical picture and confirmation using PCR. Transmission is probably tick-borne.

The disease is not transmissible between humans.

3.82 *Vibrio parahaemolyticus*

Vibrio parahaemolyticus causes a gastrointestinal infection that is particularly associated with consumption of contaminated seafood.

Suggested on-call action

If other cases known to you or reporting clinician/microbiologist then consult local outbreak plan.

Epidemiology

V. parahaemolyticus food poisoning is rare in north and west Europe, e.g. 20–25 cases p.a. are reported in England and Wales. It is, however, responsible for over half of food-borne disease in Japan in summer months and is also relatively common during summer months in coastal areas of the United States, the Caribbean Islands, Bangladesh and south-east Asia. Most cases in the UK are in travellers returning from warmer countries. All ages are susceptible.

Clinical features

The illness is characterized by explosive watery diarrhoea, usually accompanied by abdominal cramps. Nausea, vomiting and headache are common. Fever and chills occur in a minority of cases and occasionally there is bloody diarrhoea. The illness usually lasts 1–7 days (median of 3). Death is rare but may occur in very young children or elderly people with underlying disease.

Laboratory confirmation

Diagnosis is dependent upon isolation of the organism from culture of stool specimen or rectal swabs on selective media (i.e. warn the laboratory if organism suspected). All pathogenic *V. parahaemolyticus* are 'Kanagawa-positive' (complete lysis of human erythrocytes) but most environmental isolates (and *V. cholerae*) are 'Kanagawa-negative'.

The organism may also be cultured from food: 10^3 organisms per gram would be expected. There are numerous serotypes but isolates from both food and faeces often contain a mixture of types.

Transmission

V. parahaemolyticus is ubiquitous in coastal waters of temperate and tropical countries (it has been demonstrated in both the UK and the Netherlands). During the warm season (water $>10\,°C$), the organism is found free in water, fish and shellfish.

Transmission to humans is food-borne via consumption of raw or undercooked seafood (particularly in Japan), or food contaminated after cooking, e.g. by washing with seawater. The organism multiplies rapidly at room temperature: most outbreaks appear to involve a stage in which the food was held for several hours without refrigeration, to allow formation of an infective dose.

The organism is killed by temperatures of $80\,°C$ for 15 min and refrigeration is effective at controlling multiplication.

Pathogenesis

- The incubation period is dependent upon the ingested dose: extremes of 4–96 h have been reported, with the median for most outbreaks being 13–23 h.
- The organism is non-communicable between humans.
- The minimum infectious dose is 10^6 organisms.
- Immunity does not appear to develop in response to infection.

Prevention

- Cook seafood so that all parts reach $80\,°C$ for 15 min, or irradiate before eating raw.
- Avoid cross-contamination from raw seafood in kitchen. Do not use raw seawater to wash food.

Surveillance

Report to local public health departments (notify as 'suspected food poisoning' in UK) and to national surveillance systems.

Response to a case

- Obtain details from case on foods consumed

in 48 h before onset, especially seafood. Any history of travel?
- Although person-to-person transmission unusual, PHLS guidelines suggest cases in risk groups 1–4 (Table 2.2.1) excluded from work/school for 48 h after first normal stool.

Investigation of a cluster

- Plot epidemic curve: if all cases within 48 h then single exposure likely. If not, assume continuing source as secondary spread unlikely.
- Obtain food (especially seafood) and travel/recreation history for 48 h before onset of each case.
- Organize laboratory testing of suspect foods.

Control of an outbreak

- Identify and rectify any of the following faults:
  processes risking undercooking of seafood;
  processes risking cross-contamination from seafood;
  consumption of raw seafood without adequate temperature control;
  use of raw seawater.
- Re-inforce food hygiene and handwashing.
- Report any suspected commercially produced food to relevant authority, e.g. Food Standards Agency in UK.

Suspected case-definition for use in outbreak

Confirmed: diarrhoea or abdominal cramps with *V. parahaemolyticus* identified in stool sample.
Clinical: watery diarrhoea and abdominal pain with onset 4–48 h after exposure to suspect meal.

3.83 Viral haemorrhagic fevers

Viral haemorrhagic fevers (VHF) are severe, life-threatening viral infections of high mortality which commonly present with haemorrhagic manifestations. They are endemic in a number of parts of the world: Africa, S. America and some parts of Asia, the Middle East and eastern Europe. About 35 cases of viral haemorrhagic fever have been reported in England and Wales over the past 10 years. The environmental conditions in the UK and western Europe do not support the natural reservoirs or vectors of these diseases. The risk of epidemic spread in the general population is negligible.

There is a risk of secondary infection from four types of VHF (Lassa, Ebola, Marburg and Crimean/Congo haemorrhagic fevers), particularly among those who might be exposed to body fluids particularly from needlestick injury or by contamination of broken skin or mucous membranes. High rates of secondary disease in those caring for cases in developing countries have been reported.

Epidemiology

Each of the viruses grouped together here has a different epidemiology. They are found in rural areas.

Surveillance

Viral haemorrhagic fevers are notifiable in most countries, including the UK. Local and national public health authorities should be informed of cases immediately on clinical suspicion.

Response to a case

The response to a case in England and Wales is laid out in the Guidelines of the Advisory Committee on Dangerous Pathogens (see Appendix 2).

Strict infection control precautions are required to protect those who may be exposed. In England and Wales the Control of Substances Hazardous to Health (COSHH) Regulations 1994 require employers to assess risks to employees and others in the work place including, when appropriate, an assessment of the risk of VHF infection occurring at work.

Patient assessment and risk categorization

VHF should be considered in any patient presenting with a pyrexia of unknown origin (PUO) shortly after having returned from abroad. In most cases this can be dismissed on epidemiological grounds; most patients suspected of VHF will be suffering from malaria. Laboratory tests to exclude or confirm malaria should be undertaken as soon as possible for minimum and moderate risk patients. A checklist of enquiries to help identify patients at risk is available in the Guidelines. A risk assessment where patients are assigned to one of three risk groups: minimum, moderate or high should be undertaken to ensure appropriate management for the patient and protection for the laboratory and clinical staff. Clinicians should seek the help and advice of a specialist in infectious diseases or tropical medicine.

Minimum risk

This category includes febrile patients who have:
• not been in known endemic areas before the onset of illness;
or
• been in endemic areas (or in contact with a known or suspected source of a VHF), but in whom the onset of illness was definitely more than 21 days after their last contact with any potential source of infection.

Moderate risk

This category includes febrile patients who have:
• been in an endemic area during the 21 days before the onset of illness, but who have none of the additional risk factors which would place him or her in the high risk category;
or
• not been in a known endemic area but who may have been in adjacent areas or countries during the 21 days before the onset of illness, and who have evidence of severe illness with organ failure and/or haemorrhage which

Table 3.83.1 Viral haemorrhagic fever

Virus	Lassa fever virus
Family	Arenaviridae
Epidemiology	Rural areas of W. Africa Animal reservoir: Multi-mammate rat
Clinical diagnosis	Gradual onset, malaise, fever, sore throat Pharyngeal exudates common Hypotension and shock Albuminuria 15–20% case fatality rate for hospitalized cases
Laboratory diagnosis	Reduced platelet count Virus can be isolated from blood, urine, and throat washings IgM may be detectable by ELISA or IFA Specimens must be handled in a Category 4 laboratory
Transmission	Contact with urine of infected rat Person-to-person transmission via contact with bodily secretions (including sexual contact)
Pathogenesis	Incubation period: 6–21 days Infectious period: Virus is present in body secretions, including the pharynx during the acute illness, and may be excreted in the urine for 2–3 months
Prevention	Avoid contact with rat excreta Strict isolation of clinical case Strict handling of body fluids

Virus	Ebola
Family	Filoviridae
Epidemiology	Rural areas of W. and Central Africa Animal reservoir: Not known: Monkey? Primate?
Clinical diagnosis	Sudden onset, malaise, fever, myalgia, diarrhoea Hypotension and shock 50–90% case fatality rate for hospitalized cases Multisystem involvement
Laboratory diagnosis	IgG detection by IFA, ELISA, Western blot Viral nucleic acid detection in skin snip Specimens must be handled in a Category 4 laboratory
Transmission	Contact with infected monkeys? Person-to-person transmission via contact with bodily secretions (including sexual contact)
Pathogenesis	Incubation period: 2–21 days Infectious period: Virus is present in body secretions, including the pharynx during the acute illness, may be excreted in semen for 2–3 months
Prevention	Strict isolation of clinical case Strict handling of body fluids

Table 3.83.1 *Continued*

Virus	Marburg
Family	Filoviridae
Epidemiology	First described when laboratory workers became infected following exposure to body fluids of tissues from African green monkeys from Uganda
Clinical diagnosis	Sudden onset, malaise, fever, myalgia, diarrhoea Hypotension and shock 50–90% case fatality rate for hospitalized cases Multisystem involvement
Laboratory diagnosis	IgG detection by IFA, ELISA, Western blot Viral nucleic acid detection in skin snip Specimens must be handled in a Category 4 laboratory
Transmission	Contact with infected monkeys Person-to-person transmission via contact with bodily secretions (including sexual contact)
Pathogenesis	Incubation period: 3–9 days Infectious period: Virus is present in body secretions during the acute illness
Prevention	Strict isolation of clinical cases Strict handling of body fluids

Virus	Crimean–Congo haemorrhagic fever (CCHF)
Family	Nairovirus
Epidemiology	Africa, Asia, former USSR and SE Europe Tick-borne
Clinical diagnosis	Sudden onset, malaise, fever, headache, anorexia Petechial rash, purpura Haemorrhage 2–50% case fatality rate for hospitalized cases
Laboratory diagnosis	Reduced platelet count Virus can be isolated from blood, urine, and throat washings IgM may be detectable by ELISA or IFA Specimens must be handled in a Category 4 laboratory
Transmission	Bite of infected tick Butchering infected animals Person-to-person transmission via contact with bodily secretions (including sexual contact)
Pathogenesis	Incubation period: 3–12 days Infectious period: Virus is present in body secretions during the acute illness
Prevention	Avoid tick bites and contact with rat excreta Strict isolation of clinical case Strict handling of body fluids

could be due to a VHF and for which no alternative diagnosis is currently evident.

High risk

This category includes febrile patients who:
1 Have been in an endemic area during the three weeks before illness and:
   • have lived in a house or stayed in a house for more than 4 h where there were ill, feverish persons known or strongly suspected to have a VHF;
   or
   • took part in nursing or caring for ill, feverish patients known or strongly suspected to have a VHF, or had contact with the body fluids, tissue or the dead body of such a patient;
   or
   • are laboratory, health or other workers who have, or have been likely to have come into contact with the body fluids, tissues or the body of a human or animal known or strongly suspected to have a VHF;
   or
   • were previously categorized as 'moderate' risk, but who have developed organ failure and/or haemorrhage.
2 Have not been in an endemic area but during the three weeks before illness they:
   • cared for a patient or animal known or strongly suspected to have a VHF or came into contact with the body fluids, tissues or dead body of such a patient or animal;
   or
   • handled clinical specimens, tissues or laboratory cultures known or strongly suspected to contain the agent of a VHF.

Initial management

Decisions on the management of a suspected case should be taken with an infectious disease specialist. An incident/outbreak control group should be convened to ensure that formal guidance is implemented correctly.

Minimum risk patients may be admitted (if requiring hospitalization) under standard isolation and infection control procedures. Moderate risk patients should be admitted to a high-security infectious disease unit or intermediate isolation facilities and, apart from the malaria test, specimens should only be sent to a high security laboratory. High-risk patients must be admitted to a high security infectious disease unit, samples should only be sent to a high security laboratory and close contacts should be identified. Special precautions (ambulance category III) are required to transport moderate and high-risk patients.

The CCDC will wish to ensure the following.
• The patient is in the category of accommodation appropriate to risk.
• Any ambulance staff have been appropriately advised (liaise with ambulance control unit).
• Hospital staff have been appropriately advised (liaise with infection control doctor).
• Cases or contacts in other districts are followed up (liaise with other CCDC).
• Any specimens or contaminated material from before diagnosis suspected are dealt with appropriately.
• Contacts of are identified and followed up appropriately.
• Any necessary disinfection of domestic and primary care premises is carried out.
• The body of any deceased case is appropriately dealt with.
• Appropriate agencies (DH and CDSC in England and Wales) are informed.
• Arrangements are made for dealing with the media.

Laboratory confirmation

Obtaining and handling laboratory specimens (blood, urine, etc.) is the most common cause of cases of VHF in healthcare settings: blood and body fluids from high-risk VHF patients are likely to contain high concentrations of virus. Therefore most laboratory tests are discouraged in the initial assessment. Good laboratory practice guidelines must be in place and specimens must be taken and examined by experienced staff in appropriate facilities.

UK guidance is that specimens for virological investigations from moderate or high-risk cases must be sent to a viral diagnostic laboratory equipped to handle Hazard Group 4 biological agents. In the UK, appropriate high-security laboratories are the Central Public Health Laboratory at Colindale, and the Centre for Applied Microbiology and Research at Porton Down. The appropriate specimen and investigation should be discussed first. Virus can be detected in body fluids. Newer techniques involve the detection of viral nucleic acid.

Post-mortem examination is a potential risk: if further tests necessary to confirm the diagnosis, specialist advice should be sought.

Management of contacts

Close contacts of a high risk or confirmed case should be kept under daily surveillance for a period of 21 days from the last possible date of exposure to infection. Close contacts are those who after the onset of the patient's illness:

• Had direct contact with the patient's blood, urine or secretions, or with clothing, bedding or other fomites soiled by the patient's blood, urine or secretions (not including saliva).
• Cared for the patient or handled specimens from the patient—for example, household members, nurses, laboratory staff, ambulance crew, doctors or other staff.
• Had direct contact with the body of a person who died of viral haemorrhagic fever, either proven or in high or moderate risk categories, before the coffin was sealed.
• Had direct contact with an animal infected with VHF, its blood, body fluids, or corpse.

There need be no restriction on work or movement within the UK but the contact's temperature should be recorded daily and enquiry made about the presence of any suspicious symptoms. Those suffering any rise of temperature above 38 °C should be kept under observation at home, and if fever persists for more than 24 h, advice should be sought from a consultant in infectious or tropical diseases regarding the need for admission to an isolation unit.

When contact with a VHF patient has not been close, the risk of infection is minimal. Therefore there is no need to trace and/or follow up contacts that are not in the categories listed above.

3.84 Warts and verrucae

Warts are caused by human papilloma viruses (HPV). These may occur anywhere on the body and usually regress spontaneously. There is interest in certain types of HPV as causes of genital tract, skin and respiratory malignancies.

Suggested on-call action
None.

Epidemiology

Warts are common in childhood, with 4–20% of schoolchildren having warts at any one time.

Clinical features

Four types of wart are recognized.
1 Common warts (verrucae vulgaris); flesh-coloured or brown, keratotic papules 2–10 mm in diameter with rough surface, may be filiform, paring reveals thrombosed capillaries.
2 Plantar warts (verrucae plantaris); grow inwards and are painful; common in adolescents and children.
3 Flat or planar warts (verrucae planae); smaller, flat topped, non-scaling, papules, cluster on hands, neck or face.
4 Condylomata acuminata (genital warts); occur in the genital tract, transmitted sexually (see Chapter 3.25).

Laboratory confirmation

The diagnosis can be confirmed histologically.

Transmission and pathogenesis

Warts spread by direct contact or indirectly via contact with contaminated floors. Auto-inoculation occurs as a result of scratching. The incubation period is 2–3 months and the person will remain infectious as long as the warts persist. Warts are more common in immunocompromised people.

Prevention

Health education, environmental hygiene in swimming pools and other communal areas and avoiding direct contact with warts where practicable may reduce spread.

Surveillance

Case reporting is not necessary.

Response to a case

Nearly all warts resolve spontaneously in time. Children with warts do not have to stay away from school. Affected children can go swimming. Plantar warts should be covered if practicable in swimming pools, gymnasia and changing rooms.

3.85 Whooping cough (pertussis)

Whooping cough is an acute bacterial respiratory infection caused by *Bordetella pertussis*. Its public health importance lies in the severity of the disease, particularly in young infants, and its preventability by vaccination.

Suggested on-call action

- Start antibiotic treatment (erythromycin).
- Exclude from nursery or school for five days from starting antibiotic treatment.

Epidemiology

Pertussis is well controlled in countries with good immunization coverage. Where coverage is low, the disease has a cyclical pattern, with epidemics occurring at 3–4 yearly intervals. These epidemics affect young children; infants under 6 months are particularly at risk.

There were large epidemics in the UK during the 1970s and 1980s when vaccine coverage fell due to (unfounded) concerns about vaccine safety. Vaccine coverage has since risen to over 90%, and in 1999 only 1139 cases were notified in England and Wales. Epidemics of pertussis also occurred in Sweden, where pertussis vaccine was discontinued altogether for some years. Germany, the Netherlands and France have also experienced resurgences of pertussis in recent years. The reported case fatality rate is 1 per 1000 overall, although it is higher than this in young infants, in whom pertussis is often not recognized. Enhanced surveillance identified 18 deaths from whooping cough in England and Wales between 1995 and 1997, of which 83% were in infants under 4 months of age.

Clinical features

The initial illness starts with cough, cold and a fever. Over the next week, the cough gradually becomes paroxysmal; there are bouts of coughing which are terminated by the typical whoop, or by vomiting. The cough often lasts for two to three months. Young infants do not usually whoop, and coughing spasms may be followed by periods of apnoea. Adults have a milder illness that lasts two to three weeks. Pertussis is being increasingly recognized as a cause of chronic cough in adults.

Laboratory confirmation

The classical method is culture from a pernasal swab, although the organism is difficult to grow, so sensitivity is low (although specificity is high). The sensitivity has been greatly improved by the recent advent of PCR diagnosis (specialist laboratory only). Serology (EIA) is also available.

Transmission

Man is the only reservoir. Transmission is by droplet spread from an infectious case, often an older sibling or parent. Carriers do not exist. Mild or subclinical cases among vaccinated individuals are also a source of infection.

Pathogenesis

_21|7

The incubation period is 7–10 days, by may occasionally be up to three weeks. A case is highly infectious during the early stage of the illness, before the typical cough; infectiousness then decreases and the case is normally not infectious three weeks after the onset of paroxysmal cough, although in a proportion of cases (up to 20%) infectivity may persist for up to 6 weeks. The period of communicability may be shortened by erythromycin treatment. An attack of pertussis usually confers immunity, although second cases do sometimes occur.

Prevention

Pertussis vaccine is 80–90% effective at preventing illness, although its role in limiting transmission is less clear. Pertussis vaccine has also been shown to reduce the incidence of sudden infant death syndrome.

There are two types of pertussis vaccine: killed whole-cell preparations and subunit acellular vaccines. Many countries in Europe have recently switched from whole cell to acellular vaccines because of the lower incidence of side-effects with acellular vaccine. Both types of vaccine are currently used in the UK, where the recommended schedule is three doses (as part of DTP/Hib vaccine) at 2, 3 and 4 months of age. In most European countries (although not the UK) a fourth dose is given in the second year of life and in some countries there is a fifth dose at school entry. This is based on evidence of waning immunity in older children and adults.

It is important that pertussis vaccine is not delayed in infants, and that older siblings and parents are fully vaccinated. The only true contraindication is a severe reaction to a previous dose.

Surveillance

Pertussis is notifiable in most countries, including the UK. Laboratories should also report all clinically significant infections to the local and national surveillance.

Response to a case

• Isolate, with respiratory precautions, in hospital.
• Start antibiotic treatment (erythromycin) and exclude from nursery or school for five days after treatment has started (course to continue for 14 days).
• Arrange for laboratory confirmation.
• Check vaccination status of case and household contacts, and arrange for vaccination if any are unvaccinated.
• Erythromycin prophylaxis may be of value for unvaccinated household contacts, particularly infants under six months of age, if given within 21 days of onset of case.

Investigation of a cluster and control of an outbreak

Obtain laboratory confirmation, including serotyping. Look for unvaccinated individuals and consider community-wide vaccination if coverage is low (NB three doses of vaccine are required for protection, so vaccination is a long-term outbreak control measure).

Outbreaks in institutions can be controlled by a combination of case-finding, antibiotic treatment, and case exclusion.

Suggested case-definitions for an outbreak

Clinical: 14 days or more of cough plus one of:
  epidemiological link to a confirmed case,
or one of
  paroxysms, whoop, or postcoughing vomiting.
Confirmed: compatible symptoms with *B. pertussis* infection confirmed by culture, PCR, or serology.

3.86 Yellow fever

An imported, acute flavivirus infection, which may be severe.

On-call action
None usually necessary.

Epidemiology

Yellow fever is endemic in Central Africa and areas of South and Central America. The mosquito vector does not occur in Europe, but the disease is a potential risk to travellers to endemic areas.

Clinical features

Cases are classified as inapparent, mild, moderately severe, and malignant. Onset is sudden, with fever of 39–40 °C. The pulse, rapid initially becomes slow for the fever. In mild cases, the illness ends after 1–3 days. In moderately severe and malignant cases, the fever falls suddenly 2–5 days after onset, and a remission of several hours or days ensues. The fever then recurs, albuminuria, and epigastric tenderness with haematemesis appear. Oliguria or anuria may occur and petechiae and mucosal haemorrhages are common. In malignant cases, delirium, convulsions, and coma occur terminally.

Up to 10% of clinically diagnosed cases die, but overall mortality is actually lower, since many infections are undiagnosed.

Laboratory confirmation

Diagnosis is confirmed by virus isolation from blood, by a rising antibody titre (in absence of recent immunization and after exclusion of cross-reactions to other flaviviruses), or at autopsy. Antigen or genome detection tests may be available.

Transmission

In sylvatic yellow fever, the virus is acquired from wild primates and transmitted by forest canopy mosquitoes. In urban yellow fever, the virus is acquired from a viraemic patient within the previous 2 weeks and transmitted by the *Aedes aegypti* mosquito.

Pathogenesis

Incubation lasts 3–6 days.

Prevention

Active immunization with the live, attenuated vaccine effectively prevents cases.

Vaccination requirements vary by country; information and addresses of vaccination centres can be obtained from public health authorities.

Eradication of urban yellow fever requires widespread mosquito control and mass immunization.

Surveillance

Yellow fever is a notifiable disease and should be reported to local public health authorities and to WHO.

Response to a case

• The case should be reported urgently to WHO and the country of origin.
• The case should be transferred to suitable isolation facilities and strict procedures such as those laid down by the Advisory Committee on Dangerous Pathogens (UK) followed.
• In an area where there is potential for further mosquito transmission, patients should be isolated in a screened room sprayed with residual insecticide.
• Hospital and laboratory personnel should be aware of the risk of transmission from inoculation.

Investigation of a cluster and control of an outbreak

Control of an outbreak is through mass immunization and vector control.

Suggested case-definition
Clinically compatible case confirmed by fourfold rise in antibody titres or demonstration of virus, antigen or genome.

3.87 Yersiniosis

Non-plague yersiniosis has emerged in recent years as an important cause of intestinal infection in many countries. *Yersinia enterocolitica* causes predominantly enterocolitis, whereas *Yersinia pseudotuberculosis* mainly causes an appendicitis-like illness.

Suggested on-call action
• Exclude symptomatic cases in high-risk groups.   • If you or reporting microbiologist/ clinician know of other cases, consult outbreak control plan.

Epidemiology

Although documented in temperate regions in all continents, *Y. enterocolitica* is more common in northern Europe and Canada, where it appears to be responsible for 2–4% of cases of diarrhoea. All ages are susceptible, but most cases occur in those under 10. Peak incidence in Europe is in autumn and winter. Infection may be more common in rural areas and amongst those exposed to pigs or their carcasses. Reported cases have fallen over the last decade in England and Wales from over 500 in 1990 to fewer than 100 in 1999.

Y. pseudotuberculosis has a worldwide distribution but is more commonly reported from Europe. Most cases are aged 5–20 years and males are more commonly affected. Peak incidence is in winter.

Clinical features

Y. enterocolitica enteritis presents with diarrhoea accompanied by fever and abdominal pain in two-thirds of cases, and vomiting in one-third. The duration of illness is usually 2–3 weeks, slightly longer than for most enteric pathogens. Bloody diarrhoea occurs in approximately 20–25% of affected children. Post-infectious problems include reactive arthritis and erythema nodosum. Other presentations include pharyngitis, appendicitis-like syndrome in older children, and septicaemia in the infirm.

Y. pseudotuberculosis usually presents as mesenteric adenitis causing fever and right lower abdominal pain. Many cases result in appendicectomy. Erythema nodosum may occur, but enteritis and septicaemia are uncommon.

Carriage of *Yersinia* species in studies of asymptomatic individuals ranges from 0 to 2.9%.

Laboratory confirmation

Serological diagnosis is available for both species. *Y. enterocolitica* can be diagnosed by stool culture but grows slowly on routine culture media and would not be routinely ascertained by most laboratory. If yersiniosis is suspected on epidemiological grounds then enrichment and highly selective media can be used, but this takes several days. Small numbers of organisms may continue to be excreted for 4 weeks.

Y. enterocolitica are divided into six biotypes, of which types 2, 3 and 4 are the most common, and over 50 serotypes, of which O3 and O9 are the most common in Europe. A phage-typing scheme also exists.

Y. pseudotuberculosis is usually confirmed by isolation from an excised mesenteric lymph node. All strains are biochemically homogenous and, although there are six serotypes, most human cases are serotype 1.

Transmission

The most important reservoir of *Y. enterocoliti-*

ca in Europe is asymptomatic carriage in pigs. Other hosts are rodents, rabbits, sheep, goats, cattle, horses, dogs and cats. *Y. pseudotuberculosis* is found in a number of mammals and birds, particularly rodents and poultry. Humans usually acquire the infection orally via:

1 Food: especially pork or pork products. Pork is easily contaminated in the abattoir and if eaten raw or undercooked may cause illness. Refrigeration offers little protection as the organism can multiply at 4 °C. Milk has also been implicated in *Y. enterocolitica* outbreaks, probably due to contamination after pasteurization, although pasteurization failure is possible. Vegetables such as tofu or bean sprouts have become contaminated from growing in contaminated water. The optimum temperature for growth is 22–29 °C.

2 Person to person: evidence for transmission to household contacts is conflicting, but outbreaks have occurred in nurseries, schools and hospitals in which person-to-person spread is likely to have played a part. Respiratory transmission from cases with pharyngitis appears unlikely.

3 Direct contact with animals: human cases have been reported after contact with sick puppies and kittens.

4 Blood-borne: contaminated blood in blood banks has led to severe disease and several deaths in recipients. Not all donors were unwell. The ability of the organism to replicate in refrigerators is likely to be relevant.

Pathogenesis

The incubation period is usually 4–7 days with a range of 2–11.

The infectious dose is likely to be high, perhaps 10^9 organisms.

Secondary infection appears to be rare: it may be best to assume that the infectious period extends until 48 h after the first normal stool.

Natural infection confers immunity although the extent and duration is unclear. Maternal antibodies protect the newborn.

Prevention

• Avoidance of consumption of raw meats, particularly pork products.

• Reduction of contamination of raw pork by improved slaughtering methods, improved husbandry or irradiation of meat.

• Avoidance of long-term refrigeration of meat (maximum 4 days). Growth should not occur at freezer temperatures under −2 °C.

• Pasteurization of dairy products and subsequent separation from unpasteurized milk-handling processes.

• Chlorination of drinking water.

• Exclusion of blood donors with recent history of diarrhoea or fever.

• General measures to protect against gastrointestinal infection, including handwashing, safe disposal of human and animal/pet faeces, food hygiene and exclusion of cases with high risk of onward transmission.

Surveillance

• Cases of yersiniosis should be reported to local public health departments (notify as suspected food poisoning in UK) and to national surveillance.

• Clinicians should inform the local public health department of any increase in cases of mesenteric adenitis or appendicectomy, especially in autumn and winter.

Response to a case

• Give hygiene advice to case (enteric precautions).

• Exclude case and symptomatic contacts if in risk group (Box 2.2.1) until 48 h after first normal stool. No microbiological clearance necessary.

• Obtain history of consumption of pork or pork products, raw or undercooked meat, milk or water. Ask about sick pets, blood transfusions and exposure to animals/carcasses.

Investigations of a cluster

• Discuss case finding with local laboratory:

need to change testing policy for routine specimens?

• Discuss further microbiological investigations of existing cases to discover if all one serotype or phagetype.

• Conduct hypothesis-generating study. Questionnaire should include consumption of pork and pork products; consumption of raw or undercooked meats; source of milk; source of water; all other food consumed in last 11 days; contact with other cases; blood or blood product transfusions; hospital treatment; occupation; contact with animals (wild, agricultural or pet).

Control of an outbreak

• Exclude symptomatic cases in high-risk groups and ensure enteric precautions followed.

• Reinforce food hygiene and handwashing.

• Look for ways in which food could have become contaminated (especially cross contamination from raw pork), undercooked or stored too long in a refrigerator. Check that pasteurized milk could not become contaminated in dairy.

• Prevent use of unpasteurized milk. Prevent use of raw vegetables grown in untreated water, unless subsequently cleaned adequately.

Suggested case-definition for outbreak

Clinical: diarrhoea *or* combination of fever and right lower abdominal pain with onset 4–7 days after exposure.

Confirmed: isolate of outbreak strain or serological positive with one of diarrhoea, fever, abdominal pain, or vomiting beginning 1–11 days after exposure.

3.88.1 Helminths

Intestinal roundworms
(Table 3.88.1a)

Most intestinal nematodes are not passed directly from person to person, and so spread is rare in developed countries. Control is based on enteric precautions and early treatment of cases. The main exception is threadworm infection (see Chapter 3.74).

Tapeworms (cestodes)
(Table 3.88.1b)

Humans are the only definitive host for the tapeworms *Taenia saginata* and *Taenia solium* and may also be accidental intermediate hosts for *T. solium*, giving rise to cysticercosis, and for *Echinococcus granulosus*, giving rise to hydatid disease.

Eggs, or whole detached segments (proglottids), are evacuated in the faeces of the definitive host and disseminate in the environment. Following ingestion by a suitable intermediate host they develop into invasive larvae in the gut, migrate through the tissues and settle as cysts at sites determined by the tropism of the parasite. When the intermediate host is eaten by a definitive host, allowing the cysts to develop into adults, the life cycle is completed.

Filariae
(Table 3.88.1c)

Filariae produce larvae called microfilariae directly without an egg stage, and have a life cycle involving an arthropod intermediate host, usually a biting insect which acts as a vector for the dissemination of the disease. At least 10 species infect man. The incubation period is prolonged and may be more than a year. There is no person-to-person spread; individuals remain infectious for the insect vector if microfilariae are present. The insect vectors are not present outside the endemic range of the diseases.

Table 3.88.1a Intestinal roundworms

Disease and organism	Mode of transmission	Epidemiology	Clinical	Investigation	Public health action
Ascariasis *Ascaris lumbricoides*	Humans are reservoir but transmission is indirect. Non-infective eggs excreted in faeces become infectious after 2–3 weeks in soil and may survive many months. Infective eggs ingested from soil or foods contaminated by soil Eggs hatch in duodenum. Larvae migrate in blood and lymphatics to lung and oropharynx where swallowed to develop into adult worms in small intestine. Adults live 6–12 months	Worldwide but concentrated in tropical and subtropical areas with poor sanitation. Estimated that more than 1 billion persons are infected, making ascariasis the world's most prevalent intestinal helminth infection	Migrating larvae may produce an eosinophilic pneumonia Asymptomatic patient may pass an adult worm by vomiting or per rectum Heavy infection may produce abdominal cramps and may cause intestinal obstruction Even moderate infections can lead to malnutrition in children	Diagnosis is made by detection of the eggs in stools Occasionally, adult worms are passed in the stool or vomited	Uncooked and unwashed vegetables should be avoided in areas where human faeces (night soil) is used as fertilizer There is no risk of transmission from a case in Europe if basic hygienic precautions are taken
Whipworm infection *Trichuris trichiura*	Humans are only reservoir, but transmission is indirect. Noninfective eggs excreted in faeces to	The parasite is found principally in the tropics and subtropics	Infection is often asymptomatic. Heavy infections cause abdominal pain, anorexia,	Identification of the eggs in faeces	Prevention rests upon adequate sanitation and good personal hygiene

Continued on p. 220

Table 3.88.1a *Continued*

Disease and organism	Mode of transmission	Epidemiology	Clinical	Investigation	Public health action
	develop in soil over 10–14 days. Ingested from soil or via contaminated food or water. No migration to other tissues. Adult worms may live 7 to 10 years		and diarrhoea and may retard growth. Rarely weight loss, anaemia, and rectal prolapse may occur		
Hookworm infection *Ancylostoma duodenale* or *Necator americanus*	Eggs passed in human stool hatch in 1 to 2 days and release larvae, which mature over 5 to 8 days and may then penetrate human skin (often on feet), migrate to the lungs via blood vessels, ascend to epiglottis, and are swallowed. Adult worms may live 2 to 10 years. Occasionally cat and dog hookworms may infect humans	*A. duodenale* is widely distributed in the Mediterranean, India, China, Japan, and South America. *N. americanus* is the predominant hookworm of Central and South America, southern Asia, Melanesia, the Caribbean and Polynesia. About 25% of the world's population are infected with hookworms	Most cases are asymptomatic. Migration of larvae may cause an eosinophilic pneumonia. Adult worms in the intestine may cause colicky pain, and non-specific symptoms. Chronic infection may lead to iron-deficiency anaemia and hypoproteinaemia	Depends upon recognition of the eggs in fresh stool	Preventing defecation where others may come into contact with the stool. Avoiding direct skin contact with the soil. Wearing shoes Periodic mass deworming may be effective in high-risk populations
Strongyloidiasis *Strongyloides stercoralis*	Adult worms live in the duodenum and jejunum. Released eggs hatch immediately and release larvae that are passed in	Endemic throughout the tropics and subtropics	Most cases are asymptomatic. There may be non-specific abdominal symptoms. An enteritis, protein-losing	Larvae can be identified in stool 25% of the time. Repeat examination of concentrated stool is necessary	Prevention of primary infections is as for hookworms

faeces. After a few days the larvae mature and can penetrate the skin of humans, migrate through the lungs, and reach the intestine, where they mature in about 2 weeks

Filariform larvae can bypass the soil phase and directly penetrate the colon or the skin

Transmission is often due to exposure of bare skin to larvae in contaminated soil in unsanitary conditions

Faecal–oral transmission may occur in mental institutions and day care centres

Self-reinfection may occur and can result in extremely high worm burdens (hyperinfection syndrome)

enteropathy, urticaria and pulmonary symptoms are seen less frequently. Larva currens, a serpiginous, migratory, urticarial lesion, is pathognomonic

Hyperinfection produces serious gastrointestinal symptoms including haemorrhage, pulmonary infiltration, and hepatitis and may involve the CNS. Even with treatment the mortality is over 50%

The hyperinfection syndrome and disseminated strongyloidiasis are seen in persons with impaired immunity

Immunosuppression may lead to overwhelming hyperinfection in persons with previously asymptomatic infection

To prevent the serious hyperinfection syndrome, patients with possible exposure to *Strongyloides* (even in the distant past) should undergo several stool examinations and, if necessary, a string test or duodenal aspiration before receiving immunosuppressive therapy, including steroids

Continued on p. 222

Table 3.88.1a Continued

Disease and organism	Mode of transmission	Epidemiology	Clinical	Investigation	Public health action
Trichinosis *Trichinella* spp., especially *T. spiralis*	From eating undercooked meat from infected carnivores. Larvae develop in the small intestine, penetrate the mucosa, and become adults in 6 to 8 days. Mature females release living larvae for 4–6 weeks, before dying or being expelled. Newborn larvae travel to striated muscle cells, where they encyst over 1 to 3 months. The cycle continues when encysted larvae are ingested by another carnivore	Trichinosis occurs worldwide. The life cycle is maintained by animals that feed on (e.g., pigs) or that hunt (e.g., bears, boars) other animals whose striated muscles contain encysted infective larvae (e.g., rodents). There have been outbreaks in Europe associated with imported horsemeat	Gastrointestinal symptoms are absent or mild; nausea, abdominal cramps, and diarrhoea may occur during the first week. The characteristic syndrome of periorbital oedema, myalgia, fever, and subconjunctival haemorrhages and petechiae appears in weeks 2–3 Soreness may affect the muscles of respiration, speech, mastication, and swallowing. Heavy infection may cause severe dyspnoea, multi-system disease, or fatal myocarditis Most symptoms and signs resolve by the 3rd month	There are no specific tests for the intestinal stage of trichinosis. Eosinophilia usually begins when newborn larvae invade tissues, peaks 2 to 4 weeks after infection, and gradually declines. Muscle enzymes are elevated in 50% of patients A muscle biopsy may disclose larvae, inflammation and cysts. Serologic tests can give false-negative results, especially if testing is done early. Serologic tests are of most value if they are initially negative and then turn positive	Trichinosis is prevented by cooking meat thoroughly (55°C [140° F] throughout). Larvae can also be killed by freezing at −15°C (5°F) for 3 weeks or −18°C (0° F) for 1 day Meat should be inspected before being sold There is no person-to-person spread Investigate clusters for a common contaminated food source

Table 3.88.1b Tapeworms (cestodes)

Disease and organism	Mode of transmission	Epidemiology	Clinical	Investigation	Public health action
Taeniasis *T. saginata* *T. solium*	Infection is acquired by eating undercooked infected pork or beef	Occurs in most countries where beef or pork is eaten undercooked. Rare in NW Europe	Adult *T. saginata* (beef tapeworm) may grow to 10 m and *T. solium* (pork tapeworm) to 4 m, but infection is usually asymptomatic Abdominal pains are sometimes reported. Detached motile segments (proglottids) of *T. saginata* may be noticed as they emerge from the anus	Infections are usually diagnosed because of eggs or proglottids in the faeces	Basic hygienic precautions Exclusion of cases of pork tapeworm in risk groups 1–4 (see Box 2.2.1) until treated Regular deworming of pets
Dwarf tapeworm *Hymenolepsis nana*	Eggs excreted in human faeces are infectious. May spread faeco–orally or via contaminated food. May be autoinfection	Imported from Asia, SE Europe, Africa or Latin America Occasionally found in institutions or immunocompromised	Asymptomatic or mild abdominal discomfort. May be anorexia, dizziness, diarrhoea	Identification of characteristic eggs in stool	Basic hygiene precautions Exclusion of risk groups 1–4 until treated Consider screening household
Fish tapeworm *Diphyllobothrium latum*	Acquired by eating undercooked fish	Worldwide, rare in NW Europe	Causes B12 deficiency	Identification of eggs in the faeces	Avoiding raw, smoked or undercooked fish

Continued on p. 224

Table 3.88.1b *Continued*

Disease and organism	Mode of transmission	Epidemiology	Clinical	Investigation	Public health action
Cysticercosis: Disease due to the pork tapeworm (*T. solium*)	If eggs excreted by a human carrier of the pork tapeworm are ingested the cysticerci preferentially settle in skeletal muscle and central nervous system, where they act as space occupying lesions	Occurs in most countries where beef or pork is eaten undercooked and person-to-person transmission occurs. Rare in NW Europe	Clinical features may include epilepsy, raised intracranial pressure and chronic basal meningitis	Diagnosis has been much advanced by modern brain imaging techniques, which may be supported by serology or by evidence of cysticerci in other tissues. Definitive identification of parasite segments and eggs, and serology is available from reference laboratory	
Hydatid disease: Disease due to the dog tapeworm *Echinococcus granulosus*, or *E. multilocularis*	Humans acquire hydatid cysts, the metacestodes of *Echinococcus* spp. by ingesting eggs excreted in the faeces of an infected dog	Found in most sheep- and cattle-raising parts of the word	The commonest sites for hydatid cysts are liver, lung and bone. The cysts expand slowly over several years. Occasionally leaks occur which may cause hypersensitivity phenomena such as generalized urticaria and can seed further cysts at distant sites. Symptoms are most often due to the mass effect of the lesion	An appropriate imaging technique, such as ultrasound of the abdomen, will reveal the diagnosis, and may be supported by serology	Treatment of hydatid disease and cysticercosis should be undertaken by specialists. Most cases will be acquired. Poor hygiene and close contact with infected animals and ingestion of undercooked infected meat are all risk factors
Sparganosis *Spirometra*	Infection by larvae of *Spirometra* tapeworm	Human infection results from use of flesh of an infected frog as poultice (SE Asia), or exposure to contaminated water	Larvae develop into cysts in subcutaneous tissue		Avoid frog poultices

Table 3.88.1c Filariae

Disease and organism	Mode of transmission	Epidemiology	Clinical	Investigation	Public health action
Lymphatic filariasis (elephantiasis), *Wuchereria bancrofti, Brugia malayi*	Adult worms inhabit the lymphatics, and the microfilariae, which have a strong diurnal periodicity, appear briefly in the peripheral blood around midnight when they can be ingested by mosquitos which are the vectors	*Wuchereria bancrofti* has a widespread distribution in South Asia, the Pacific islands, tropical Africa and some parts of South America. Two species of *Brugia*, restricted to South-East Asia, give rise to a similar syndrome	Cause of elephantiasis. Fever and lymphangitis may occur early in the disease. The most serious consequences are the chronic sequelae of lymphatic damage caused by dying worms. Gross lymphoedema, most often of the legs or genitals, and chyluria are typical features	Definitive diagnosis is by recognition of the microfilariae in a midnight sample of blood. Serology provides supportive evidence but there may be cross-reactions with other nematode infections	Eliminating vector breeding sites
Onchocerciasis (river blindness), *Onchocerca volvulus*	Microfilariae in the skin are ingested by a black fly of the genus *Simulium*. These are the insect vectors	Primarily an African disease although there are some foci in Central America	The adult *Onchocerca* lives in the subcutaneous tissues. Clinical consequences are caused by the inflammation resulting from death of the microfilariae. In the skin this causes a chronic dermatitis. Most significant is damage to the eye. The inflammatory process may involve all the structures between the cornea and the optic nerve. Blindness occurs after 20 years or more of heavy infection	Diagnosis depends on detecting microfilariae in superficial snips of skin	Eliminating vector breeding sites

Continued on p. 226

Table 3.88.1c *Continued*

Disease and organism	Mode of transmission	Epidemiology	Clinical	Investigation	Public health action
Loiasis *Loa loa*, (African eye worm)	Adult *Loa loa* are migratory and roam widely in the subcutaneous tissues and may become visible on passing under the conjunctiva of the eye. The microfilariae appear with a diurnal periodicity in the blood around midday	Rain forests of West and Central Africa	Many cases asymptomatic, symptoms include 'Calabar swellings', diffuse areas of subcutaneous oedema, usually distally on the limbs, which last a few days	Diagnosis is by recognizing the microfilariae in midday blood	Eliminating vector breeding sites
Dracontiasis *Dracunculus medinensis* (Guinea worm)	The disease is acquired by drinking water containing *Cyclops* which harbour larvae. These invade, develop into adults and mate. The gravid female, about 60 cm long, then makes her way to the lower extremities where she penetrates to the surface, giving rise to an irritating ulcer. Contact with water causes her to release larvae through this defect where they may be able to infect new *Cyclops*	Indian subcontinent, Africa	The chronic ulceration, and associated secondary infection, may be a severe problem in conditions of poor hygiene. Death of the worm causes intense inflammation	Recognition of larvae or adult worm	Provision of clean drinking water

3.88.2 Protozoa
(Table 3.88.2, pp. 228–230)

Leishmaniasis oriental sore

Leishmania are flagellate protozoan parasites. The major species are *L. donovani*, the causative agent of kala-azar, *L. tropica* and *L. major*: causing Old World cutaneous leishmaniasis and *L. brazilienzis*, the agent of New world cutaneous (American) leishmaniasis.

Trypanosomiasis

There are three trypanosomes that are pathogenic to man. *T. brucei* gambiense and *T. brucei* rhodesiense are transmitted to man through the bite of a blood-sucking fly of the *Glossina* genus (tsetse fly). *T. cruzi* infects man by inoculation of faeces from its blood-sucking insect vector, the triatomid bug.

Babesiosis

Infection with bovine or rodent *Babesia* spp., which cause a malaria-like illness.

3.88.3 Fungi
(Table 3.88.3, pp. 231–232)

In addition to the common superficial fungal infections, a number of fungal species are implicated in deep-seated disease processes. These include ubiquitous organisms, such as *Candida* and *Aspergillus*, which are only invasive in an immunocompromised host; specifically in neutropenia or T-cell defects. Others occur as specific infectious entities in apparently otherwise healthy individuals, often within a confined geographical range; these primary deep pathogens are usually acquired by the respiratory route. Almost all fungal pathogens can cause opportunist infections.

None of these agents spread person to person.

Table 3.88.2a Protozoa

Disease and organism	Incubation period	Infectious period	Mode of transmission	Epidemiology	Clinical	Investigation	Public health action
Visceral leishmaniasis	Usually 2–4 months 10 days to 1 year	As long as there are parasites present, this may be many years. Person-to-person spread is reported	Transmitted to man by the bite of a sand fly. Infective blood meals may come from another man or an animal reservoir host. This may be a dog or rodent, depending on the species of *Leishmania*.	Tropical and subtropical areas. Mediterranean, Middle East, Indian sub-continent	A primary lesion resembling cutaneous leishmaniasis may occur. The onset is usually insidious. Patients present with anorexia malaise and weight loss, and may complain of abdominal discomfort due to splenic enlargement. Anaemia and cachexia are present and the liver and spleen are enlarged. Fever is intermittent and undulant with often two spikes in one day. Untreated patients undergo a slow decline and die usually from secondary infections after about 2 years	Amastigotes of *Leishmania donovani* may be found by direct microscopy of bone marrow or splenic aspirate. Occasionally amastigotes may be demonstrated in the buffy coat cells. The leishmanin reaction is usually negative, due to failure of cell-mediated immunity	Measures to break transmission cycle. Cover the cutaneous lesion. No isolation required. Rare direct person-to-person spread
Cutaneous leishmaniasis	A few days to more than 6 months		Direct person-to-person spread may occur		The lesions begin as a small itching papule with increasing infiltration of the dermis. The lesion becomes crusted which, when scratched, produces a shallow discharging ulcer. A variety of different clinical courses follows	Laboratory diagnosis is made by split skin smear, with culture on Schneider's insect medium. Antibody titres using indirect fluorescent antibody test may also be helpful. Culture in special medium should also be performed	

Table 3.88.2b Trypanosomiasis

Disease and organism	Incubation period	Mode of transmission	Epidemiology	Clinical	Investigation	Public health action
African trypanosomiasis *Trypanosoma brucei gambiense*	Few days to months	Bite of the tsetse fly	Man is the main reservoir of infection; it is an infection of river and lakeside areas of West and Central Africa	The symptoms and signs are similar. Gambiense infection runs a chronic course and can last several years. Rhodesiense infection: acute, untreated infection can cause death in a few months and usually before one year. Initial sign is a papule that develops into an indurated nodule (chancre) at the bite site. The diagnosis should be suspected in a patient with fever and lymphadenopathy who has recently resided in an endemic area. Death occurs as a result of encephalitis, which may be insidious	Parasites may be demonstrated by Giemsa-stained films of the peripheral blood during the early stages of infection, in the CSF, and sometimes in a lymph node aspirate. Serologic tests (immunofluorescent assay [IFA], enzyme-linked immunosorbent assay [ELISA], card agglutination) are useful.	Control strategies are based on the elimination of the tsetse flies. There are no control implications outside endemic areas. No person-to-person spread
Trypanosoma brucei rhodesiense	Few days to two to three weeks	Bite of the tsetse fly	Found in Southern and Eastern Africa. The reservoir of infection is in wild antelope, particularly the bushbuck			
South American trypanosomiasis *Trypanosoma cruzi* is the aetiological agent of South American trypanosomiasis or Chagas disease	1–2 weeks for acute disease Many years for chronic	Triatomid bugs live in cracks in poorly constructed houses in South America and excrete infective organisms in their faeces. These are inoculated into the bite when the victim scratches. Trypanosomes can also be transmitted by transfusion of blood and blood products		In many instances acute infection is asymptomatic or unrecognized. A local inflammatory reaction at the site of the bite with regional lymphadenopathy, generalized adenopathy and hepatomegaly may also be found. Acute infection is complicated by myocarditis in about 15% of cases, and most deaths are due to this complication. The latent stage follows and this asymptomatic period may last for up to 25 years. The final stage, Chagas disease, is characterized by cardiomyopathy, and intractable congestive cardiac failure	Examination of Giemsa-stained preparations of peripheral blood for parasites. Parasites may be concentrated by centrifugation and lysis of the red cells. *T. cruzi* may be cultured *in vitro* or in mice. In xenobiotic culture laboratory-reared triatomid bugs are fed on the patient with suspected disease. After 30 days the bugs are killed and trypomastigotes are sought in the insect's gut. An ELISA is available to detect antibodies to *T. cruzi* in serum—this is most useful in excluding Chagas disease in patients who have lived in endemic countries, and in seroepidemiological surveys	South American trypanosomiasis may be controlled by improving the quality of housing construction, thus removing vector breeding sites, together with spraying of houses with residual insecticide. There are no control implications outside endemic areas. No person-to-person spread

Table 3.88.2c Babesiosis

Disease and organism	Incubation period	Mode of transmission	Epidemiology	Clinical	Investigation	Public health action
Babesia spp.	1–2 weeks	Voles are the principal natural reservoir, and deer ticks the usual vectors	Endemic in parts of the USA (New England, Wisconsin, Georgia, and California). Other *Babesia* spp. infect humans in some parts of Europe (Ireland, Yugoslavia). Babesiosis can also be transmitted by blood transfusion	Malaise, fatigue, rigors, myalgia, and arthralgia. Hepatosplenomegaly with jaundice, mild to moderately severe haemolytic anaemia, mild neutropenia, and thrombocytopenia may occur. Infection may be life-threatening in asplenic persons	Diagnosis is made by finding *Babesia* in blood smears. Methods to detect parasite DNA in blood after PCR are available	Asplenic persons should avoid endemic areas. Use insect repellents. Wear protective clothing. Search the body for ticks after exposure. No person-to-person spread

Table 3.88.3 Fungi

Disease and organism	Incubation period	Mode of transmission and reservoir	Epidemiology	Clinical	Investigation	Public health action
Aspergillosis	Days to weeks	Inhalation of organism Found in damp hay and decaying vegetation	Occurs worldwide, including UK	Chronic pulmonary disease. Invasive disease in the immunocompromised	Serum precipitins Microscopy of sputum. Culture confirmation	Some species produce carcinogenic aflatoxins on foods. Clusters of cases may occur where immunocompromised patients are gathered together. Environmental investigation should be carried out to determine the source
Blastomycosis	Weeks to many months	Inhalation of organism	Central and SE USA, Central and S. Africa, India, Near and Middle East	Picture similar to TB	Microscopy. Serology may be misleading because of cross-reactions with other fungi	Identify likely exposure—often not determined
Coccidioidomycosis	Weeks to years	Inhalation of organism	N & S America Arid and desert areas. Occupational exposure in farmers etc.	Reactivations seen in HIV-positive individuals	Culture Laboratory should be warned if suspected	Anti-dust measures in endemic areas
Histoplasmosis	Weeks to years	*Histoplasma capsulatum* can be found in soil and in bird and bat droppings. Infection is acquired by the inhalation of spores; bat caves are sometimes identified as the source	Principally a disease of the Americas	Asymptomatic infection is very common in endemic areas. Illness may take the form of an acute pneumonia, a chronic, often apical, chest infection mimicking tuberculosis or, in the immunocompromised, a fulminant disseminated infection. Resolution of the pneumonia may leave multiple miliary calcifications visible on the chest X-ray	Culture Laboratory should be warned if suspected	Identify likely exposure—often not determined

Continued on p. 232

Table 3.88.3 *Continued*

Actinomycosis and nocardiosis	Actinomycetes are a group of bacteria that were formerly classified with fungi because they can be cultured on fungal media and they form long branching chains. Species of *Actinomyces* are amongst the causes of mycetoma (see below). *Actinomyces israelii* typically causes multiple abscesses around the mouth, in the chest, or at the terminal ileum. *Nocardia asteroides* causes severe systemic opportunistic infections and occasionally chronic chest infections in the immunocompetent	No particular public health action
Mycetoma	Localized chronic granulomatous infections with multiple discharging sinuses and slowly progressive destruction of underlying structures including bone occur in many tropical countries and are known collectively as mycetomas. They may be caused by true fungi such as *Madurella mycetoma*, or by actinomycetes (see above) such as *Streptomyces somaliensis* or *Nocardia brasiliensis*. Organisms are inoculated through the skin, typically by thorns. After some delay, a painless swelling appears which subsequently breaks down and discharges pus. A network of sinuses and chronic inflammatory tissue extends over a period of months, destroying surrounding structures. Bacterial secondary infection commonly exacerbates the problem. The commonest site for mycetoma is the foot. Drug treatment will differ markedly according to the organism so that accurate microbiological diagnosis is essential	No particular public health action
Opportunistic mycoses	Fungal infection is associated with immunosupression. Immunosupression may be due to underlying disease, malignancy, diabetes mellitus or HIV, or pharmacological. Patients are being treated for an increasing variety of conditions with immunosuppressive agents. In these patients the diagnosis of fungal infection is frequently made post-mortem. Fungal infection should be considered in all immunosuppressed patients with an unexplained fever. Diagnostic tests for fungi are improving and mycological advice should be sought early so that appropriate specimens are sent. *Candida* septicaemia in a transplant recipient or periorbital mucormycosis in a diabetic require prompt treatment if the patient is to survive	
Aspergillosis	Invasive aspergillosis most frequently involves the lungs and sinuses. This fungus may disseminate and involve the brain, kidneys, liver, heart, and bones. Neutropenia due to cytotoxic chemotherapy and systemic corticosteroids are predisposing factors for invasive aspergillosis	No particular public health action
Candidiasis	*Candida albicans* is the most common cause of candidiasis. Candidiasis may be classified as superficial or deep. The alimentary tract and intravascular catheters are the main routes of entry for visceral candidiasis. The main predisposing factors are prolonged courses of broad-spectrum antibiotics, vascular catheters, cytotoxic chemotherapy, and corticosteroids	No particular public health action
Cryptococcal meningitis	Principally a disease of the immunosuppressed and now occurs most commonly in AIDS. Clinically it is in many ways analogous to tuberculous meningitis with a similar subacute onset and CSF findings. Cryptococcal yeast cells can often be demonstrated on direct microscopy by India ink staining but antigen detection is also routinely available and is more sensitive	No particular public health action
Zygomycosis/ mucormycosis	Due to *Rhizopus, Rhizomucor, Absidia, Mucor* species, causes invasive sinopulmonary infections such as the rhinocerebral syndrome, which occurs in diabetics with ketoacidosis	No particular public health action

3.88.4 Rare viruses

(see the Table below)

Table 3.88.4 Rare potentially imported viral infections

Viral species	Infection	Clinical	Incubation period	Public health action	Vector/ transmission	Geographical spread
Arenaviridae	Junin, Machupo, Sabia virus	Fever, prostration and haemorrhagic features	7–16 days	Rare person-to-person spread	Wild rodents	S America
	Lymphocytic choriomeningitis	Menin-goencephalitis	8–13 days	Look for source No person-to-person spread	Common house mouse, hamster, cell lines	US, S America, Europe
Bunyaviridae	Bunyamwera virus	Fever, headache, non-specific	3–12 days	No person-to-person spread	Mosquito	All continents except Australia and Antarctica
	Oropouche	Fever, headache, non-specific	3–12 days	No person-to-person spread	Midge	Central & S America
	Phleboviruses: Sandfly fever	Fever, headache, non-specific	3–12 days	No person-to-person spread	*Phlebotomus* flies and mosquitoes	Africa and some parts of Asia Mediterranean
	Rift Valley fever	Fever, haem-orrhagic features	3–12 days	No person-to-person spread ACDP guidelines	Handling animal tissues	Central Asia Africa
	California encephalitis LaCrosse virus	Meningo-encephalitis	5–15 days	No person-to-person spread	Mosquito	Mid-west US
Flaviviridae	Powassan encephalitis (POW)	Fever, encephalitis	7–14 days	No person-to-person spread	Tick-borne (*Ixodes*)	US, Canada, Russia
	Russian spring–summer encephalitis	Fever encephalitis	7–14 days	No person-to-person spread	Tick-borne (*Ixodes*)	Russia
	Louping III	Fever encephalitis	7–14 days	No person-to-person spread	Tick-borne (*Ixodes*)	UK
	St. Louis encephalitis	Encephalitis, hepatitis	5–15 days	No person-to-person spread	Mosquito	Americas
	Omsk haemorrhagic fever	Fever, diarrhoea, vomiting, haemorrhage	3–8 days	No person-to-person spread	Tick bite	Far East
	Kyasanur Forest disease	Fever, diarrhoea, vomiting, haemorrhage	3–8 days	No person-to-person spread	Tick bite	Far East
	West Nile fever	Fever, meningism	3–12 days	No person-to-person spread	Mosquito	Eastern Europe, East Mediterranean, eastern USA

Continued on p. 234

Table 3.88.4 *Continued*

Viral species	Infection	Clinical	Incubation period	Public health action	Vector/ transmission	Geographical spread
Paramyxo-viridae	Hendra virus Nipah virus	High fever, myalgia, respiratory disease, encephalitis	4–18 days	No person-to-person spread	Horses Pigs ?Fruitbats	Australia Malaysia
Poxviridae	Monkeypox	Fever, rash	?	Occasional person-to-person transmission	? Monkeys and squirrels	Central Africa
Togaviridae	Eastern equine encephalitis Western equine encephalitis	Fever, encephalitis	5–15 days	No person-to-person transmission	Mosquito	US and Canada
	Venezuelan equine encephalitis	Fever, chills, encephalitis	2–6 days	No person-to-person spread	Mosquito	S and Central americas

3.88.5 Bites, stings and venoms

Epidemiology

Although western Europe has few indigenous venomous species, the pet trade has increased the likelihood of exposure to exotic animals which may bite or sting.

Bites

Human, dog and cat

These bites frequently become infected. The bite should be cleaned and dead tissue removed. Infecting organisms are usually derived from the oral flora; these may include streptococci, *Pasteurella* and anaerobes. Antibiotics covering the likely organisms should be given if there is evidence of infection.

Venomous snakes

There are few venomous snakes in Europe; however, bites may arise from imported snakes. Venomous snakebites are medical emergencies; a poisons centre should be contacted. The symptoms and signs depend upon the species and size of snake, the volume of venom injected, the location of the bite (central bites tend to be more severe than peripheral), the age, size and health of the victim.

The victim should avoid exertion and be urgently moved to the nearest medical facility. Rings, watches, and constrictive clothing should be removed and the injured part immobilized in a functional position just below heart level. Tourniquets, incision and suction are contraindicated.

Attempts should be made to identify the snake so that the appropriate antivenom can be provided.

Spiders

Venomous spiders may be introduced as novelty pets. In the event of a bite every attempt should be made to identify the spider and a poisons centre should be contacted.

Other arthropods

There are a large number of other biting

arthropods, mosquitoes, fleas, lice, bedbugs sand flies, horseflies, none of these are venomous. The lesions produced vary from small papules to large ulcers, dermatitis may also occur, bites can be complicated by sensitivity reactions or infection; in hypersensitive persons, they can be fatal.

Ticks

Ticks may transmit infection such as Lyme disease or relapsing fever. Ascending flaccid paralysis may occur when toxin-secreting ticks remain attached for several days. Symptoms and signs include anorexia, lethargy, weakness, incoordination, and ascending flaccid paralysis. Tick paralysis may be confused with Guillain–Barré syndrome, botulism, myasthenia gravis, or spinal cord tumour. Bulbar or respiratory paralysis may develop.

Tick paralysis is rapidly reversible on removal of the tick (or ticks) and may require only symptomatic treatment.

Mites

Mite bites are common. Chiggers are mite larvae that feed in the skin, causing a pruritic dermatitis. There may be sensitization.

Centipedes and millipedes

Some centipedes can inflict a painful bite, with some localized swelling and erythema. Lymphangitis and lymphadenitis are common. Millipedes may secrete a toxin that can cause local skin irritation and, in severe cases, marked erythema, vesiculation, and necrosis. Some species can spray a secretion that causes conjunctival reactions.

Stings

Bees, wasps

The average person can tolerate c. 20 stings/kg body weight. One sting can cause a fatal anaphylactic reaction in a hypersensitive person.

Stings may remain in the skin and should be removed. An ice cube will reduce pain. Persons known to be hypersensitive should carry epinephrine with them.

Scorpions

Stings from pet scorpions should be treated as potentially dangerous as the species may be difficult to determine. The victim should be observed. Information on antivenoms should be obtained from a poisons centre.

3.88.6 Chemical food-borne illness

Scombrotoxin fish poisoning

Caused by excess histamine, leading to diarrhoea, flushing, headache and sweating, sometimes accompanied by nausea, abdominal pain, burning in the mouth, tingling and palpitations. Onset is 10 min to 2 h after consumption and symptoms usually resolve over 12 h. Antihistamines may reduce severity. Excess histamine typically results from inadequate refrigeration of tuna, mackerel and other fish. Histamine level of fish can be tested.

Paralytic shellfish poisoning

Caused by saxitoxins produced by certain algae. Causes neurological symptoms: dizziness, tingling, drowsiness and muscular paralysis. Severe cases may suffer respiratory failure and death. May occasionally be gastrointestinal symptoms. Onset is 30 min to 2 h after consumption. Usually due to consumption of filter-feeding bivalve shellfish or crustacea (e.g. mussels, clams, oysters, scallops and crabs) that have consumed the algae, sometimes after 'red tides'. Saxitoxins can be measured in shellfish by specialist laboratory.

Diarrhetic shellfish poisoning

Caused by okadaic acid and other toxins

in algae. Causes diarrhoea, nausea, vomiting and abdominal pain, with onset 30 min to 12 h after consumption. Illness lasts 3–4 days. Usually associated with eating shellfish, often after 'red tides'. Toxin may be detected in shellfish.

Phytohaemagglutinin poisoning

Due to inadequate preparation of pulses such as red kidney beans, butter beans and lentils. Causes nausea and vomiting, followed by abdominal pain and diarrhoea, with onset 30 min to 12 h after consumption.

Mushroom poisoning

Due to cyclopeptides and amatoxins consumed in *Amanita phalloides* (death cap), *Amanita verna*, *Amanita virosa* and some *Galerina* and *Lepiota* species. Causes colic, nausea, vomiting and diarrhoea, which after apparent recovery may be followed by liver or kidney failure with appreciable mortality. The advice of a regional poisons centre is vital for both investigation and treatment.

Others

• Gastrointestinal illness due to heavy metal poisoning (e.g. from food containers).
• Intoxication (alcohol-like) due to mushrooms.
• Gastrointestinal, liver and renal illness due to aflatoxins (e.g. fungal contamination of cereals).
• Neurological illness due to pesticides.
• Ciguatera fish poisoning (Americas, Australia, Pacific).
• Amnesiac shellfish poisoning (North America).
• Puffer fish poisoning (Japan).

3.88.7 Bioterrorism agents

(see the Table below)

Table 3.88.7 Potential bioterrorism organisms and toxins

Agent (disease)	Potential source	Ability to cause disease	Incubation period	Ability to spread from person to person	Prophylaxis	Further details
Bacillus anthracis (anthrax)	Aerosol (spores)	Moderate	2–7 days	None	Penicillin Ciprofloxacin Doxycycline	Chapter 3.2
Brucella spp. (brucellosis)	Aerosol Food	High	5–60 days	None	Ciprofloxacin Doxycycline	Chapter 3.5
Burkholderia (melioidosis)	Aerosol	High	1–7 days	Negligible	Ciprofloxacin Doxycycline	Stable agent of variable severity
Chlamydia psittaci (psittacosis)	Aerosol	Moderate	6–15 days	Negligible	Doxycycline	Chapter 3.9
Clostridium botulinum toxin (botulism)	Food/water Aerosol	High	2 hours to 10 days	None	Antiserum	Chapter 3.4
Coccidioides immitis (coccidioidomycosis)	Aerosol	High	1–2 weeks plus	None	Fluconazole	Table 3.88.3
Coxiella burnetii (Q fever)	Aerosol Food supply	High	14–39 days	Negligible	Doxycycline	Chapter 3.59
Ebola/Lassa/ CCHF (viral haemorrhagic fevers)	Aerosol	High	2–21 days	Moderate (body fluids)	None	Chapter 3.82
Francisella tularensis (tularaemia)	Aerosol	High	3–14 days	None	Doxycycline	Chapter 3.79
Hantavirus	Aerosol	High	4–42 days	None	None	Chapter 3.26
Histoplasma capsulatum (histoplasmosis)	Aerosol	High	1–2 weeks plus	None	Fluconazole	Table 3.88.3
Influenza virus	Aerosol	High	1–5 days	High (respiratory)	Amantadine (A) Zanamivir (A/B)	Chapter 3.38
Rickettsia prowazekii (typhus)	Aerosol Infected vectors	High	1–2 weeks	None	Doxycycline	Chapter 3.81
Rickettsia rickettsii (Rocky Mountain spotted fever)	Aerosol Infected vectors	High	3–14 days	None	Doxycycline	Table 3.81.1
Rickettsia tsutsugamushi (scrub typhus)	Aerosol Infected vectors	High	6–21 days	None	Doxycycline	Table 3.81.1

Continued on p. 238

Table 3.88.7 *Continued*

Agent (disease)	Potential source	Ability to cause disease	Incubation period	Ability to spread from person to person	Prophylaxis	Further details
Salmonella spp. (gastro-enteritis)	Food Water	Low	6–72 hours	Moderate (faeco–oral)	Ciprofloxacin	Chapter 3.66
Salmonella typhi (typhoid)	Food/water Aerosol	Moderate	1–3 weeks	Low (faeco–oral)	Ciprofloxacin	Chapter 3.80
Shigella spp. (dysentery)	Food Water	High	12–96 hours	High (faeco–oral)	Ciprofloxacin	Chapter 3.68
Variola virus (smallpox)	Aerosol	High	10–17 days	High (aerosol)	Vaccine	Chapter 3.69
Staphylococcal enterotoxin B	Sabotage Aerosol	High	1–7 hours	None	None	Chapter 3.71
Vibrio cholerae (cholera)	Food/water Aerosol	Low	6–48 hours	Low (faeco–oral)	Ciprofloxacin Doxycycline	Chapter 3.11
VTEC (haemorrhagic gastroenteritis)	Food Water	High	1–9 days	High (faeco–oral)	None	Chapter 3.23
Yersinia pestis (plague)	Aerosol Vectors	High	1–6 days	High (pneumonic)	Ciprofloxacin Doxycycline	Chapter 3.56

Section 4
Services and organizations

4.1 Administrative arrangements for communicable disease control

Communicable disease control in the community is a complex activity which relies on co-operation and collaboration between many different agencies and individuals. Individuals and organizations listed in Table 4.1.1 are a source of surveillance data, they diagnose and treat infections, they implement control of infection measures, they take action to prevent infections, they give advice and they enforce legislation. In turn they need information, advice, practical assistance and training. The key agencies for each European country are given in the relevent chapter of section 5.

Health authorities

In England and Wales there are 105 health authorities serving populations that vary in size between 170000 and 1000000. Health authorities are public bodies appointed by and accountable to the Secretary of State for Health. They are responsible for assessing the health needs of their resident population and commissioning an appropriate range, quantity and quality of services to meet those needs. Health authorities, in collaboration with other agencies, protect public health by controlling communicable disease and infection and managing the human health aspects of other environmental hazards. This includes ensuring the following.
• They appoint a Consultant for Communicable Disease Control (CCDC) within their department of public health. The CCDC is responsible for the surveillance, prevention and control of communicable disease and infection within the health authority boundaries. They should have administrative support and may employ a scientist and a community infection control nurse (CICN).
• There are satisfactory and properly re-sourced arrangements for the surveillance, control and prevention of communicable diseases within the community, including general practice.
• There are up-to-date joint plans with the local authority for managing communicable disease incidents and outbreaks.
• There are adequate infection control arrangements within local hospitals.
• There are named co-ordinators for immunization and HIV services.

Primary Care Groups (PCGs) started work in April 1999. PCGs are groupings of general practices serving areas with populations of about 100000. Their role is to improve health, reduce inequalities, improve the quality of primary and community health services and to commission hospital services. They also have responsibility for some preventative services, including immunization. PCGs are assuming many of the functions of health authorities and in time they will become Primary Care Trusts (PCTs). PCTs in partnership with schools, local authority departments and local employers will play an increasingly important part in health improvement.

Health authorities will continue as strategic bodies. At the present time it is planned that they will retain responsibility for communicable disease control, genito-urinary medicine (GUM) services and tuberculosis services.

Hospital and community trusts

NHS healthcare providers are run as non-profit making trusts and include acute hospitals and trusts providing healthcare in the community.

Hospital trusts have agreements with health authorities which require satisfactory infection control arrangements. Arrangements in community trusts vary but they should have an infection control doctor (ICD) and infection control team (ICT) cover. They may employ a CICN or by agreement receive a service from the CCDC and his/her team.

The CCDC

The CCDC is a source of advice on all aspects of

Table 4.1.1 Agencies, individuals and organizations involved in communicable disease control

Health authority community	Consultant for Communicable Disease Control, Infection Control Nurse
Hospitals	Medical microbiologist, Infection Control Doctor, Infection Control Nurse, infectious disease specialist, TB specialist, genito-urinary medicine specialist
Community trusts	Health visitors, district nurses, school health nurses and doctors, TB nurse advisers
Local authority departments (environmental health, education, social services)	Environmental health officers, proper officer (usually the CCDC), teachers, social workers, home carers, residential home managers, safety managers
Local public health laboratory	Medical microbiologist
Public Health Laboratory Service	Medical microbiologist
PHLS Communicable Disease Surveillance Centre	Consultant epidemiologist, regional or national
Primary care	General practitioners, practice nurses and other practice staff, community pharmacists, general dental practitioners
Private nursing homes, residential homes	Managers, nursing staff, carers
Occupational health departments	Occupational health doctors and nurses
Day nurseries	Managers, nursery nurses
General public	Citizens, newspapers, radio, TV
Food Standards Agency	Meat hygiene service
NHS Executive	Regional and national officers, including Regional Director of Public Health
Department of Health	Medical officers
Ministry of Agriculture, Fisheries and Food	State Veterinary Service
Health and Safety Executive	Inspectors
Water companies	Quality managers

the control and prevention of infection and has full responsibility for infection control in the community. Through contracts and professional collaboration with the ICT and ICD, the CCDC will ensure that there are effective arrangements for infection control in hospitals and community trusts. He/she will be a member of the local hospital infection control committee and will co-operate with the ICT and outbreak control group in the investigation and management of outbreaks of infection in hospitals.

The key tasks of the CCDC include securing the support of hospitals and local authorities in implementing infection control within the community, ensuring that surveillance data and information are communicated to those who need to know, ensuring compliance with statutory requirements, following Department of Health (DH) and other relevant guidelines and ensuring that residential homes, nursing homes and schools have access to infection control advice and assistance (see Table 4.1.2).

Table 4.1.2 Responsibilities of CCDCs and their staff (including CICN)

Core activities	Non-core activities
Setting up and maintaining surveillance systems	District Immunization Co-ordinator
Analysing trends in infectious disease incidence	District HIV Prevention Co-ordinator
Investigation and control of outbreaks	Tuberculosis contact tracing
Proper officer for Public Health legislation	Port health
Liaison with others involved in control of infectious disease	Chemical incident planning and management
Advice to local authorities, primary care staff and public	Investigation of environmental hazards
Infection control advice and support to nursing and residential homes and schools	Emergency planning
Advice to health authority on commissioning services to prevent, control and treat infection	National Assistance Act (Section 47)
Prevention and health promotion programmes	Rehousing on medical grounds
Teaching and training	
Continuing education, audit and research	

The CCDC will usually establish a District Infection Control Committee to review and advise on district-wide infection control strategies and policies, encourage collaboration between different providers, purchasers, local authorities and other agencies and to assist the CCDC in his/her work.

General practitioners

General practitioners provide care for patients with infection including diagnosis and treatment. They notify cases of infection to the local authority proper officer, who is usually the CCDC. They advise on hygiene and other measures that patients can adopt to limit the spread of infections, they are a source of travel health advice and deliver immunization programmes.

Community nurses

Community nurses are employed by community trusts and work alongside general practitioners, usually as members of a primary healthcare team. They are a source of information on infection problems within the community and in turn need access to infection control advice. This may be provided by the CICN, the CCDC or the hospital ICT.

Local government

Local government in England and Wales is based on democratically elected councils, which are accountable to the residents that they serve. They are not directly accountable to central government but exercise their responsibilities within a broad legal framework. They are funded both by central government and locally raised revenue, the council tax.

There are 39 county councils whose functions include police, fire, education, social services, waste disposal, civil defence, highways, consumer protection and planning.

There are around 400 district councils whose functions include environmental health, housing, planning, refuse collection, cemeteries and crematoria, markets and fairs, licensing activities and leisure and recreation.

Some district councils, particularly those covering the large cities and London boroughs, also carry out county council functions (unitary authorities).

Councils consist of elected members or councillors and exercise their powers through committees, subcommittees or delegation to salaried officers. Officers acting on behalf of a council must ensure that the powers and responsibilities they exercise have been lawfully delegated to them by the elected members. Often legislation requires that the council exercises its power through a specific officer, usually referred to as the proper officer. For some public health legislation the proper officer would be the CCDC.

Environmental health departments

The responsibilities of environmental health departments include food safety, air quality, noise, waste, health and safety, water quality, port health controls at air and sea ports, refuse collection and pest control.

Environmental health officers

Environmental health officers (EHOs) are typically university graduates who have completed a period of practical training. EHOs investigate outbreaks of food and water-borne infections, they advise on and enforce food safety legislation, they routinely inspect food premises, and they investigate complaints and provide food hygiene training. EHOs liase with a wide range of other professionals including the CCDC, general practitioners, teachers, microbiologists and veterinarians.

The Public Health Laboratory Service

The PHLS aim is *to protect the population from infection*. The PHLS comprises of a network of approximately 50 public health laboratories organized into nine regional groups, together with two national centres, the Central Public Health Laboratory (CPHL) and the Communicable Disease Surveillance Centre (CDSC),

both located with the PHLS headquarters at Colindale, London.

PHLS provides information and advice to government departments to support the development of policies for the prevention and control of communicable disease.

Nearly all the public health laboratories are based in NHS Trust hospitals where they provide clinical diagnostic microbiological services to their host Trusts and local GPs. In addition, PHLSs undertake public health microbiology including the testing of food, water, milk and environmental samples for local environmental health departments and the investigation of clinical specimens from outbreaks. There are structured programmes for the microbiological surveillance of food and water.

The CPHL is the major British reference centre for microbiology, offering specialized tests and identification of unusual or difficult organisms and epidemiological typing.

CDSC was set up within PHLS in 1977, becoming the main surveillance centre, collecting, analysing and disseminating data on the occurrence and spread of communicable disease and responding rapidly to national outbreaks or international threats of infection. CDSC includes a regional services division that provides regional epidemiological services to the NHS Executive under contract (see below). CDSC provides advice and support to CCDCs, conducts national surveillance, publishes the weekly *Communicable Disease Report* (CDR) and the monthly *Communicable Disease and Public Health* and provides training and teaching in communicable disease control.

CPHL and CDSC play a leading role in international surveillance and prevention of communicable disease.

The Department of Health

In addition to its general responsibility for the provision of health services and social services the Department of Health (DH) has specific responsibility for public health, communicable disease surveillance and control, and microbiological safety of food, water and the environment. The DH makes policy, drafts legislation and issues guidance on legislation. The DH should be informed of any serious incident or outbreak of infection and will co-ordinate the national response to any hazard including food, medical supplies or drugs. This may include issuing appropriate hazard warning notices.

The National Health Service Executive

The National Health Service Executive (NHSE) is a government executive agency with overall responsibility for ensuring health services are available at local level. Regional offices of the NHS Executive provide support for the control of communicable disease through a contract for regional epidemiology services with PHLS and should be informed of significant incidents or outbreaks of infection in hospitals or the community.

The Health Development Agency

The Health Education Authority, the statutory body responsible for health education in England was replaced by a new organization, the Health Development Agency (HDA) in April 2000. The HDA's role is to raise standards in public health, and its main functions will be research, evidence, standard setting and capacity development. The HDA will not carry out direct public education. Some of the HEA's public education work, including immunization and sexual health, will transferred to a new unit, Health Promotion England.

Health and Safety Commission and Executive

The Health and Safety Commission (HSC) and Health and Safety Executive (HSE) are statutory bodies whose aims are to protect those at work and those who may be affected by any work-related activity. In particular, the HSE is the enforcement agency for the Health and Safety at Work, etc. Act 1974, the Control of Substances Hazardous to Health (COSHH) Regulations 1994 and the Management of

Health and Safety at Work (MHSW) Regulations 1994. The COSHH regulations require employers to assess the risk of infection for their employees and others, for example waste disposal workers, engineers and members of the public. The MHSW regulations require an assessment of risks to health, provision of health surveillance if appropriate and information for employees. The Reporting of Incidents, Diseases and Dangerous Occurrences Regulations 1985 (RIDDOR) require employers to report acute illness requiring medical treatment where there is reason to believe that this resulted from an exposure to a pathogen or infected material.

The CCDC may work with staff from the local HSE office when investigating cases of infection (e.g. *Legionella* infection) that may be linked to a particular workplace.

Occupational Health Services

Occupational Health Services (OHSs) advise managers and employees about the effect of work on health and of health on work. They devise risk management programmes to ensure that the hazards which staff face during their work are minimized. Within the NHS, OHSs are responsible for ensuring that at-risk staff are immunized against hepatitis B.

Food Standards Agency

A Food Standards Agency was set up in the UK in April 2000 to protect public health from all risks connected with the consumption of food. It will do this by providing independent advice and information to the public and to Government on food safety, nutrition and diet. It will also monitor food safety and enforce standards throughout the food chain and promote accurate food labelling.

The Meat Hygiene Service

The Meat Hygiene Service (MHS) is an executive agency of the Food Standards Agency with responsibility for hygiene and animal welfare inspection and enforcement in slaughterhouses and meat cutting plants.

Ministry of Agriculture, Fisheries and Food

The main public health objectives of the Ministry of Agriculture, Fisheries and Food (MAFF) are listed below.

• To protect public health in relation to farm produce and zoonoses (in conjunction with the Food Standards Agency).

• To ensure that farmed animals and fish are protected by high welfare standards and do not suffer unnecessary pain or distress.

• To reduce risks to public health and the environment from flooding and coastal erosion.

• To safeguard the continuing availability of adequate supplies of wholesome, varied and reasonably priced food and drink.

State Veterinary Service

The State Veterinary Service (SVS) is MAFF's veterinary body dealing with all animal health and welfare matters.

4.2 Surveillance

The effective management of infectious disease depends on good surveillance. This is true whether infection occurs in hospital or the community. Surveillance has been defined as the continuing scrutiny of all aspects of the occurrence and spread of a disease through the systematic collection, collation and analysis of data and the prompt dissemination of the resulting information to those who need to know so that action can result. Surveillance has been described as information for action. To allow effective control, surveillance systems should be ongoing, practicable, consistent, timely and have sufficient accuracy and completeness.

The purpose of surveillance

• Surveillance allows individual cases of infection to be identified so that action can be taken

to prevent spread (e.g. the measures taken to limit spread following a case of tuberculosis, meningococcal infection or food-borne infection affecting a food handler).

• Surveillance measures the incidence of infectious disease. Changes in incidence may signal an outbreak which may need further investigation and the introduction of special control measures (e.g. food-borne infection, *Legionella* infection).

• Surveillance tracks changes in the occurrence and risk factors of infectious disease and can indicate if sections of the population are at increased risk of infection as a result of environmental or behavioural factors (e.g. travel-associated infections in persons of minority ethnic origin). This allows specific interventions to be targeted at those groups.

• Surveillance allows existing control measures to be evaluated, and if new control measures are introduced, continuing surveillance will allow their effectiveness to be measured (e.g. routine surveillance of vaccine-preventable infections allows the effectiveness of immunization programmes to be judged). A fall in the incidence of an infection may allow existing control measures to be relaxed.

• Surveillance allows the emergence of new infections of public health importance to be detected. It allows the epidemiology of these infections to be described and will produce hypotheses about aetiology and risk factors (e.g. HIV, vCJD).

The principles of surveillance

A good surveillance system consists of the following key steps.

• There should be a case-definition which includes clinical and/or microbiological criteria (e.g. food poisoning is defined as disease of an infectious or toxic nature caused by or thought to be caused by the consumption of food or water). Case-definitions have been published by the Public Health Medicine and Environmental Group in the UK and the Charter Group (State Epidemiologists from EU countries).

• Cases of infection are identified from a variety of sources including reports from clinicians and laboratories.

The case or an informant, who may be a relative, friend or medical or nursing attendant, is contacted by a member of the communicable disease control team by telephone, visit or letter, depending on the degree of urgency. A data set is collected for each case. The data that are collected depend on the nature of the infection. For all infections, the following minimum data set is usually collected: name; date of birth; sex; address; ethnic group; place of work; occupation; name of GP; recent travel; immunization history; date of illness; clinical description of illness.

For food-borne infections, food histories and food preferences may be recorded. For infections that are spread from person to person the names and addresses of contacts may be requested, and for infections with an environmental source such as Legionnaires' disease places visited and routes taken may be recorded. For some infections where intervention is required additional data are collected. For example, in the case of meningococcal infection the names of close household contacts may be recorded so that chemoprophylaxis and immunization may be offered.

For rare or novel infections, or where there is a need to find out more about the epidemiology, an enhanced data set may be collected or there may be a request for laboratory data to confirm the diagnosis. An example of this is the serological confirmation of clinical reports of measles, mumps and rubella using salivary antibody testing.

• Data are recorded on specially designed data collection forms and collated in a computerized database (e.g. CoSurv). Data may also be downloaded from databases used for patient management.

• One of the first uses of the data is to ensure that the cases satisfy the case-definition. The database then allows analysis of the data and the production of summary statistics including frequency counts and rates, if suitable denominators are available. This permits the epidemiology of the infection to be described in terms of person, place and time. Local data can be shared and merged to produce datasets at national or even international level.

• Interpretation of the data and summary statistics leads to information on trends and risk factors, which are disseminated so that action can be taken. Dissemination can take place in a variety of ways, including local and national newsletters, the Internet, electronic bulletin boards such as Epinet™, letters from the Chief Medical Officer and journals such as *Mortality and Morbidity Weekly Report* (MMWR), *Weekly Epidemiological Record* (WER), the *Communicable Disease Report* (CDR) *Communicable Disease and Public Health and Euro-Surveillance, the European Communicable Disease Bulletin.*

• Output of surveillance data is increasing all the time and much is available on the Internet as well as in paper form (see Section 5 for country-specific details).

• Feedback to local data providers is important. It demonstrates the usefulness of the data and creates reliance on it. This in turn will lead to improvement in case ascertainment and data quality. Many CCDCs publish a regular newsletter which may be sent to GPs, hospital clinicians, microbiologists and EHOs.

• There should be continuing surveillance to evaluate the effect of interventions.

Sources of surveillance data

A number of data sources are available for the surveillance of infectious diseases.

Many cases of infection are subclinical. These cases can only be detected by serological surveys. Clinical infection that does not lead to a medical consultation can be measured by population surveys. Cases that are seen by a doctor may be reported via a primary care reporting scheme or statutory notification system. Cases that are investigated by laboratory tests may be detected by a laboratory reporting system, and those that are admitted to hospital will be counted by a hospital information system. Finally the small proportion of infections that result in death will be detected by the death notification system.

When designing a surveillance system it is important to ensure that the most appropriate data source is utilized. For example it is not sensible to rely on laboratory reports for the surveillance of pertussis, which is only rarely diagnosed by the laboratory. In England and Wales the main routine data collecting systems are as follows.

Statutory notifications of infectious disease

The system for each European country is described in the relevent chapter of section 5. The current list of notifiable infectious diseases in England and Wales is shown in Table 4.2.1. Any clinician suspecting these diagnoses is required to notify the proper officer of the local authority, who is usually the CCDC. The proper officer sends a return to the Office of National Statistics (ONS) every week. These are published weekly in the *Communicable Disease Report* (CDR). There are also quarterly and annual reports, such as the ONS *Population and Health Monitor*. Statutory notifications are an important way of monitoring trends in infectious disease, such as measles and whooping cough, where the diagnosis is rarely confirmed by laboratory test.

Laboratory reporting system

Public Health Laboratories, NHS hospital laboratories and private laboratories should be able to offer a full diagnostic service for all common pathogenic micro-organisms. If the laboratory is unable to carry out the work, then specimens are forwarded to a suitable reference labora-tory. Medical microbiologists ensure that results of clinical significance are notified to the requesting clinician.

Micro-organisms of public health significance are also notified to the CCDC in accordance with previously agreed arrangements. This should be covered by a written policy. Typical arrangements for reporting to the CCDC are shown in Table 4.2.2. The method of reporting will vary depending on the urgency with which public health action is required. Increasingly, electronic reporting is recommended, but telephone, facsimile and letter are alternatives.

In England and Wales reports are also sent to CDSC; electronic reporting via CoSurv is now gradually replacing the old paper reporting system, and should allow significant improvements in quality and timeliness of surveillance without increasing the burden to laboratories. These data are collated and analysed and are reported regularly in the *Communicable Disease Report* or are available on request. Regular regional reports are also available. Although the data are usually of high quality, they are limited to infections for which there is a

Table 4.2.1 Statutorily notifiable infectious diseases in England and Wales

Very rare infections	Rare infections	Common infections
Anthrax	Leptospirosis	Food poisoning
Leprosy	Yellow fever	Viral hepatitis
Typhus	Cholera	Whooping cough
Relapsing fever	Diphtheria	Tuberculosis
Plague	Poliomyelitis	Malaria
Smallpox	Typhoid fever	Meningitis
Viral haemorrhagic fever	Paratyphoid fever	Meningococcal septicaemia
	Rabies	Ophthalmia neonatorum
	Tetanus	Measles
	Encephalitis	Mumps
		Dysentery (amoebic and bacillary)
		Rubella
		Scarlet fever

Table 4.2.2 Reporting of infectious diseases to the CCDC in England and Wales

During working hours
Telephone CCDC as soon as possible for

Typhoid fever	Paratyphoid fever	*E. coli* O157
Meningococcal infection	All meningitis	Hib infection
Acute hepatitis B	Legionnaires' disease	Diphtheria

Also, less commonly:

Acute poliomyelitis	Anthrax	Botulism
Psittacosis	Cholera	Leprosy
Relapsing fever	Tetanus	Typhus
Viral haemorrhagic fever	Yellow fever	

CoSurv, telephone, fax or send notification form to CCDC or Environmental Services Department for

Campylobacter	Shigellosis	Salmonellosis
Other food poisoning	Amoebic dysentery	Malaria
Mumps	Rubella	Measles
Tuberculosis	Ophthalmia neonatorum	Pertussis
Viral hepatitis (other than 'B')	Cryptosporidium	

Out of hours and at weekends
Contact on-call Public Health Physician as soon as possible for the following infections

Typhoid fever	Paratyphoid fever	Hib infection
Meningococcal infection	Toxin-producing diphtheria	

suitable laboratory test. Infections which are easy to diagnose clinically tend to be poorly covered. Trends are difficult to interpret, since the data are sensitive to changes in testing or reporting by laboratories. In addition, because data are based on place of treatment rather than place of residence, denominators are not usually available and because negatives are not reported, neither the number of specimens tested nor the population at risk is known with certainty.

Reporting from general practice

In both England and Wales there are systems which collect data on initial consultations from a limited number of volunteer general practices. The data can be related to a defined population so that rates can be calculated for a selection of common diseases which are not notifiable, for which laboratory confirmation is not usually obtained and which do not usually result in admission to hospital. These are listed in Table 4.2.3. The data are published in

the ONS *Population and Health Monitor*. Around 70 general practices participate, covering a population of 600 000. This population is too small for the surveillance of less common diseases and may not be representative of the country as a whole. However, the system is particularly useful for monitoring seasonal trends in respiratory infections such as influenza.

Hospital data

Data are available from district and regional information systems on infectious diseases that result in admission to hospital. This is a useful source of data on more severe diseases likely to result in admission to hospital, for example, brucellosis and meningitis, although data are often not sufficiently timely for some routine surveillance functions.

Sexually transmitted diseases

Form KC60 records number of initial contacts at all genito-urinary medicine (GUM) clinics

Table 4.2.3 Infections that are covered by the GP reporting system

Acute otitis media	Infectious intestinal disease
Common cold	Scarlet fever/sore throat
Flu/flu-like illness	Whooping cough
Acute tonsillitis	Meningitis/encephalitis
Laryngitis/acute tracheitis	Rubella
Pneumonia/ pneumonitis	Chicken pox
Acute bronchitis	Herpes zoster
Pleurisy	Mumps
Asthma	Infectious hepatitis
Allergic rhinitis	Infectious mononucleosis
	Scabies

and is sent quarterly to CDSC on behalf of the Department of Health. Data are aggregated by age-group, sex and diagnosis. Male patients who are thought to have acquired their infections through homosexual contact, and age-group, are recorded for selected infections. Since clinics do not service defined catchment populations these data are of limited use below regional or national level. At local level clinics may provide anonymized non-aggregated data that can be used for service planning.

Death certification and registration

Mortality data on communicable disease are of limited use since communicable diseases rarely cause death directly. Exceptions are deaths due to influenza, AIDS and TB. However, not all deaths due to infection are coded as such, and data may not be sufficiently timely for all surveillance functions.

International surveillance

Communicable disease surveillance in Europe was given considerable impetus by the World Health Organization (WHO) programme *Health for All*, first agreed in 1982. The programme includes targets such as the elimination of measles, polio, congenital rubella, diphtheria, congenital syphilis and malaria. Surveillance of communicable disease is undertaken by individual European countries and collation of data from these countries is carried out on behalf of the WHO regional office for Europe in Copenhagen by WHO collaborating centres or WHO and European Union surveillance projects. Surveillance is undertaken for food-borne infections, rabies, travel-associated legionellosis, AIDS and HIV infection, influenza, tuberculosis and meningitis (see Chapter 5).

Enhanced surveillance

For England and Wales, CDSC has established enhanced surveillance systems which use multiple sources of data for infections of particular public health importance, including meningococcal disease and tuberculosis.

Other sources of data

• CDSC co-ordinates a national surveillance scheme for general outbreaks of infectious intestinal disease. These are outbreaks affecting members of more than one private residence or residents of an institution. They are distinct from family outbreaks, which affect members of the same private residence only. When an outbreak is over, the CCDC or lead investigator is asked to complete a structured questionnaire. The output from this scheme is reported regularly in the CDR.
• The Medical Officers of Schools Association reports illness in children in approximately 55 boarding schools in England and Wales weekly to CDSC. This is useful in the surveillance of influenza.
• The surveillance unit of the College of Paediatrics and Child Health (formerly the British Paediatric Surveillance Unit) co-ordinates surveillance of uncommon paediatric conditions. A reporting card is sent each month to consultant paediatricians in the UK. They indi-

cate if they have seen a case that month and return the card. An investigator then contacts the paediatrician for further information. Conditions of infective origin that are under surveillance include AIDS/HIV in childhood, congenital rubella, subacute sclerosing panencephalitis, congenital syphilis and Hib infection.

- Cases of HIV infection in England and Wales are reported to CDSC on a structured report form by clinicians participating in a voluntary confidential reporting system. The form requests demographic, behavioural and clinical data.
- Active surveillance of selected occupationally acquired infections is carried out by the Surveillance of Infectious Diseases at Work (SIDAW) Project at the Centre for Occupational Health at the University of Manchester.
- CDSC have carried out surveillance of childhood immunization uptake since 1987. The system is known as COVER (Cover of Vaccination Evaluated Rapidly) and results are reported regularly in the CDR. Local data can be compared with regional and national averages.
- Increasingly surveillance data is shared via the Internet and e-mail. Other local reporting arrangements may include histopathology laboratories (for TB), haematology laboratories (for malaria), pharmacies, GUM clinics, chest clinics and drug teams. The CCDC should agree a local surveillance protocol, publicize case definitions and remind clinicians annually of their responsibility to report infections.

4.3 Managing infectious disease incidents and outbreaks

An infectious disease incident may be defined in one of the following ways.

- Two or more persons with the same disease or symptoms or the same organism isolated from a diagnostic sample, who are linked through common exposure, personal characteristics, time or location.
- A greater than expected rate of infection compared with the usual background rate for the particular place and time.
- A single case of a particular rare or serious disease such as diphtheria, rabies, viral haemorrhagic fever or polio.
- A suspected, anticipated or actual event involving microbial or chemical contamination of food or water.

The first two of these categories may also be described as an outbreak. The control of an outbreak of infectious disease depends on early detection followed by a rapid structured investigation to uncover the source of infection and the route of transmission. This is followed by the application of appropriate control measures to prevent further cases.

Outbreaks of infectious disease are usually investigated and managed by an informal team comprising the CCDC, a medical microbiologist from the local hospital or public health laboratory and an EHO from the local authority. If the outbreak affects a large number of people, if it is a serious infection, if it affects a wide geographical area or if there is significant public or political interest, then consideration should be given to convening an *outbreak control team* to oversee the management of the episode. A written *outbreak control plan* detailing the steps that should be taken is an essential requirement. In an incident with a large number of cases, a particularly pathogenic organism, the potential for spread and a high level of public interest, it will be worthwhile setting up an incident control room. Potential areas for use as incident rooms within local authority or health premises should be identified in the outbreak control plan. In circumstances where there are likely to be significant numbers of enquiries from members of the public—for example during a look-back exercise following identification of a healthcare worker infected with hepatitis

B—a dedicated telephone helpline may be established. Telephone helplines can deal with large numbers of people needing information, counselling or reassurance and they can be used for case finding. Setting up an incident room and telephone helpline are useful parts of an outbreak exercise or simulation (see Box 4.3.1).

Detection

An outbreak will be recognized by case reports, complaints or as a result of routine surveillance.

An outbreak of haemorrhagic colitis due to consumption of cold turkey roll contaminated with E. coli O157 was discovered when several people who had attended the same christening party were admitted to the infectious disease ward at a local hospital.

An outbreak of gastro-enteritis due to Salmonella panama infection due to the sale of contaminated cold meats from a market stall was detected when the local public health laboratory isolated this unusual organism from several faecal samples sent in by GPs from patients with diarrhoea.

An outbreak of food-borne viral gastro-enteritis affecting people who had attended a wedding reception at a hotel came to light when affected guests complained to the local environmental health department.

An outbreak due to the common strain of Salmonella enteritidis PT4 was uncovered when environmental health officers questioned several people, initially reported as sporadic cases by clinicians and laboratories, with this infection in a Midlands town. They all reported buying and eating bakery products from a mobile shop. Further investigations revealed that custard mix used in the preparation of trifle had become contaminated with raw egg.

Systematic investigation

A systematic approach to the investigation of an outbreak comprises the following stages.
- Establishing that a problem exists.
- Confirming the diagnosis.
- Immediate control measures.

- Case finding.
- Collection of data.
- Descriptive epidemiology.
- Generating a hypothesis.
- Testing the hypothesis.

Often several of these stages will be occurring simultaneously.

Establishing that a problem exists

A report of an outbreak of infection may be mistaken. It may result from increased clinical or laboratory detection of cases, changes in reporting patterns, changes in the size of the at-risk population or false-positive laboratory tests.

Increases in the number of cases of tuberculosis in recent years following many years of decline may be due to increases in the size of certain population subgroups that are at increased risk of tuberculosis. These would include the elderly, the homeless, and those that have migrated from areas of the world where the incidence of tuberculosis remains high.

An outbreak of cryptosporidiosis was due to false-positive laboratory tests. The microbiology technician mistook fat globules for oocysts of the protozoon Cryptosporidium parvum in faecal smears.

Other pseudo-outbreaks due to laboratory contamination were recognized because cases, despite having identical microbiological results, had no detectable epidemiological links, inconclusive clinical diagnoses and were only reported by one laboratory.

Confirming the diagnosis

Cases can be diagnosed either clinically or by laboratory investigations. At an early stage it is important to produce and adhere to a clear case-definition. This is particularly important with previously unrecognized diseases in which proper definitions are needed before epidemiological studies can proceed.

In 1989, an investigation was started into an outbreak of atypical pneumonia affecting men of working age in the Birmingham

Box 4.3.1 Setting up an incident room and telephone helpline

The incident room
- Dedicated use
- 24-h access and security
- Large enough for the incident team their equipment and files
- Sufficient telephone lines
- A dedicated fax machine
- Computer with access to the internet and e-mail
- Access to photocopying facilities
- Filing systems for storing all communications, minutes of meetings, notes of decisions, etc.

Helpline
- Decision taken by the outbreak control team
- Part of the local emergency plan
- A subgroup should take responsibility for planning and establishing the helplines
- The group should include a public health physician; a person with the authority to make financial decisions; a telecommunications expert; administrative support
- The purpose of the helpline must be clear
- List of staff needed to staff the line
- Needs of minority ethnic groups and the hearing impaired should be considered
- Early liaison with clinical specialists to ensure that staff are properly briefed
- Question and answer and frequently asked question sheets should be developed
- Mechanisms to deal with unexpected calls or complex queries
- Training to deal with obscene, silent, or threatening calls
- Staff may have to deal with anxious and distressed callers and should be properly supported
- Facilities to call back may be required
- Briefing materials and procedures should be reviewed regularly to identify any inadequacies
- All calls should be logged
- A minimum data set would include date and time of call; sex, age, and postcode of caller; and the appropriateness of the call
- Further data collection would depend upon the nature of the helpline
- Headsets rather than handsets should be provided so that helpline workers can keep their hands free to make notes or use computer terminals
- Media can be used to publicize the helpline
- It can be difficult to estimate the number of telephone lines required; the limiting factor may be the number of people available to staff the lines. Most calls arrive in the first few days, so the maximum number of lines should be available at the start of an incident; excess lines can then be closed down
- Calls can first be screened by an experienced person who then allocates them appropriately- or calls can be taken by a first-line person, who passes on difficult calls
- Four-hour shifts are generally used, some may be able to do two shifts
- A supervisor is needed for each shift to deal with briefings and administration and cover staff breaks.
- The hours that the helpline is open will depend on circumstances
- It should include the evening so that those working shifts or with children can call for example from 8 a.m. to 9 p.m.
- Hours may need to be adjusted to cope with anxieties raised by media coverage, for example keeping the helpline open until midnight if the issue is covered in the evening
- An answering machine message giving the opening hours should be available when closed
- After the incident the helpline should be reviewed; lessons learned can be recorded and a formal report prepared for the health authority

area. Four weeks elapsed before the laboratory confirmed the diagnosis as Q fever and progress could be made with the epidemiological investigation.

Immediate control measures

Control measures involve either controlling the source of infection, interrupting transmission or protecting those at risk.

Case finding

In an episode of infection, the cases that are first noticed may only be a small proportion of the total population affected and may not be representative of that population. Efforts must be made to search for additional cases. This allows the extent of the incident to be quantified, it allows a more accurate picture of the range of illness that people have experienced, it allows individual cases to be treated and control measures to be taken, and it provides subjects for further descriptive and analytical epidemiology.

There are several ways of searching for additional cases.
• Statutory notifications of infectious disease.
• Requests for laboratory tests and reports of positive results.
• People attending their GPs, the local accident and emergency department, hospital inpatients and outpatients.
• Reports from the occupational health departments of large local businesses.
• Reports from schools of absenteeism and illness.
• Household enquiries.
• Appeals through TV, radio and local newspapers.
• Screening tests applied to communities and population subgroups.

In a local outbreak of Salmonella panama infection a fax message was sent to all microbiologists in the region asking them to report isolates of Salmonella panama to the investigating team.

In the 1989 outbreak of Q fever local GPs were telephoned and local occupational health departments were contacted to enquire about cases of atypical pneumonia or unexplained respiratory disease.

CCDCs and microbiologists can be alerted by a note on the front page of the weekly CDR or by a message sent by fax or e-mail. In the past they have been asked to report cases of Legionnaires' disease associated with a Midlands industrial site, cases of meningitis associated with a university hall of residence and food-borne infection associated with hotels and social gatherings.

Collection of data

A set of data is collected from each of the cases. This includes name, age, sex, address, occupation, name of GP, recent travel, immunization history, date of illness and clinical description of illness.

Data should also be collected about exposure to possible sources of the infection. In the case of a food-borne infection this would include a recent food history. In the case of infection spread by person-to-person contact the case would be questioned about contact with other affected persons. In the case of an infection spread by the air-borne route, cases would be questioned about places they had visited.

It is preferable to collect these data by administering a detailed semi-structured questionnaire in a face-to-face interview. This allows the interviewer to ask probing questions which may sometimes uncover previously unsuspected associations between cases. Telephone interviews or self-completion questionnaires are less helpful at this stage of an investigation.

In an investigation of a possible national outbreak of Salmonella newport infection that was thought to be food-borne, very detailed questioning was undertaken about the food that had been consumed in the seven days prior to illness. This included asking specifically about a whole range of different food items, where they had been purchased and the brand that had been purchased.

In the investigation of an outbreak of Legion-

naires' disease thought to have an environmental source, cases were asked to indicate on a map the exact places they had visited in the 10 days prior to illness.

It may be necessary to re-interview early cases to ask about possible exposures that are reported by later cases.

In the investigation of the Salmonella panama outbreak, it was not until the seventh case was interviewed that the market stall was mentioned for a second time. The early cases were questioned again and all but one reported buying or receiving items that could be traced to this stall.

Descriptive epidemiology

Cases are described by the three epidemiological parameters of time, place and person. Describing cases by person includes clinical features, age, sex, occupation, social class, ethnic group, food history, travel, leisure activity. Describing cases by place includes home address and work address. Describing cases by time involves plotting the epidemic curve, a frequency distribution of date or time of onset. This may allow the incubation period to be estimated which, with the clinical features, may give some clues as to the causative organism (see Table 2.2.1). The incubation period should be related to events that may have occurred in the environment of the cases and which may indicate possible sources of infection.

In a national outbreak of Salmonella ealing infection, those affected were mainly infants. This suggested a connection with a widely distributed infant food. Dried baby milk was subsequently found to be the source of infection.

A national outbreak of Salmonella napoli infection affecting mainly children was found to be due to contaminated chocolate bars.

Figure 4.3.1 is the epidemic curve that would occur in a milk-borne *Campylobacter* outbreak due to delivery and consumption of contaminated milk on one particular day (point source outbreak). Figure 4.3.2 is the epidemic curve in a similar outbreak in which contaminated milk was consumed at the school over several days (continuing source outbreak). Figure 4.3.3 is the epidemic curve in a community outbreak of measles where the infection is spread from person to person (propagated outbreak). There is a smooth epidemic curve with distinct peaks at intervals of the incubation period.

Generating a hypothesis

A detailed epidemiological description of typical cases may well provide the investigators with a hypothesis regarding the source of infection or the route of transmission. A description of atypical cases may also be helpful.

Testing the hypothesis

Finding that consumption of a particular food, visiting a particular place or being involved in a certain activity is occurring frequently among cases is only a first step. These risk factors may also be common among those who have not been ill. To confirm an association between a risk factor and disease, further microbiological or environmental investigations may be required, or an analytical epidemiological study may be necessary. This can be either a cohort study or a case–control study.

Case–control study

A case–control study compares exposures in people who are ill (the cases) with exposure in people who are not ill (the controls). Case–control studies are most useful when the at-risk population cannot be accurately defined (e.g. when cases are laboratory reports of infection in the general population). Controls can be selected from a GP's practice list, from the health authority patient register, from the laboratory that reported the case, from people nominated by the case or from neighbours selected at random from nearby houses.

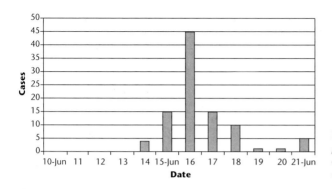

Figure 4.3.1 Outbreak of *Campylobacter* gastro-enteritis associated with consumption of unpasteurized milk (point source).

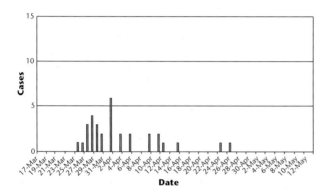

Figure 4.3.2 Outbreak of *Campylobacter* gastro-enteritis associated with consumption of unpasteurized milk (continuing source).

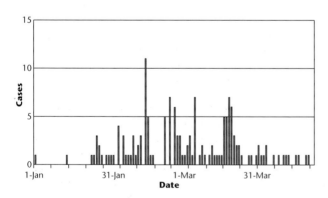

Figure 4.3.3 Outbreak of measles in a community (propagated outbreak).

Cohort study

The cohort study is a type of natural experiment in which a proportion of a population is exposed to a factor, while the remainder is not. The incidence or attack rate of infection amongst exposed persons is compared with the rate amongst unexposed persons. For example, following a food poisoning outbreak at a social gathering, thought to be due to consumption of contaminated chocolate mousse, the cohort (all those who attended) is divided into those who ate the mousse (the exposed) and those who did not (the unexposed).

Collecting the data

A set of data is collected from both cases and control or from the exposed and unexposed persons within the cohort. A case-definition should be agreed and sample size calculation should be performed to ensure that the study has adequate statistical power. To avoid any bias the data must be collected from each subject in exactly the same way. Usually this is done by questionnaire. Unlike the hypothesis-generating questionnaire, the questionnaire for an analytical study is often shorter, more structured and uses mostly closed questions. It may be administered at interview, by telephone or it may be a self-completion postal questionnaire. Questionnaires should be piloted before use. If several interviewers will be used they should be adequately briefed and provided with instructions to ensure the questionnaire is administered in a consistent way.

Analysis

In both cohort and case–control studies initial analysis is by a 2×2 table. In cohort studies the ratio of incidence in exposed to incidence in unexposed is calculated. This is the relative risk. In case–control studies the odds of exposure in the cases is compared with the odds of exposure in the controls. This is the odds ratio, which usually approximates the relative risk.

Confidence intervals for these estimates can be calculated and tests of statistical significance applied. Computer programmes (e.g. Epi-Info) are freely available which will perform these calculations.

In an outbreak of cryptosporidiosis in Kent at the end of 1990, the hypothesis was that infection was associated with the consumption of cold drinking water supplied by the local water company. This was tested using a case–control study. Cases were defined as people living locally who had had a diarrhoeal illness between 1 December 1990 and 31 January 1991, with oocysts present in a faecal sample. Cases were excluded if they had travelled abroad or if another household member had diarrhoea in the four weeks before the onset of their illness. The names and addresses of controls were obtained from the patient list held by the health authority. They were matched with the cases for sex, age group and GP or health centre. They were excluded if they had been abroad within four weeks of the onset of illness in their matched cases or if they themselves had diarrhoea since 1 December 1990. Five names and addresses of controls were obtained for each case. For each case and control a questionnaire was completed by a member of the investigating team during a telephone interview. The questionnaire asked about illness and consumption of various food items, including milk, salad, meat and cheese. Participants were also asked about the consumption of cold tap water both at home and outside the home, consumption of untreated, filtered or bottle water and exposure to recreational water. The results are shown in Table 4.3.1. There was a dose–response relationship with the quantity of tap water consumed.

An outbreak of Salmonella enteritidis phage type 4 infection affected a party of 136 elderly people staying at a hotel on the south coast of England over Christmas and New Year 1988/89. The hypothesis was that illness was associated with consumption of contaminated food items served in the hotel restaurant. This was tested with a cohort study. The cohort was guests and staff at the hotel. Cases were defined as members of staff or guests who had gastrointestinal symptoms between 23 and 29 December. All members of the cohort were asked to complete a questionnaire during an interview with an EHO, which enquired about symptoms and food eaten in the hotel. Attack rates for those who did and didn't eat certain food items were compared and relative risks were calculated. Consumption of three food items (Table 4.3.2) were significantly associated with illness. All these items contained fresh egg, the presumed source of infection in this outbreak.

Table 4.3.1 Cryptosporidiosis in Kent, December 1990. Odds ratios for exposure to selected factors

	Case		Control		Odds	95% CI on
	Y	N	Y	N	ratio*	odds ratio
Unpasteurized milk	0	29	0	80	N/A	N/A
Lettuce	16	11	51	29	0.83	0.31–2.22
Fresh raw vegetables	2	6	56	23	1.51	0.5–5.12
Unpasteurized cheese	0	29	10	69	0	0–1.15
Contact with farm animals	0	27	0	80	N/A	N/A
Tap water Y=>1 cup/day, N=<1 cup/day	19	7	33	47	3.87[†]	1.35–12.03[‡]
Water consumed outside the home	15	10	23	51	3.33	1.18–9.49
Water filter	0	29	8	72	0	0–1.57
Bottled water	0	29	16	64	0	0–0.63[§]
Swimming pool	5	23	16	64	0.87	0.22–2.87
Rivers	2	26	1	79	6.08	0.3–363

Notes:

* The odds ratio is the odds of exposure in the cases divided by the odds of exposure in the controls. An odds ratio of 1 indicates no association.

[†] Consumption of tap water is nearly four times as likely in cases as in controls.

[‡] The 95% confidence interval does not include 1, indicating that this is a significant association that is unlikely to be due to chance.

[§] Controls are significantly more likely than cases to have been exposed to bottled water, i.e. there is a protective effect.

Table 4.3.2 *Salmonella* infection in a south coast hotel, Christmas 1988. Relative risk of infection for consumption of selected foods (significant items only)

	Ill		Not ill		Relative	95% CI on
Food	Ate	Did not eat	Ate	Did not eat	risk*	relative risk
Chocolate mousse	66	2	21	14	6.07[†]	1.65–2.31[‡]
Lemon mousse	60	4	25	12	2.82	1.2–6.67[§]
Crème caramel	55	9	24	13	1.7	1.01–2.57[§]

* The relative risk (RR) is the risk of illness in the exposed divided by the risk of illness in the unexposed. A RR of 1 indicates no difference and therefore no association between illness and exposure. The relative risk can only be calculated for cohort or cross-sectional studies.

[†] Illness is six times more likely in those who ate chocolate mousse.

[‡] The 95% confidence interval does not include 1, so the results are unlikely to have occurred by chance.

[§] There are weaker but none the less significant associations between illness and lemon mousse and crème caramel.

4.4 Community infection control

The community can be defined as all environments that are outside hospital. This includes nursing and residential homes, hostels, day care centres, schools, colleges and nurseries, factories, offices and other workplaces, leisure centres, hotels, restaurants, shops, cinemas, theatres and other places of entertainment, open spaces and communal areas, transport and finally people's own homes and gardens.

Control measures for community infection

To prevent the spread of infection, measures can be taken to control the source of infection and the route of transmission, and susceptible people can be offered protection with antibiotics or immunization.

These measures are directed at the person or case, his or her contacts, the environment and the wider community. The control measures that are adopted should be of proven effectiveness. If not, they should at least be rational. As in hospital infection control, there can be no place for infection control rituals.

Person

The case is contacted by visit, telephone or letter and details are recorded on a specially designed case report form. Diagnostic samples may be requested, for example faecal samples in the case of suspected gastrointestinal infections.

An assessment is made of the risk that the case may spread infection. Guidelines are available to assist with this risk assessment. For example, with gastrointestinal infections the case may be assigned to one of four risk groups: food handler, health or social care worker, child aged less than five years or older child or adult with low standards of personal hygiene (Box 2.2.1). Factors such as type of employment, availability of sanitary facilities and standards of personal hygiene should be taken into account. The risk assessment will help to determine the control measures that are needed.

The case may be isolated until no longer infectious. The extent of this isolation will vary. Usually isolation at home will be sufficient. However, strict isolation for highly infectious or virulent infections that spread by both the airborne route as well as direct contact may necessitate admission to an infectious diseases unit. It may be necessary to exclude infectious cases from school or work.

The case may be kept under surveillance, examined clinically or undergo laboratory investigations. The case may be treated to reduce the communicable period. The case, his or her family and household contacts and medical and nursing attendants may be advised to adopt certain precautions to reduce the risk of transmission. Precautions that are advised to prevent transmission of blood-borne pathogens include advice not to share personal items, careful use and disposal of needles and other sharp instruments, careful disposal of clinical waste, safe sex and careful attention to blood spillages. Enteric precautions for gastrointestinal infections may comprise use of gloves and gowns, sanitary disposal of faeces and babies' nappies, attention to personal hygiene including handwashing, regular cleaning and use of appropriate disinfectants. The case may be advised to restrict contact with young children and others who may be particularly susceptible to infection. He or she may be advised not to prepare food for other household members.

Advice should be reinforced with written material such as leaflets, or a video may be available. Legal powers are available, but these are rarely used.

Public health law

The Public Health (Control of Disease) Act 1984 and the Public Health (Infectious Diseases) Regulations 1988 give UK local authorities wide ranging powers to control communicable disease. Local government authorities exercise these powers in one of two ways: either by direct action or through the *proper officer*. The proper officer is an officer appointed by the local authority for a particular purpose. For communicable disease control issues, the proper officer is usually the CCDC.

Some powers, such as those which deal with the notification of diseases, are purely administrative. However, there are powers to control things, premises and people. This includes preventing the sale of infected articles, preventing infected people from using public transport, cleaning and disinfection of premises, excluding people from work and school, offering immunization, compulsory examination, removal to hospital and detention in hospital and obtaining information from householders and schools in order to prevent the spread of disease.

There are four pieces of legislation concerned with diseases that can be transmitted sexually. The Venereal Disease Act 1917 makes treatment and advertising treatment for STDs other than by designated clinics an offence. The National Health Service (Venereal Diseases) Regulations 1974 and the National Health Service Trusts (Venereal Diseases) Directions 1991 give limited confidentiality to patients and the AIDS (Control) Act 1987 requires information about AIDS to be sent to the Secretary of State.

There are public health regulations covering aircraft, ships and international trains that pass through the Channel Tunnel (see Chapter 4.15). These deal with infectious persons or infectious animals or material on board.

Contacts

Contacts of a case of infectious disease may be at risk of acquiring infection themselves, they may risk spreading infection to others, or they may be the source of infection. It is important to have a definition of a contact and conduct a risk assessment.

For example, a contact of a case of gastrointestinal infection is someone who has been exposed to the excreta of a case. With typhoid this definition would be extended to those exposed to the same source as the case, such as those who were on the same visit abroad. A contact of a case of meningococcal infection is someone who has spent a night under the same roof as the case in the seven days before onset, or has had mouth kissing contact.

Contacts may be subjected to clinical or laboratory examination. For example, in the case of diphtheria and typhoid, they may be offered advice, placed under surveillance or offered prophylaxis with antibiotics or immunization. In some circumstances contacts may be excluded from school or work (legal powers are available).

Environment

In some circumstances it may be appropriate to investigate the environment of a case of infection. This may involve inspection and laboratory investigation of home or work. Examples are food-borne infections, gastrointestinal infections and Legionnaires' disease. There are legal powers to control the environment, including powers to seize, destroy and prohibit the use of certain objects. This may be necessary in the event of infection caused by a contaminated foodstuff. It may be appropriate to advise on cleaning and disinfection.

Community

The occurrence of cases of infection will have an effect on the wider community. For example, a case of Legionnaires' disease or tuberculosis may generate considerable anxiety in the workforce. Meningitis and hepatitis B will have a similar effect in schools on staff, pupils and parents. Scabies in day care centres and head lice in schools are other examples.

It is helpful to keep all sections of the community informed about certain cases of infection. This can be done by letter or public meeting. In some circumstances it may be appropriate to set up a telephone advice line. In addition it can be helpful to inform local newspapers, radio, television and politicians. All sections of the community have information needs with respect to the prevention and control of infectious disease. Advice is available from a range of health professionals. This can be reinforced by leaflets, videos and through the media.

In community settings such as schools, nursing homes, residential homes and primary care it is helpful to make available written guidelines on infection control in the form of a manual or handbook. These materials can subsequently from the basis for training and audit in infection control. Examples are available from the Public Health Medicine Environmental Group in the UK.

Prevention of infectious disease

Activity to prevent infection can be directed at the host or the environment.

Host

Risk behaviour may be changed by health education campaigns. These may be national or local, and may be aimed at the general population or targeted at those who are particularly at risk.

Infections that have been the subject of national health education campaigns include HIV infection, STIs, *Salmonella*, *Listeria*, and *E. coli* VTEC infection. For example, the Chief Medical Officer has given the following food safety advice:

"Avoid eating raw eggs or uncooked dishes made from eggs. Pregnant women, the elderly, the sick, babies and toddlers should only eat eggs that have been cooked until both the yolk and the white are solid. To avoid listeriosis, pregnant women and those people with decreased resistance to infection are advised to avoid eating soft ripe cheeses such as Brie, Camembert and blue vein varieties and to avoid eating paté. These groups are also advised to re-heat cook-chilled meals and ready-to-eat poultry until piping hot rather than eat them cold. Beefburgers should be cooked thoroughly throughout until the juices run clear and there are no pink bits inside."

Health services offer diagnosis, screening, treatment, prophylaxis and immunization. Examples are routine and selective immunization, services for tuberculosis screening, treatment for newly arrived immigrants and services for STIs.

Environment

Local authority environmental health departments have responsibilities and legal powers to ensure that supplies of food and water are wholesome and will not harm health and that there are adequate arrangements for the disposal of sewage, waste collection and disposal and pest control.

The Food Safety Act 1990 provides a framework for a range of food hygiene regulations that govern the activity of food businesses and implement European Union (EU) directives. The enforcement of food law is usually the responsibility of local authorities. There are statutory codes of practice which provide guidance.

The Food Safety (General Food Hygiene) Regulations 1995 apply to all types of food businesses, from a hot dog van to a five star restaurant. They do not apply to food cooked at home for private consumption. They require food businesses to identify all steps that are critical to food safety and ensure adequate safety controls are in place, maintained and reviewed. This is the formal system known as Hazard Analysis and Critical Control Points (HACCP). Guidance notes and explanatory booklets are available. The 1995 Regulations changed the arrangements governing food handlers' fitness to work in the UK. The aim of the changes is to prevent the introduction of infection into the food business workplace, by advising staff of their obligation to report to management any infectious or potentially infectious conditions and to immediately leave the workplace if they should have such a condition. The conditions are diarrhoea and vomiting, gastrointestinal infections, enteric fever and infected lesions of skin, eyes, ears and mouth. Before returning to work following illness due to gastrointestinal infection there should be no vomiting for 48h, a normal bowel habit for 48h and good hygienic practices, particularly hand-washing.

Other regulations include the Food Safety (Temperature Control) Regulations 1995 which detail the temperatures at which particular types of food should be stored before consumption. There are also a range of product specific regulations covering fresh meat, wild game, minced meat and shellfish aimed at dairies, meat processors or wholesale fish markets.

The government and local authorities carry out publicity campaigns on food safety and food hygiene aimed at food businesses and the general public.

There is a comprehensive food surveillance programme, with over 140000 analyses carried out each year for a wide range of food contaminants. The annual EC co-ordinated food control programmes require member states to carry out inspection and sampling of specified categories of food items, for example refrigerated salads for *Listeria*.

4.5 Hospital infection control

Hospital infection control comprises a range of activities which aim to prevent hospital-acquired infection (HAI) and limit the spread of community-acquired infection in hospitals. HAI, which is also called *nosocomial infection*, is infection found to be active or requiring treatment which was not present or incubating when a patient was admitted to hospital.

Hospital-acquired infection includes:
• urinary tract infection;

• surgical wound infection;
• lower respiratory tract infection;
• skin infection;
• gastro-enteritis;
• bacteraemias.

The main micro-organisms that cause HAI include:
• methicillin-resistant *Staphylococcus aureus* (MRSA);
• *Clostridium difficile*;
• *Klebsiella* and other Gram-negative organisms;
• coliforms and other intestinal bacteria;
• *Pseudomonas*.

Community-acquired infections typically affect a different range of sites and are caused by different micro-organisms.

Whilst most cases of HAI are sporadic, outbreaks and clusters can occur, since infection spreads readily within hospitals amongst patients who may be more susceptible to infection as a result of illness or treatment.

The importance of HAI

Despite the use of antibiotics, HAI is an important cause of death, disability and ill health. In one UK study 7.8% of patients developed HAI and 19% of those who did not reported symptoms of infection after leaving hospital. Patients with HAI on average incurred additional hospital costs of £2917 and remained in hospital for an extra 11 days. It is estimated that in England HAI costs the hospital sector £930 million annually in inpatient costs alone. Costs are also borne by community health services, the individual and his or her family. It is estimated that 1% of patients with HAI will die as a result of their infection and a further 3% will die with HAI as a contributory cause.

There is evidence that up to a third of hospital infections may be avoided. In a large US study, programmes of hospital infection surveillance and control were associated with a 32% reduction in infection rates. Most would agree that at least a 10% reduction in HAI is still achievable in the UK. Such a reduction would result in the release of considerable resources which could be used for other aspects of patient care.

There are legal duties to take appropriate steps to protect patients, staff and visitors from harm. As well as the common-law duty of care there are legal regulations such as the Control of Substances Hazardous to Health (COSHH) Regulations and the Food Safety Act which demand that hospital infection control is an important part of a hospitals risk management and clinical governance programme. HAI is also an indicator of the quality of patient care. Outbreaks of HAI may result in adverse publicity.

Risk factors for HAI

Compared with the general population, hospital patients are more susceptible to infection because of the following.
• Immunosuppression as a result of age (the very young and the very old), other medical conditions and medical and surgical treatment.
• Exposure to other patients with infections as a result of being nursed on the same ward and being cared for by the same staff.
• Modern medical practice, involving more invasive procedures.
• Improved chances of survival of high-risk patients which increase their risk of infection.
• The frequent need for antibiotics that encourage the emergence in hospitals of resistant bacteria.

Surveillance of HAI

Prevalence studies measure the proportion of hospital patients who at a given point in time have HAI. This may be done by carrying out a census of patients on a particular day or week to determine if they have HAI. Such a census was carried out in 1993/94, and 9% of 37 111 patients from 157 centres were found to have HAI. Incidence studies measure the rate of new cases of HAI.

Surveillance of HAI comprises the collection, collation, analysis and dissemination of data on cases of infection. Case-definitions should be agreed for conditions or infections of clinical, economic or public health importance within the hospital. Cases can be identified in the following ways.
• Laboratory-based surveillance of *alert organisms* (see Table 4.5.1) detected in clinical specimens.
• Other laboratory-based surveillance: blood cultures, CSF, vascular catheters, postoperative wound swabs, urine samples, etc.
• Surveillance by ward staff of *alert conditions* such as diarrhoea and vomiting, food poisoning, pyrexia of unknown origin, soft tissue infections, childhood exanthemata, etc.
• Targeted surveillance by ICT members through liaison with special units and wards (intensive care, oncology, etc.) or particular subgroups of patients to enquire about infections, incidents and outbreaks.

The Nosocomial Infection National Surveillance Scheme (NINSS) was established by the Department of Health and the Public Health Laboratory Service in response to the need for a national surveillance system of hospital-acquired infection. The primary objectives of NINSS are to develop standard methods of data collection and to provide national data for comparison with local results. The scheme has already carried out surveillance of surgical site infection and hospital-acquired bacteraemia. Regular reports are published.

On each episode of infection the following data set should be collected: patient identifier, age, sex, ward, specialty, date of admission, date of onset of symptoms or signs of infection, site of infection, organism, antibiotic sensitivities, date and type of invasive procedure. Since many patients are discharged home early after surgery, the data collection process may need to be extended into the community.

Data should be collated using a computerized database to allow data retrieval and analysis. Weekly, monthly and annual totals and antibiotic resistance patterns should be reported. Infection rates may be calculated using appropriate denominators (admissions, discharges, deaths, patient days, days of device usage, etc.) for surgical wound infection, urinary tract infection, respiratory tract infection and bloodstream infections. Surveillance data

Table 4.5.1 Alert organisms

Bacterial isolates	Methicillin-resistant *Staphylococcus aureus*
	Other highly resistant *Staphylococcus aureus* strains (e.g. gentamicin/ fusidic acid resistance)
	Streptococcus pyogenes
	Penicillin-resistant *Streptococcus pneumoniae*
	Beta-lactamase producing enterococci
	Clostridium difficile and/or detection of its toxins
	Legionella spp. (including serology results)
	Verotoxin-producing strains of *Escherichia coli* (e.g. *E. coli* O157)
	Salmonella or *Shigella* species
	Gentamicin-resistant, extended spectrum, beta-lactamase resistant and quinolone-resistant Gram-negative rods
	Other multi-antibiotic resistant Gram-negative rods
	Other bacteria isolates with unusual antibiotic resistance (e.g. *Haemophilus influenzae* resistant to ampicillin and trimethoprim)
	Pseudomonas aeruginosa
	Strenotrophomonas maltophilia (*Xanthomonas maltophilia*)
Viral isolates/positive antigen tests	Rotavirus
	Respiratory viruses—respiratory syncytial virus, influenza, etc.
	Varicella-zoster
	Parvovirus B19
Fungi	In special units, *Candida* species, *Aspergillus*

should be widely circulated and discussed. An annual report should be compiled and presented to and discussed by the Hospital Infection Control Committee.

Management arrangements for the control of HAI

Arrangements for infection control in hospitals should be a key part of governance, risk management and quality assurance. Overall responsibility for infection control in hospitals and trusts rests with the chief executive. There should be an infection control team (ICT) comprising an infection control doctor (ICD) and one or more infection control nurses (ICN) and, if the ICD is from another specialty, a consultant medical microbiologist. The number of ICNs should be appropriate to the number of beds, number of hospitals, the area over which they are located and the patient case mix. It is recommended that there should be at least one trained

ICN for every 250 acute beds. There should be a multidisciplinary infection control committee (ICC).

The function of the ICT

The ICT is responsible for the prevention, control and surveillance of hospital infection. The ICT should agree an annual programme of activity, which may include the following.
• Surveillance.
• Developing policies and procedures.
• Educating staff.
• Carrying out audits.
• Advising on proposed building constructions and the purchase of equipment and consumables to ensure they conform with infection control requirements.
• Advising on tenders for other services.
   Written infection control policies should cover:
• handwashing;
• antibiotic usage;

- clinical procedures;
- disposal of waste;
- outbreaks and incidents;
- decontamination, sterilization and disinfection;
- management of patients at risk of acquiring or transmitting infection;
- use of isolation facilities;
- management of specific communicable diseases;
- laundry, catering (including food hygiene) and domestic cleaning;
- mortuary procedures;
- engineering and building services (including *Legionella* infection);
- equipment purchasing;
- new building;
- staff immunization (hepatitis B, influenza, BCG) and other aspects of occupational health;
- sharps injuries;
- operating theatres;
- transfer and discharge of patients;
- pest control.

These written policies should be collated in an infection control manual which should be available on every ward. Policies should be reviewed and updated regularly.

Infection control audits should cover:
- hand hygiene;
- clinical practices (isolation, protective clothing, catheter care);
- environmental cleaning and hygiene;
- ward kitchen areas;
- waste disposal;
- sharps management;
- care of linen;
- decontamination of equipment.

Outbreak and incident control plans should be exercised if not in regular use, and regularly updated.

Hospital infection control committee

Each hospital should have a hospital infection control committee (HICC) which advises and supports the infection control team. Membership of this committee should include the hospital chief executive or a director-level deputy, the CCDC and the occupational health physician. The HICC should meet at least twice a year and its meetings should be documented.

Communication, liaison and reporting

The consultant microbiologist and CCDC should agree which isolations of microorganisms and other results will be reported by the laboratory to the CCDC and by what means (see Table 4.2.2). In general electronic reporting using a system such as CoSurv should be encouraged. Food poisoning thought to originate from hospital premises must be reported to the local authority environmental health department. The CCDC should be informed of any problem within the hospital that may have implications for the community. In return the CCDC will inform the ICT about any relevant community infection problems.

Relationships with community health services and primary care

Hospital-acquired infection (HAI) may present after a patient has been discharged from hospital. Hospitals are responsible for passing relevant information to the GP and to community nurses and midwives. In turn they should provide feedback to the hospital, both to the ICT and the consultant who has treated the patient, both for surveillance purposes and to alert the ICT when a potentially infected patient is to be admitted to hospital. Collaboration between community staff, the ICT and the CCDC is encouraged by the appointment of a community ICN.

The role of the CCDC

The CCDC's role in hospital infection control is: to advise the health authority and primary care groups on contractual issues; to be a member of the HICC; to liaise with the ICT; and to provide epidemiological advice when it is needed.

The role of the district health authority

The health authority has responsibility for the quality of healthcare services and, with the local authorities, for protecting public health by controlling communicable disease and infection and managing the human health aspects of other environmental hazards. Specific responsibilities with respect to HAI are summarized in Table 4.5.2.

How would the CCDC recognize a problem in a particular trust with HAI or lack of investment in infection control?

High infection rates, outbreaks and other incidents would be picked up by the CCDC through regular liaison with the ICT and attendance at HICC meetings. Further enquiries may uncover a wider problem or lack of commitment to infection control.

Surveillance data and the results of audits should be tabled at HICC meetings. These are multidisciplinary meetings. Problem areas would be highlighted and a programme of investigation and remedial action agreed.

National or regional surveillance may identify any hot spots in local hospitals and lead to enquiries and investigations.

The CCDC is involved in the investigation of infectious disease incidents in hospitals and community trusts, and any failures to implement effective infection control policies would rapidly come to light. Complaints from patients and their relatives may reveal infection control deficiencies such as standards of cleaning, catering and laundry.

Outbreaks of infection in hospital

Infectious diseases can spread readily within hospitals amongst staff and patients who may be more susceptible to infection as a result of illness or treatment.

Although a proportion of HAI is preventable, from time to time—despite high standards of infection control practice—outbreaks of infection or infectious disease incidents may occur.

Outbreaks of the following infections are reported regularly in UK hospitals.
- Infectious intestinal disease, usually due to SRSV or *Clostridium difficile*.
- Methicillin-resistant *Staphylococcus aureus*.
- Vancomycin-resistant enterococci.
- Multiple antibiotic-resistant Gram-negative organisms.
- Tuberculosis.
- Hepatitis B.
- *Streptococcus pneumoniae*.

In 1995 and 1996, of 1568 general outbreaks of infection reported to CCSC, 518 were in hospital and 473 in a residential institution. Of the hospital outbreaks 474 (91%) involved person-to-person transmission, mainly due to SRSV.

Recognition of an outbreak

An outbreak is an incident in which two or

Table 4.5.2 Health authority responsibilities for HAI

Advice to GPs on infection control in their surgery premises

Agreement with healthcare providers for adequate arrangements for infection control

The establishment of an infection control team and hospital infection control committee

Staffing, funding levels and cover for ICD and ICN

Compliance with statutory requirements including notification of infectious diseases, food safety, health and safety, clinical waste management, etc.

Compliance with relevant guidance, e.g. on *Legionella*, sterilization of instruments, sharps disposal, hepatitis B immunization, etc.

Hospital plans for managing infectious diseases outbreaks and incidents

Participation in the work of infection control committees and implementation of policies and programmes more people who are thought to have a common exposure experience a similar illness or proven infection. Outbreaks in hospital are either detected by the laboratory or by nursing or medical staff. Cases of infection and outbreaks are reported to the infection control team (ICT).

Action

Hospitals should have written plans for responding to infectious disease incidents. These should cover:
• Recognition of an outbreak.
• Circumstances in which the ICD or CCDC would take the lead.
• Initial investigation by ICD and ICN which determines whether or not an outbreak exists.
• If the outbreak is confined to hospital, whether it can be dealt with by the ICT or if an outbreak control group is needed. A major outbreak is one in which large numbers of people are affected, where the organism involved is particularly pathogenic or where there is potential for spread within the hospital and the community.
• Outbreak report to be sent to CDSC for national surveillance purposes.
• If the outbreak is not confined to hospital the CCDC would be involved and the district outbreak plan would be implemented as appropriate.
• The CCDC has responsibility to inform the Chief Medical Officer and CDSC. The PHLS should also be informed.

Outbreaks of limited extent will be dealt with by the ICT along with the relevant clinicians and nurses. It would be usual for the CCDC to be informed, although he or she may already know of the outbreak through regular contact with the ICD. If the disease involved is statutorily notifiable, the medical staff responsible for the patient(s) must notify the CCDC as proper officer of the local authority. In any infectious disease incident where food or water is implicated, a local authority environmental health officer should be informed. In large outbreaks an outbreak control team would be convened.

Initial investigation of a hospital outbreak

This should consist of the following.
1 Collect information on all cases occurring on all wards and units.
2 Establish a case definition; request laboratory tests.
3 Ensure provision of medical and nursing care for affected patients, including appropriate precautions to prevent secondary spread.
4 Consider antibiotic prophylaxis or immunization if appropriate (not usually applicable for gastrointestinal infections).
5 Consider catering arrangements, disinfection, handwashing, laundry, food samples, environmental samples and microbiological or serological screening of those at risk.
6 If a food-borne or water-borne infection is suspected, the EHO will conduct an environmental investigation, including inspection of kitchen, food handling and storage practices, review of illness amongst staff, requesting faecal samples from members of staff if necessary, review of menus, waste handling and pest-control.
7 Implement control measures, for example:
   • patient isolation/cohort nursing;
   • restriction of transfers and/or discharges;
   • staff education in infection control procedures;
   • clear instructions and information for ward staff, cleaners, etc.;
   • information to patients' relatives and visitors.
8 Decide when the outbreak is over.
9 Communicate with DH, CDSC, and media as appropriate.

Community outbreak affecting the hospital

Hospitals should have plans for responding to a major community outbreak affecting the hospital.

Major outbreaks of infectious disease in the community may place heavy demands on hospital services. Acute outbreaks developing over a few hours are generally toxin-mediated. Non-acute outbreaks, due for example to influenza, develop over days or weeks.

The ICT role would include advising on the collection of microbiological samples and advising on any control of infection measures. In many circumstances the patients will not be infectious. In non-acute outbreaks it is suggested that an outbreak control group is convened. The hospital response to an event of this kind will generally involve clinical and managerial staff. Consideration should be given to: admissions policy; appropriate management of patients; opening up additional beds; consequences of staff illness; communications with media, community staff and general practitioners, etc.

4.6 Risks to and from healthcare workers

Healthcare workers (HCWs) are at risk of acquiring infectious disease because of exposure during their work. They are also a potential source of infection for those whom they are caring for, particularly when working with those with impaired resistance to infection.

Healthcare workers can be considered according to the level of probable exposure to infectious disease risks. Target groups for preventative interventions can then be identified following a risk assessment based upon the likelihood of transmission.

Category I. Clinical and other staff, including those in primary care, who have regular, clinical contact with patients.

Category II. Laboratory and mortuary staff who have direct contact with potentially infectious clinical specimens.

Category III. Non-clinical ancillary staff who have social contact with patients, but not usually of a prolonged or close nature.

Category IV. Maintenance staff, e.g. engineers, gardeners.

Preventative interventions for healthcare staff are identified in Table 4.6.1.

Lookback studies

Purpose

The purposes of lookback studies are listed below.

• Determine who are at risk of acquiring a communicable disease following an exposure, usually related to healthcare.

• Inform exposed individuals about the risk to which they have been exposed.

• Determine who, amongst those exposed, has been infected.

• Prevent further transmissions.

• Provide appropriate interventions (treatment, counselling, etc.) for those exposed, both infected and uninfected.

• Advance understanding about reducing and quantifying exposure risks.

Context

Lookback exercises are usually carried out following exposure, or suspected exposure to blood-borne viruses (hepatitis B, hepatitis C virus or HIV) within a healthcare setting. Similar exercises may be recommended for potential exposures to other infections, such TB and vCJD. When lookback studies are being undertaken there may well be heightened media interest. Procedures for dealing with this should be established early. The importance of preserving the confidentiality of the healthcare worker and contacts should be emphasized. There may well be concern from the 'worried well', and mechanisms for providing reassurance may need to be established.

Table 4.6.1 Preventative interventions for healthcare staff

Infection	Target group (see p. 268)	Rationale	Comments
Diarrhoea	Category I	Personal and patient protection	Staff with diarrhoea should report to occupational health
Diphtheria	Category I staff caring for patients with diphtheria Category II staff	Personal protection	National immunization programme should ensure immunity. Category II staff should have immunity checked
Hepatitis A	Category I staff working in institutions for patients with learning disabilities Category II laboratory staff who may handle the virus Category IV maintenance staff exposed to sewage	Personal protection	Immunization may be offered following a risk assessment
Hepatitis B	Category I and II staff with exposure to blood, blood-stained body fluids and tissues	Personal and patient protection	Immunization may be offered to other groups of staff following a risk assessment
Hepatitis C	Category I and II staff with exposure to blood, blood-stained body fluids and tissues	Personal and patient protection	See section on lookback exercises
HIV	Category I & II staff	Personal and patient protection	See section on lookback exercises Risk assessment to be undertaken, particularly if exposure to TB
Influenza	Category I staff	Personal and possibly patient protection	Annual immunization should be offered by occupational health service
Poliomyelitis	All HCWs	Personal protection	National immunization programme should ensure immunity
Rabies	Those directly caring for rabid patients	For their own protection	Immunization

Continued on p. 270

Table 4.6.1 *Continued*

Infection	Target group	Rationale	Comments
Rubella	Category I HCWs working in maternity departments	For patient protection	National immunization programme should ensure immunity. HCWs in high-risk areas should have documented immunity
TB	Important for all Category I & II staff	Personal and patient protection	Staff without a BCG scar or documented BCG immunization should be tuberculin-tested and offered BCG Staff should report possible TB symptoms promptly
Tetanus	Category III staff at higher risk of tetanus-prone wounds, e.g. gardeners	Personal protection	National immunization programme should ensure immunity
Varicella	Category 1 HCWs working in high-risk clinical areas such as maternity and oncology	Patient protection	Varicella-zoster vaccine not licensed in the UK. Varicella-zoster antibodies to be checked. Non-immune staff to be excluded from high-risk areas between days 7–21 following exposure

HIV

Guidance on lookback exercises is given by the UK Expert Advisory Group (EAGA): Expert Advisory Group on AIDS. *AIDS/HIV infected healthcare workers: practical guidance on notifying patients.* London: HMSO, 1993; UK Health Departments. *AIDS/HIV infected healthcare workers: guidance on the management of infected healthcare workers and patient notification.* London: Department of Health 1998.

When to carry out a look back
EAGA recommends 'that all patients who have undergone an exposure-prone procedure (EPP) where the infected healthcare worker

was the sole or main operator should, as far as practicable, be notified of this'.

What is an EPP?
A procedure in which there is a risk that injury to the heathcare worker may result in exposure of the patient's open tissues to the blood of the healthcare worker. This usually involves operations in which the HCW's fingers are not visible whilst exposed to sharp objects (Table 4.6.2).

Methods
- Establish incident management team.
- Ensure overall co-ordination is clear.
- Establish helplines.

Table 4.6.2 Classification of procedures by risk of transmission of bloodborne virus

Risk of exposure	Definition	Examples
Higher	Major operations	Vaginal or abdominal hysterectomy, caesarean section, prolapse repair, salpingectomy
Low	Other procedures, suturing or sharp instruments	Laparoscopy, forceps delivery, episiotomy repair, incision of Bartholin's abscess
None	Procedures that do not involve suturing or sharp instruments	Manual removal of placenta, dilatation and curettage, cystoscopy, spontaneous vaginal delivery

From *Commun Dis Public Health* 1999; **2**: 127.

- Ensure GPs kept informed.
- Define exposure-prone procedure. It may be necessary to define high- and low-risk procedures in order to concentrate resources on those most at risk.
- Identify those exposed. This may involve extensive searches through hospital records, operating theatre registers, etc.
- Contact exposed patients—this may be personally by GPs or their staff, or by letter. The method will need to be sensitive to the risk, and to the need of those contacted for support and counselling.
- It is important to ensure that helplines/counselling is in place, and that there are clear algorithms for the care of those identified.
- Ensure close liaison with press office throughout.

Transmission risk

A number of lookback studies have been carried out following exposure to HIV-infected healthcare workers. Studies of over 30 000 patients (about half of whom have undergone testing) have shown no evidence of transmission of HIV to patients. Two incidents—a Florida dentist who transmitted infection to 6 patients and a French orthopaedic surgeon who infected one patient—have been reported.

The risk of transmission from an HIV-infected healthcare worker to a patient following an EPP is likely to be low.

Sources of further advice

- Expert Advisory Group on AIDS.
- CDSC.
- Department of Health.

Hepatitis B

Healthcare workers who carry hepatitis B virus may infect patients who become exposed to their serum.

The UK Health Departments require all HCWs who undertake exposure-prone procedures to be vaccinated against hepatitis B virus, and their subsequent immunity to be documented. Non-responders to vaccination should be investigated for evidence of chronic HBV infection.

HCWs who are hepatitis e antigen—positive may not undertake EPPs (see Table 4.6.2) because of the significant risk they pose to patients.

In spite of the recommendations for immunization and restriction placed upon practice, a number of events have still occurred where patients have been exposed to an infected healthcare worker, or to the risk of transmission in a healthcare setting.

When to carry out a look back

There is no formal guidance. However, the recommendations given by EAGA for HIV lookback exercises are helpful. Notification exercises should not extend beyond 12 months unless high rates of transmission have been documented.

What is an EPP?
As for HIV.

Methods
As above. The incubation period for hepatitis B virus (2–6 months) is such that exposed patients may be identified during the period before seroconversion. Serum should be taken from patients on identification and they should be retested six months after exposure to identify seroconversions. DNA sequencing of fragments of HBV DNA may be useful to establish transmission.

Interventions
Hepatitis B immunoglobulin is effective up to one week after exposure and should be offered to individuals at risk. The value of hepatitis B vaccination is unclear, and there is probably little merit in using hepatitis B vaccine more than two weeks after exposure. Systems will need to be put in place for ensuring that those who do not clear the virus are followed up and if appropriate offered treatment for chronic hepatitis B.

Transmission risk
Transmission rates identified in incidents involving surgical staff in the UK from 1975 to 1990 have ranged from 0.9 to 20%, depending on the procedures and other factors.

Sources of further advice
- Expert Advisory Group on hepatitis.
- CDSC.
- Department of Health.

Hepatitis C

Guidance on the risks and management of occupational exposure to hepatitis C was issued by the PHLS in December 1999 (M.E. Ramsay,

Guidance on the investigation and management of occupational exposure to hepatitis C. *Commun Dis Public Health* 1999; **2**: 258–62), also available on http://www.phls.org.uk/advice/other.htm).

Healthcare workers who carry hepatitis C virus may infect patients who become exposed to their serum; however, the risk of transmission is much lower than the risk of transmission for hepatitis B from an e antigen—positive surgeon. Healthcare workers are not restricted in carrying out exposure-prone procedures unless they have been shown to transmit hep-atitis C. They should be advised on adherence to precautions for the control of blood-borne infection by the occupational health department.

When to carry out a look back
As for hepatitis B.

What is an EPP?
As for HIV.

Methods
Serum should be taken from those exposed on identification. Advice should be sought on when repeat testing should be performed. It is recommended that serum is obtained from healthcare workers exposed to a known positive source at baseline, 6, 12 and 24 weeks and tested for HCV RNA at 6 and 12 weeks and anti-HCV at 12 and 24 weeks. Genotyping may be useful to establish transmission.

Interventions
Although there is some disagreement over the effectiveness of early treatment in preventing progression of disease, most experts favour treatment of patients with acute hepatitis C.

Sources of further advice
- Expert Advisory Group on hepatitis.
- CDSC.
- Department of Health.

4.7 Co-ordination of immunization services

The role of the Immunization Co-ordinator

Each health authority should delegate a particular person (or persons) to take on special responsibility for implementing improvements to immunization programmes at local level. The separation of commissioning and delivery of service in the UK usually results in the need for two individuals to be involved in co-ordination: the most obvious candidates being a CCDC and a community paediatrician.

The main functions of the Immunization Co-ordinator are as follows:

• To ensure that an appropriate strategy, with the aim of ensuring that every child (in the absence of genuine contraindications) receives immunization, is devised and implemented.

• To ensure that appropriate resources are in place to support the strategy.

• To ensure that appropriate local policies and procedures, based on models of good practice, are in place to support the strategy.

• To act as a local source of advice and information on immunization issues for both the public and professionals.

• To co-ordinate the role of all those involved with immunization in primary care, child health services, hospitals, educational establishments, and elsewhere, and to gain their commitment to the strategy and its aim.

• To chair the district immunization committee and ensure delivery of its identified responsibilities (see below).

• To ensure that training and updating of all staff involved in immunization is available.

• To ensure that up-to-date and reliable figures on immunization uptake rates are available.

• To ensure that non-immunized children are identified and followed up.

• To investigate the reasons for poor uptake figures and to promote appropriate methods to overcome identified problems.

• To ensure that appropriate audit is carried out on the availability, effectiveness and efficiency of local immunization services.

Box 4.7.1 UK immunization schedule

Age	Vaccine
Neonates	BCG (certain groups only)
	Hepatitis B (certain groups only)
2, 3, 4 months	*3 dose primary course of:*
	Diphtheria/tetanus/pertussis (DTP)
	Oral polio
	Hib
	Meningococcus C
12–15 months	*1 dose primary course of:*
	Measles/mumps/rubella (MMRI)
3–5 years	*1 dose booster of:*
	Diphtheria/tetanus (DT)
	Oral polio
	Measles/mumps/rubella (MMRII)
10–14 years	BCG
13–18 years	*Booster doses of:*
	Diphtheria (low dose)/tetanus (Td)
	Oral polio
Adult	Boosters for tetanus and polio if appropriate
	Vaccines for occupational or lifestyle risks
65 years	Influenza
Any age	Influenza, pneumococcus (medical risk groups)
	Travel vaccines

The district immunization committee (DIC)

The Immunization Co-ordinator should be supported by a DIC. An appropriate membership might be any of the following:

Box 4.7.2 How to rectify a poor vaccine uptake rate

First check how accurate the figures are. In our experience recorded figures can underestimate true uptake by 3–4%.
• Check denominator against most up-to-date register of population. The immunization database should be regularly updated from the general practitioner (formerly 'FHSA') register in the UK.
• Check the numerator by sending lists of apparently unvaccinated children to their GPs to verify. In the UK, the date for submission of claims for payment is later than that for calculating uptake figures. It may be useful to carry out this exercise every quarter.
• Is information being received on children who are immunized in neighbouring districts (e.g. resident of district A registered with GP in district B)?

Consider the following actions to increase the number vaccinated:
• Calculate uptake rates by each general practice. Low performers may benefit from assistance with organizing routine clinics or opportunistic vaccination (e.g. prompts on medical notes) or input from a facilitator.
• Look for GPs with good uptake for most vaccines, but low uptake for pertussis or MMR. These practices may benefit from a visit by a community paediatrician (e.g. to educate on true contraindications) and access to an advice line or special clinic for children with 'problem histories'.
• Encourage other staff (e.g. hospital paediatricians, A & E staff, health visitors) to identify and refer non-vaccinated children.
• Consider domiciliary vaccination and opportunistic vaccination at routine health checks for non-attenders. This may also reduce inequalities in vaccine uptake.
• Organize CPD sessions for staff from targeted practices.
• Ensure nurses are trained to give immunizations without a doctor present.
• Organize public education on severity of illness and safety of vaccines via local media.
• Systems generally associated with good uptake involve a computerized system of routine appointments, personal letters from the patients' own doctor, target payments for GPs and arrangements for opportunistic or domiciliary immunization. GP clinics tend to have higher uptake than health authority clinics.

Other points of interest:
• A major predictor of low uptake of MMR and preschool vaccinations is failure to attend for the primary immunization course.
• A reminder card based on the health belief model led to a higher uptake in one Australian study.
• Particular problems may be identified with late immunization of preterm infants, and low uptake of BCG and hepatitis B in target groups. These problems are usually due to organizational failures. There also may be language difficulties for parents of some of the targeted groups.

• CCDC.
• Community paediatrician.
• Information manager (child health/immunization database).
• Community services manager.

• Community services commissioner.
• General practitioner.
• Practice nurse.
• Pharmacist.
• Health promotion officer.

The terms of reference of the DIC could be:

• To review and advise on immunization policies within the district and to develop an integrated district-wide strategy in order to achieve the maximum immunization uptake within the district, in line with Department of Health guidelines.

• To implement and monitor the immunization programme.

• To ensure accurate information is maintained to support the immunization programme, and is shared appropriately.

• To ensure the organization of an efficient and effective recall system.

• To ensure that an accurate record of all immunizations given to any child in the district is provided to any professional caring for that child and the parent/carer.

• To ensure appropriate training and updating is available on an ongoing basis for all staff involved in the immunization programme.

• To ensure that advice is given on the appropriate systems for the storage of vaccines.

• To co-ordinate health promotion activities within the district on immunization issues.

• To ensure organization of an efficient patient recall system.

• To ensure that a source of clinical management advice concerning the immunization programme is available within the district.

• To ensure that a rapid response is possible should a particular immunization need arise.

Immunization uptake rates

The theoretical aim of immunization services is to achieve herd immunity against those diseases transmitted from person to person (e.g. measles) and to protect everyone against those with other sources (e.g. tetanus). Many countries have set general targets for immunization uptake based on the WHO approach. In the UK, these are 95% update of all primary immunizations (including MMR) by the child's second birthday.

Many districts fail to achieve these targets. These districts are often those with the highest population density, and therefore where a higher uptake than average is needed to achieve herd immunity. Many districts also vaccinate a significant proportion of their children much later than the target age: this further increases the pool of susceptibles, allowing transmission to continue. A further consequence of late vaccination is the exposure of infants to pertussis and Hib at an age at which severity of disease is highest.

Contributing reasons for low or late immunizations may be:

• Reduced public confidence in certain vaccines after media scares, e.g. MMR and pertussis. Concern may be highest in higher social class parents.

• Confusion amongst health professionals as to safety and true contraindications of vaccines, particularly pertussis.

• Factors related to social deprivation, particularly high population mobility, lone parenthood, and large family size.

• Factors relating to religion and lifestyle (particular problems in the Netherlands) and ethnicity. Children born abroad are often not up to date with vaccination.

• Problems with the way programmes are organized, delivered and remunerated.

4.8 Co-ordination of services for HIV infection in the UK

Services for HIV infection face the challenge of working with socially marginalized groups such as gay men, injecting drug users, persons of black and minority ethnic origin, prisoners and sex workers. Many of these groups are difficult to reach and influence. Prevention initiatives are needed that not only attempt to change individual behaviour but also the social context in which people are sexually active.

In the UK, public health departments have particular responsibilities for HIV services.

This public health focus is less obvious in other European countries.

In the UK, each health authority is required to appoint an HIV prevention co-ordinator (HPC) with responsibility for ensuring there is appropriate development of services for the prevention, treatment and care of HIV infection. The HPC is often the CCDC. It is important to ensure that investment in HIV services is based on a sound understanding of the epidemiology of HIV at both local and national level. Accurate and timely HIV surveillance data is the key to this.

Health authorities have a key role to play in needs assessment, and this can be particularly challenging in areas where there is currently a low prevalence of HIV infection.

Efforts should be made to involve general practice and primary care in HIV services. Community-based and self-help voluntary organizations may be better placed to carry out targeted health promotion work rather than statutory agencies.

Health authorities should ensure that HIV is covered in their health improvement programmes, which are local plans to improve health and modernize services. Local targets to tackle local priorities may be agreed.

It is anticipated that the Government will publish a national service framework for HIV infection. The National Institute of Clinical Excellence will have a role in monitoring the quality of HIV services.

Each year in England, the Government earmarks about £290m for HIV treatment and care and £54m for HIV prevention. These funds are allocated to health authorities, using a formula that is based on SOPHID data (see Chapter 3.33). In its HIV strategy, the UK Government lists key priority areas for action (Table 4.8.1) and health authority performance in investing in these areas is monitored through annual returns, which are a legal requirement under the AIDS (Control) Act 1987.

Health service arrangements vary between countries in Europe. For example in the Netherlands and Germany, municipal health services offer HIV testing and health education; treatment and care for HIV and AIDS is financed by health insurance; and treatment is provided by hospitals and individual physicians.

Table 4.8.1 UK Government priorities for HIV services

Surveillance
• Maintain existing surveillance systems

Treatment and care
• Ensure all patients with HIV infection have equal access to new antiviral therapies
• Ensure there is consistent high quality social care for people with HIV infection, particularly services for individuals and families of African origin
• Ensure there is access to high-quality confidential GUM services for the treatment of STIs and counselling and testing for HIV infection

Diagnostic testing
• Encourage voluntary confidential testing for HIV infection to reduce the proportion of infection that is undiagnosed until a clinical illness develops
• Introduce routine antenatal HIV testing to reduce the transmission of HIV from mother to infant

Health promotion to reduce transmission of HIV infection
• Ensure there is high-quality HIV health promotion for the general population
• Ensure there is targeted health promotion for gay men, in particular young gay men, bisexuals and other men who have sex with men, injecting drug users, heterosexuals at behavioural risk of acquiring STIs, men and women who travel to, or who have family links with, high-prevalence countries, particularly sub-Saharan Africa, women partners of men in the above groups and people with HIV infection

4.9 Services for tuberculosis control

In the UK, the Consultant in Communicable Disease Control (CCDC) has responsibility on behalf of the health authority to ensure that there is a comprehensive district programme for the surveillance, prevention and control of tuberculosis. This depends on the prompt recognition, confirmation and treatment of cases and the implementation of infection control measures to reduce spread of infection from infectious patients to others.

This requires a team approach and close working relationships between health professionals and others involved in the care of patients with TB including the TB physician (usually a consultant chest physician who is familiar with anti-TB drugs and who has experience of the management of TB), the microbiologist, the hospital infection control team, the TB nurse specialists, the CCDC and in some cases the HIV or GUM physician.

Good tuberculosis programmes can reduce the transmission of tuberculosis and the incidence of drug-resistant disease. Failure to maintain such programmes contributed to loss of TB control in the late 1980s in some parts of the world. Key UK guidance documents are listed in Appendix 2.

There should be a written health authority policy for tuberculosis prevention and control (Table 4.9.1).

Table 4.9.1 Health authority policy for the prevention and control of tuberculosis

Policy area	Details
Aims and objectives	• To halt and reverse the recent rise in cases of TB in the UK • To reduce avoidable mortality associated with TB • To minimize morbidity • To prevent secondary cases • To prevent emergence of drug resistant TB
Surveillance	A detailed data set should be collected on all cases of TB. A computerized register should be maintained. Regular reports should be made to CDSC. The CCDC should write an annual TB report
Identification of cases	A high level of clinical suspicion for TB should be encouraged amongst local GPs and hospital clinicians. An annual TB postgraduate education event should be considered. Surgeons, radiologists and microbiologists should discuss possible cases with the TB physician
Diagnosis	All isolates must be sent to the regional tuberculosis reference laboratory. HIV testing should be offered where appropriate
Notification	All cases of TB (including those associated with HIV infection) must be reported to the CCDC
Management of cases	Treatment of all cases must be supervised by a TB physician and specialist TB nurse
	Accurate prescribing is important. There should be early recognition and management of drug-resistant TB
	Particular skills and tactics are needed with patients who are non-compliant or who have disorganized lifestyles
	Directly observed treatment (DOT) should be used if necessary. Compulsory admission to hospital for treatment is not usually practicable

Continued on p. 278

Table 4.9.1 *Continued*

Policy area	Details
Contact tracing	Contact tracing should be undertaken promptly to minimize the risk of continuing transmission. Contacts are managed according to national guidelines
Control of infection	All hospitals caring for patients with tuberculosis should have a tuberculosis control plan drawn up in conjunction with the infection control team covering assessment of risk of infection and transmission including HIV related and drug-resistant tuberculosis, isolation room requirements, measures for the protection of healthcare workers and other contacts, including use of masks and disinfection of equipment
	When patients in a hospital have been exposed to a healthcare worker or another patient with infectious tuberculosis, the infection control team, TB physician, occupational health department and the CCDC should work jointly to agree appropriate control measures
Case finding	Case finding should be carried out by screening population groups at risk of infection and offering chemoprophylaxis and BCG where appropriate
	High-risk groups include contacts of TB cases, new immigrants, refugees and asylum seekers, rough sleepers and hostel dwellers
BCG immunization	Local immunization policies should follow national guidelines. In the UK, immunization is recommended for school children aged between 10 and 14 years, high-risk neonates, contacts of cases with active pulmonary tuberculosis, new immigrants from high-prevalence countries, those at risk of occupational exposure and those planning to travel to and stay in a high-prevalence country for more than a month
Occupational health	Employers are required to assess the risk of TB for their employees and select appropriate control measures. These may include pre-employment screening and use of BCG. Staff should be made aware of the symptoms of tuberculosis so that they can seek advice early if problems arise
Prisons and other institutions where residents may be at higher risk of tuberculosis	The CCDC should liaise with medical staff at prisons and other relevant institutions where residents may be at higher risk of tuberculosis to agree appropriate policies for staff and prisoners
Arrangements for outbreak, recognition and investigation	The identification of a single case of TB in a school or hospital or a cluster of cases of TB in a community setting requires a co-ordinated response, as with any other infectious disease incident or outbreak
Education and training	There should be appropriately targeted educational material for the general public and healthcare staff and others at higher risk of tuberculosis
Monitoring and audit	Performance targets should be set. There should be an audit of completeness of notification
Resources	The CCDC requires resources for data collection and collation in order to undertake the core functions of surveillance, outbreak investigation and policy co-ordination
	For control services, the British Thoracic Society suggests a minimum of one full-time equivalent health visitor or nurse plus appropriate clerical support for every 50 notifications. Some higher incidence districts and those with a large immigrant or homeless population may require more than this. Some elements of the TB control programme such as managing non-compliant patients, contact tracing and screening new arrivals are labour-intensive and require staff with appropriate training and expertise

4.10 Travelhealth

Up to 75% of short-term travellers to the tropics or subtropics report health problems. These are mostly minor, and less than 1% require hospitalization. Infection contributes substantially to this morbidity in travellers, particularly diarrhoeal disease, but only about 1% of deaths among this population. Individuals also carry their epidemiological risk with them; hence cardiovascular disease is the most common cause of death in travellers from Europe. Injury and accidents (motor vehicle, drowning, etc.) are the next most common cause of serious morbidity and mortality.

Travel health clinics providing up-to-date advice on risk and risk reduction can be effective in preventing ill health through simple precautions. However, the epidemiology of infectious disease risks to the traveller changes rapidly and continuously; those running travel clinics need to ensure access to up-to-date advice and current recommendations.

Prevention

Up-to-date travel advice to travellers is key to prevention. Giving appropriate advice to those with complex itineraries may be a difficult task. Opportunities should be taken to ensure that those who travel at short notice have their vaccination status reviewed regularly.

Advice should cover:
• Basic food and personal hygiene.
• Avoiding insect vectors.
• Safe sex and avoidance of potential blood-borne virus exposure.
• Avoiding dog bites and other potential rabies exposures.
• Malaria prophylaxis.
• Vaccination against specific diseases as appropriate.

Traveller's diarrhoea

Diarrhoea, usually short-lived and self-limiting, is a major cause of illness in travellers; in 20% the person is confined to bed. The main risk factor is the destination; incidence rates vary from 8% per 2-week stay in industrialized countries to over 50% in parts of Africa, Central and South America, and South-east Asia. Infants and young adults are at particularly high risk. The likelihood of diarrhoea is related to dietary indiscretions; however, few take sufficient care.

The risk of traveller's diarrhoea and other faeco–orally transmitted disease (e.g. hepatitis A and typhoid) in those who travel to developing countries can be reduced by the following:
• Washing hands after toilet and before preparing or eating food.
• Using only sterilized or bottled water for drinking, cleaning teeth, making ice and washing food (e.g. salad).
• Avoiding uncooked food (unless you can peel it or shell it yourself), untreated milk or milk products (e.g. ice cream), uncooked shellfish, food that may have been exposed to flies and any other potentially contaminated food.
• It is usually safe to eat freshly cooked food that is thoroughly cooked and still hot; hot tea and coffee; commercially produced alcoholic and soft drinks.

Malaria

It has been estimated that more than 30 000 American and European travellers develop malaria each year. The risk varies by season and place; it is highest in sub-Saharan Africa and Oceania (1 : 50–1 : 1000). An average of seven deaths per year is reported in travellers from England and Wales.

Compliance with antimalarial chemoprophylaxis regimens and use of personal protection measures are key to the prevention of malaria. However, fewer than 50% of travellers at risk adhere to basic recommendations for malaria prevention.

Measures to reduce the risk of mosquito bites include:
• Sleep in screened rooms, use knockdown insecticide in evening and use an electrical pyrethroid vaporizer overnight.
• If room cannot be made safe, use impregnated bed-nets.

- Wear long-sleeved shirts and long trousers in evening. Use insect repellent.

Advice on chemoprophylaxis has been made more difficult by the increase in chloroquine- and multidrug-resistant *Plasmodium falciparum* malaria, and primaquine- and chloroquine-resistant strains of *Plasmodium vivax*. The recommended regime will depend upon the proposed itinerary: most situations will be covered by the latest published guidance (currently *Commun Dis Rep CDR Rev* 1997; 7: R138-152), with the PHLS Malaria Reference Laboratory able to advise on specific problems (see Appendix 1).

Travellers to endemic countries should be informed of the symptoms of malaria and the need to seek urgent medical attention. Those who will be out of reach of medical services can be given stand-by therapy.

Immunization and travel

Many countries and the WHO produce recommendations for vaccination of travellers (see Appendix 2): these should be consulted.

Diphtheria, tetanus, and polio

Foreign travel is an ideal opportunity to have these immunizations updated. Diphtheria is a problem worldwide, with large outbreaks recently in the new states previously part of the Soviet Union. There are low levels of tetanus antitoxin and immunity to polio serogroups in many adults.

Hepatitis A

Hepatitis A is the most frequent vaccine-preventable infection of travellers. It is endemic in many parts of the world, including southern Europe. The risk is especially high for those who leave the usual tourist routes. Immunization is recommended for travellers to countries in Africa, Asia, Central and South America and the Caribbean, where hygiene and sanitation may be poor, and for some countries in eastern Europe, although it may be less important for short stays in good accommodation.

Hepatitis B (HBV)

Immunization against HBV should be given to all those who may come into contact with body fluids (e.g. those planning to work as healthcare workers). The incidence also appears raised in other long-stay overseas workers, perhaps as a result of medical and dental procedures received abroad. Immunization is not necessary for short-term business or tourist travellers, unless their sexual behaviour puts them at risk.

Typhoid

The risk of typhoid is especially high for those leaving the usual tourist routes, or visiting relatives or friends in developing countries. Typhoid vaccine is recommended for the same groups as hepatitis A vaccine. Vaccination against paratyphoid is not recommended.

Cholera

The risk of cholera is extremely low (approximately 1 case per 500 000 journeys to endemic areas). Cholera vaccine is not indicated for travellers. No country requires proof of cholera vaccination as a condition for entry.

Yellow fever

A yellow fever vaccination certificate is required for entry into most countries of sub-Saharan Africa and South America in which the infection exists. Many countries require a certificate from travellers arriving from, or who have been in transit through, infected areas. Some countries require a certificate from all entering travellers.

As the areas of yellow fever virus circulation exceed the officially reported zones, vaccination is strongly recommended for travel to all countries in the endemic zone (particularly if visiting rural areas), even if these countries have not officially reported the disease and do not require a vaccination certificate.

The vaccination has almost total efficacy, while the case fatality rate for the disease is more than 60% in non-immune adults. In recent years, fatal cases of yellow fever have occurred in unvaccinated tourists visiting rural areas within the yellow fever endemic zone.

Rabies

Rabies vaccination should be considered in all those who are likely to come into contact with animals where the disease is present (e.g. veterinarians), and those undertaking long journeys in remote areas.

Japanese B encephalitis

Immunization should be considered in those staying for a month or more in rural areas of endemic countries in south-east Asia and the far east.

Meningococcal disease

Immunization should be considered in those going to areas of the world where the incidence is high (e.g. the 'meningitis belt' of sub-Saharan Africa, and areas in the north of the Indian subcontinent), or to events where there may be significant exposure, such as the Hadj in Saudi Arabia.

Tick-borne encephalitis

Vaccination is recommended for those who are to walk, camp or work in late spring and summer in warm, heavily forested parts of central and eastern Europe and Scandinavia. They should also cover arms, legs and ankles and use insect repellent.

Pregnancy, infection and travel

• Dehydration resulting from diarrhoea can reduce placental blood flow, therefore pregnant travellers must be careful about their food and drink intake. They should also be aware of infections such as toxoplasmosis and listeriosis, with potentially serious sequelae in pregnancy. Women should be encouraged to breast-feed if travelling with a neonate. A nursing mother with traveller's diarrhoea should not stop breast-feeding but should increase her fluid intake.

• Malaria during pregnancy carries a significant risk of morbidity and death. Pregnant women should be advised of this increased risk if intending travelling to endemic areas. If travel is essential, then chemoprophylaxis and avoidance of bites are essential (take specialist advice).

The HIV-infected traveller

The HIV-infected traveller may be at risk of serious infection. Those with AIDS, CD4+ counts of <200/L and those who are symptomatic should seek specialist advice, particularly before going to the developing world. Those with a CD4+ cell count above 500 probably have a risk similar to a person without HIV infection.

Gastrointestinal illness

The HIV-infected traveller needs to be particularly careful about the foods and beverage consumed. Traveller's diarrhoea occurs more frequently, is more severe, protracted and more difficult to treat when in association with HIV infection. Infections are also more likely to be accompanied by bacteraemia. Organisms particularly associated with severe chronic diarrhoea in HIV-positive travellers include *Cryptosporidium* and *Isospora belli*.

Immunization

All of the HIV-infected traveller's routine immunizations should be up to date. In general, live attenuated vaccines are contraindicated for persons with immune dysfunction. Live oral polio vaccine should not be given to HIV-infected patients or members of their households. Inactivated polio vaccine (IPV) should be used. Live yellow-fever vaccine should not normally be given to HIV-infected travellers; however, if travel in an endemic area is absolutely necessary, vaccination may be considered after a risk assessment and consideration of the CD4 count. Bacille Calmette–Guérin (BCG) should not be given because of disseminated infection in HIV-infected persons.

Surveillance

Surveillance of travel-related infection is largely unsystematic and there are few good estimates of the risks of acquiring an infection when visiting a particular location. This makes basing advice on good evidence difficult.

Travel-associated infections and clusters of travel-associated infection should be reported to the public health authorities so that an improved picture of communicable disease risk can be developed.

4.11 Surveillance and investigation of environmental hazards

Surveillance of environmental hazards

Environmental health comprises aspects of human health and quality of life that are determined by physical, biological, social and psychosocial factors in the environment.

Some physical and biological factors in particular have the potential to adversely affect health, and are described as environmental hazards (Table 4.11.1). However, there are other equally important environmental determinants of health, including regeneration, transport policy, sustainable development including energy efficiency, housing policy including houses in multiple occupation and homelessness, social inclusion, planning policy, diet and nutrition policy, natural disasters,

industrial accidents and occupational health and safety.

Environmental health practice is concerned with assessing, controlling and preventing environment factors that can adversely affect health now or in the future.

The arrangements for the surveillance and management of the health aspects of non-communicable environmental hazards comprises three main areas of activity (HSG (93)56):

1 The surveillance of disease, possible causative factors and influences to identify and investigate any pattern of disease which is unusual or novel.
2 The possibility of a long-term raised level of disease in a particular area, possibly associated with a point source of continuing pollution or contamination.
3 The response to an acute incident or other accident.

Investigating the health effects of environmental hazards

Communities living near potential sources of pollution such as industrial sites and contaminated land and other environmental hazards are often concerned about possible effects on health. They may link local clusters of adverse chronic and acute health effects to exposure to these sites.

Clusters are defined as the aggregation of a number of similar illnesses in space and time and the perception that the number is excessive. Most types of health event may cluster, but cancer clusters receive the most attention. Greater significance is attached to a cluster when a site of industrial pollution is involved.

The CCDC may be asked to investigate possible clusters and other health problems associated with environmental hazards (Table 4.11.2). The investigation should start with simple but robust studies, and progress to more elaborate studies only if positive results are obtained. Often these investigations are inconclusive, and cluster investigations in particular are not usually helpful in identifying possible environmental associations. These

Table 4.11.1 Environmental hazards

Hazard	Notes
Factories and industrial processes	These may cause nuisance as a result of soiling of the environment, noise, odour or road traffic. Potential health effects may arise from chemical releases, fumes and particulates.
	The Control of Major Accident Hazards (COMAH) Regulations 1999 require the operators of major installations to carry out risk assessments and agree joint emergency plans. In the UK, COMAH sites are regulated by the Health and Safety Executive.
	Other important industries and processes are regulated by the Environment Agency under Part A of Section 1 of the Environmental Protection Act 1990. Smaller businesses are regulated by local authorities under Part B.
	Operators are required to use the best available techniques not entailing excessive cost (BATNEEC) to minimize pollution. Registers are maintained for Part A and Part B processes, although some low-level activities are not covered by this system. Emissions and pollution inventories are available.
	This system is being replaced by Integrated Pollution Prevention and Control, an EU standard incorporated into UK law.
Chemicals	There are 11 million known chemicals. 70 000 are in regular commercial use and 600 new chemicals enter the market place each month. Most chemicals have had little or no toxicological assessment. Chemicals may be released into the environment during production, storage, transport, use or disposal.
	It is helpful to identify local sites which may represent sources of major chemical hazard. This will allow action to be taken in the event of a release.
	Legislation for the control of chemicals falls under two broad headings: controls over releases of chemicals as waste to air, water and land (pollution control) and controls over the manufacture and use of chemicals (chemicals policy).
	There are 100 000 chemicals on the European Inventory of Existing Commercial Chemical Substances (EINECS), of which approximately 20 000 are currently on the market. Of these over 100 have been listed for priority attention because of their possible risk to health or the environment.
	New chemicals can only be placed on the market if the manufacturer or importer submits a notification that includes an assessment of possible harmful effects on humans and the environment.
	The EU or individual member states are able to restrict or ban dangerous substances.
	National and European activities on chemicals are part of a wider international structure under the UN Environment Programme (UNEP).
	There are also a number of international conventions and industry initiatives to restrict the use of harmful chemicals.
	The Control of Substances Hazardous to Health Regulations 1999 (COSHH) are made under the Health and Safety at Work, etc. Act 1974. They require employers to control exposure to hazardous substances to prevent ill health.

Continued on p.284

Table 4.11.1 *Continued*

Hazard	Notes
Outdoor air quality	Concentrations of outdoor air pollutants vary from region to region and from day to day. Occasionally, when concentrations are significantly raised, some adverse effects on health occur. Air quality in the UK has been improving in recent years, but further action is proposed.
	The UK Government has a National Air Quality Strategy which is under review. This sets out health-based air quality standards for a range of pollutants which represent concentrations at which there should be little or no threat to human health at a population level. The Government has set targets to improve air quality so that the air quality standards will be met in all areas by the year 2005. Local authorities have to review air quality in their areas, report, consult and decide whether to declare an Air Quality Management Zone.
	There is an extensive network of air quality monitoring stations throughout the UK and real-time data from this can be found in the national archive of UK air quality data on the Internet (http://www.aeat.co.uk/netcen/airqual).
	Pollutants such as benzene and 1,3-butadiene are carcinogens. Other air pollutants may have chronic effects on health during infancy, and may have an effect on life expectancy as a result of long-term exposure throughout life. Particulate matter, ozone and sulphur dioxide may have acute effects on susceptible members of the population, leading to premature mortality and hospital admissions in those with pre-existing respiratory disease.
Indoor air quality	Rates of respiratory disease and incidence of allergic responses such as asthma have increased in recent years, and there is concern that some of this increase may be linked to changes in the indoor environment, including allergens, tobacco smoke, oxides of nitrogen and formaldehyde.
Drinking water	Over 99% of the population in the UK receives mains water supplies; the quality of these supplies is very high and all are safe to drink.
	The basic unit of water supply is the water supply zone, which is designated by the water company, normally by reference to a source of water, and which covers a population of about 50 000 people.
	There are water quality standards, which include microbiological, chemical, physical and aesthetic parameters. Water in some water supply zones is temporarily permitted to exceed these statutory standards for certain chemicals such as lead, polycyclic aromatic hydrocarbons and pesticides. The most important source of lead in tap water is dissolution from household plumbing systems.
	Private water supplies are regulated by the local authority, but are subject to a much reduced sampling regime. Whilst covering a much smaller proportion of the population than public water utilities in the same area, substantial numbers may receive water from private supplies.
Sewerage systems and sewage	The UK has the highest percentage connection rate to sewers of any country in the EU and it also has one of the highest levels of provision of sewage treatment.
Water resources management	Under the Water Resources Act 1991 in England and Wales, the Environment Agency regulates any discharges to water to improve the quality of bathing waters.

Continued

Table 4.11.1 *Continued*

Hazard	Notes
Solid waste, reduction, regulation, collection, disposal	About 500 million tonnes of waste are produced each year in the UK. Waste management is governed by the Environmental Protection Act 1990.
Contaminated land	Contaminated land is defined by the local authority as land which by virtue of contamination may cause harm or water pollution. Contaminated land may endanger human health through the escape of contaminants from the soil.
	It is estimated that there are between 50 000 and 100 000 potentially contaminated sites across the UK, totalling between 100 000 and 200 000 hectares. However, only a small proportion of these sites pose any immediate threat to human health and the wider environment. Part II A of the Environmental Protection Act 1990 and the recent Contaminated Land (England) Regulations 2000 provide the regulatory framework for action on contaminated land.
Ionizing and non-ionizing radiation	Activities involving the use of radioactive material result in radioactive waste that has to be regulated. Radioactivity also occurs naturally. Exposure to man-made radiation gives rise to greater public concern, although natural sources, such as radon, have greater health effects.
	The body that advises on standards of protection against ionizing radiation is the International Commission on Radiological Protection (ICRP).
	Advice on radiological issues in the UK is the statutory responsibility of the National Radiological Protection Board (NRPB). In the UK, workplace exposure is regulated by the Ionizing Radiations Regulations 1985, made under the Health and Safety at Work, etc. Act 1974.
	Protection of the public and the environment from the storage, discharge or disposal of radioactive waste is covered in the UK by the Radioactive Substances Act 1993, which is policed by the Environment Agency.
	A national survey of exposure to radon in homes has shown that while radon exposure in most homes is low, there are some in which it can pose a risk to health. Monitoring should identify homes above the radon action level so that appropriate remedial action can be taken. There is concern about skin cancer in the UK resulting from exposure to solar radiation.
Noise	Noise has an important effect on the quality of life. Prolonged exposure to very loud noise can cause permanent hearing damage, but the relationship between noise and aspects of mental health is complicated.
	Road traffic noise is the most widespread form of noise disturbance, but people object most to neighbour noise. Annoyance, anger, anxiety and resentment are the most frequently reported personal consequences of exposure to noise in the home.

Table 4.11.2 How to investigate environmental hazards

Stage	Comments
Preliminary enquiries	What is the nature of the alleged health effect(s) (cancers, asthma or other respiratory diseases, admissions to hospital, deaths or birth defects)? Often a case is not clearly defined and there is a mixture of different conditions. What evidence has been cited?
	What is known about the biological causes of the health effects? Have any published epidemiological studies shown an association with environmental factors?
	What is the nature of the exposure? What is known of the toxic properties of the pollutants? Frequently no potential cause or route of exposure is obvious, or there may be many possible exposures. For example, a toxic waste site may contain hundreds of chemicals. The biological consequences of the chemicals involved are often not known.
Investigate emissions and local pollution levels	Review available emissions data and environmental monitoring data with environmental health colleagues and discuss with toxicology advisers. Consider the need for further monitoring. Enquire about the availability of tests (usually blood or urine) that may be carried out on exposed human or animal populations to quantify exposure. There are very few robust standards for chemicals.
Analyse routine health data	Agree which health events will be examined and time period for the study. Cancer registrations, causes of specific deaths, hospital admissions or GP consultations, birth defects, proportion of low birthweight births and prescriptions may be used.
	Select a study area. The study area may be defined by local concerns, or an area close to the source of pollution may be selected. Plume dispersion modelling may help to define an exposed area. The study population can be constructed using enumeration districts or postcodes. A geographical information system (GIS) can be used.
	Calculate health event rates within the exposed area. Where data are available, control for important confounding factors (age, sex, socio-economic status, smoking, clinical practice) by direct or indirect standardization. Compare exposed area with an unexposed comparison area or regional or national data.
	Ecological studies such as these are prone to bias as a result of confounding factors, which include smoking, socio-economic status and exposure to other environmental and occupational factors.
Prevalence survey	Compare the health of a representative sample of people living in the exposed area with persons living in similar social economic circumstances in an unexposed area. Health may be measured by a questionnaire which enquires about past and current respiratory symptoms, school absence, use of medication, etc., and could incorporate measurements of lung function. The survey methodology should allow adjustment for confounding factors.
	The strength of such studies is that they examine health events in the most appropriate populations at the most appropriate exposure levels. The main difficulties are the measurement of the health outcomes, the measurement of exposure and confounding factors.

Continued

Table 4.11.2 *Continued*

Stage	Comments
Communication	Often the perception of a cluster in a community may be more important than the actual presence of a cluster. In dealing with cluster reports, the public are unlikely to be satisfied with complex epidemiological or statistical arguments that deny the existence or importance of the cluster. Achieving rapport with a concerned community is critical to a satisfactory outcome.
	A mutual understanding of the limitations and strengths of available methods is crucial. It is important to respond to community suspicions and demands constructively. Once the degree of risk has been estimated, this should be communicated to the community in a sensitive, non-patronizing way.
	Co-operate with and respond to the media; provide the information they need rapidly before distortion can be introduced.
	Establishing a cause-and-effect relationship for legal purposes requires only that the preponderance of the evidence indicates the association rather than the stricter requirements of scientific proof.

investigations often serve a social rather than a scientific function.

Examples of environmental health investigations

Case study one

In a large study to determine whether particulates from open-cast coal mining had an effect on children's respiratory health, five communities close to open-cast sites were compared with five control communities matched for socio-economic and other confounding variables. There were approximately 400 children aged 1–11 years in each community. Health data were collected simultaneously from each pair of communities. These consisted of a cross-sectional health survey, daily health diaries, GP consultations, school absenteeism and medication use. Exposure was assessed by proximity to the open-cast site and by PM_{10} measurement using real-time monitors.

The effect of proximity to the open-cast site on health outcomes and PM_{10} levels was ex-amined. In addition, the association between daily PM_{10} levels and measures of ill health were examined for both open-cast and control communities.

Mean PM_{10} levels were slightly higher for the open-cast communities compared with the controls, but for much of the time, the patterns were similar despite a wide range of values. This reflects the strong regional contribution to PM_{10} levels rather than contributions from local point sources. The additional PM_{10} load around open-cast sites had a higher shale content.

Respiratory illness was similar in the open-cast and control communities, and asthmatic children in the open-cast communities did not have more or more severe asthma attacks. Respiratory symptoms reported by parents were not significantly different between the two communities, but children in the open-cast communities had more GP consultations. Small but significant positive associations between levels of PM_{10} and daily diary health events were observed in both communities, in line with previously published data. (Source: DETR 1999.)

Case study two

To examine the respiratory health of a population living near a factory producing plastic coated wallpaper where there had been concerns about the health effects of airborne emissions, a geographical information system (GIS) was used to define a set of sectors at one-kilometre intervals centred on the factory.

Asthma prevalence rates standardized for age, sex, socio-economic factors and general practice registration were calculated for each sector. The numerator, cases of asthma, was derived from a general practitioner computerized repeat prescribing system, and the denominator was obtained from health authority patient registers. Middle-aged and elderly adults living 500–1000 m in a northeasterly direction from the factory had a significantly higher prevalence of asthma. (Source: Dunn *et al.* 1995.)

Case study three

In a study to examine the health effects of living near a landfill, the health of the exposed population, defined as residents living in the five electoral wards within 3 km of the landfill, was compared with that of a comparison population from 22 other wards matched by quintiles of the Townsend deprivation score. Routinely available health outcome measures were used, including mortality, hospital admission rates, measures of reproductive health, spontaneous abortion and congenital malformations. An increased rate of congenital malformations was found in the area surrounding the landfill. (Source: Fielder *et al.* 2000.)

Case study four

In a study on the health effects of a former landfill site in the West Midlands, three exposed populations were identified after discussions with a local environmental group. The population for each of these

groups was constructed using enumeration districts, and indirectly age–sex-standardized cancer incidence ratios were calculated using data from the West Midlands Cancer Registry. The population of the West Midlands region was used as the reference population. This was stratified by Townsend deprivation score quintile to control for socio-economic confounding factors. In none of the three study sites was there a statistically significant excess of cancers. (Source: Saunders *et al.* 1997.)

4.12 Managing acute chemical incidents

There are more than 70000 manufactured chemicals in the world today (and over 11 million known chemicals in all), but for only about 7% of these is there a complete understanding of their effects on human health. About 600 new chemicals enter the workplace every month.

Potentially harmful chemicals may be released into the environment as a result of leakage, spillage, explosion, fire or inappropriate disposal. Exposure by swallowing, inhalation or contact with skin and mucous membranes may be direct or indirect, via contaminated air, food, water or soil. Chemicals can be dispersed from the site of an accident as gas, vapour or particulate cloud, by water and on clothing, equipment, livestock or vehicles (including on human casualties and on emergency service personnel and equipment).

Exposure to a harmful chemical may result either in acute injury or poisoning, or in longer-term health effects.

An acute chemical incident may be defined as an unforeseen event leading to the acute exposure of people to a non-radioactive substance resulting in illness, a potential threat to health from toxic substances or two or more

Table 4.12.1 Agencies involved in the response to an acute chemical incident

Agency	Role
The police	In overall charge Control and co-ordinate the response by the emergency services Advice to the public on protective measures such as sheltering indoors Evacuation of local residents if necessary May arrange evacuation (see below, saving life) Protection and preservation of the scene Investigation of the incident Casualty information Media enquiries

The fire service	Extinguishing fires
	Saving life, rescue of trapped casualties
	Investigation and hazard assessment
	Safety of all staff involved in the rescue work
	Making the site safe
	Minimize effect of incident on environment
	   Seal leak
	   Decontamination
	   Clean up spillage
	Arrange with contractor to remove substance, etc.

The ambulance service	Immediate care and treatment of casualties Transport to hospital
Health authorities	See below
Local authorities	Support the emergency services Support and care of the community Open emergency rest centres if necessary Co-ordinate response of other organizations, including Environment Agency and local water company Lead rehabilitation of community Restore environment

Health and Safety Executive	At sites at which chemicals are manufactured or used:
	   Inspect workplaces
	   Investigate accidents and cases of ill-health
	   Enforce good standards and legislation

individuals suffering from a similar illness which might be due to exposure to toxic substances.

Various agencies are involved in the response to an acute chemical incident (Table 4.12.1).

Health authorities are responsible for the health of their population, and have particular responsibilities for the health aspects of chemical incidents (Table 4.12.2). They must have a written plan for responding to chemical incidents and a named person to take overall responsibility. This person is often the CCDC.

Table 4.12.2 Health authority responsibilities for acute chemical incidents

Specific responsibility	Notes
Healthcare for people who have been exposed to a chemical hazard • Resuscitation • Ambulance transport to hospital • Decontamination • Treatment with antidotes, etc. • Supportive care, including intensive care	This is done on behalf of the health authority by the ambulance service and local hospitals Clinicians can obtain advice from the National Poisons Information Service
Risk assessment • Assess the toxic risk to health • Nature and quantity of the chemicals involved and known toxic effects • Routes and duration of exposure • Population that has been exposed • Number and nature of any casualties	The CCDC will have access to toxicological, environmental and chemical advice through a subscription to a local chemical incident advisory service. Advice is also available from government departments (MAFF, DH) and national agencies such as the Environment Agency and the Health and Safety Executive
Collection of biological samples	This will be done in collaboration with clinicians to indicate whether individuals have been exposed to toxic chemicals, to help in identifying the chemicals and to provide a baseline for monitoring the effects of treatment. Assays are available for solvents, metals, pesticides, drugs, cyanide, alcohols and glycol ethers
Consider the need for collection of environmental samples, including water, atmosphere, fallout, soil and food	This may be done by the chemical company, the public analyst, a water utility, a specialist agency or a contractor to identify the chemicals involved and to assess the extent and nature of the environmental contamination that has occurred
Short and long-term follow-up of persons who have been exposed	The CCDC should be prepared to set up a register and collect a dataset on those affected by the incident or exposed to the chemical(s) Those affected may require examination, testing, advice, treatment or follow-up. This will normally be carried out by local clinicians. Counselling may be considered to avoid stress-related illness
Medical advice to health and social care professionals, the public and the media	The CCDC should be prepared to provide information and advice about chemical incidents and their health consequences, the medical care of those exposed, how to avoid or minimize exposure and the probable effects of exposure
Public information	This may be sent to general practitioners, health visitors and other primary care staff; the public; the emergency services; the media; the local authority; water companies; other agencies The CCDC should reassure where there is no risk or minimal risk

Continued

Table 4.12.2 *Continued*

Specific responsibility	Notes
Control	Advise on sheltering or evacuation where there is potential for the public to be exposed to a toxic vapour cloud or where there is a risk of fire or explosion
	In the case of a gas cloud the Meteorological Office can make an assessment of local weather conditions and produce a map showing the probable shape and movement of the plume
Surveillance of incidents and hazards	The CCDC should be familiar with any databases of local sites that represent possible sources of major chemical hazards
Co-ordination	The CCDC should be prepared to co-ordinate the local response to a chemical incident and convene and chair an incident control team which has a full appropriate membership and which meets regularly during the incident
Epidemiological studies	The CCDC should be prepared to conduct or commission epidemiological studies. As a minimum there should be a descriptive study, but there may be an opportunity for an analytical study to determine the strength of any association between the chemical exposure and its health effects (see Chapter 4.11)
Incident report	The CCDC should ensure that the incident is documented and that a report is prepared and circulated for discussion

4.13 Managing acute radiation incidents

Major radiation incidents, such as accidents involving nuclear reactors, military operations and nuclear-powered satellites crashing to earth, are uncommon.

However, because of the widespread use of radioactive materials in medicine, science and industry, small-scale incidents following transportation accidents, leaks and the loss or theft of sources do occur.

In a radiation incident, radioactive material may be released into the atmosphere as a gas or particles. This forms a wind-borne plume, which is dispersed and diluted. Some material will fall to the ground, particularly if there is rain. People may be exposed by direct radiation from the plume, by inhalation, by contamination of the environment leading to direct radiation, or by consumption of contaminated food or drink.

In the UK, health services do not normally take the lead in responding to releases of radioactive materials, but they do have a role in dealing with their health effects and allaying public anxiety (Table 4.13.1). They must have a written plan to cover this and a named person to take overall responsibility. This person is often the CCDC.

Countermeasures

Intervention after a radiation accident is based on countermeasures that aim to do more good than harm. Countermeasures include sheltering, evacuation, iodine prophylaxis (in an accident involving radioactive iodine-131, 60–70% uptake of radioiodine can be blocked if potassium iodate tablets are given within three hours and 50% at approximately five hours) and banning contaminated foodstuffs.

Table 4.13.1 Radiation incidents: responsibilities in the UK

Radiation incidents arising within the United Kingdom

Civil nuclear installations	Department of Trade and Industry
	Site operators must draw up contingency plans and consult with the local health authority
	The Public Information for Radiation Emergencies Regulations (PIRER) 1992 require site operators, local authorities and fire services to provide information for the public living near nuclear installations on the action to be taken should an emergency arise. Information must also be provided if an emergency occurs. The health authority should be involved
	European Directives, which will be implemented in 2000, will result in the introduction of the Radiation (Emergency Preparedness and Public Information) Regulations (REPPIR), which will absorb the provisions of the existing PIRER Regulations
Accidents that occur during transportation of civil radioactive material	Department of Environment, Transport and the Regions, covered by the industry RADSAFE scheme. Each year there are thousands of transport movements of radioactive materials. Plans have been prepared by consignors and national authorities to deal effectively with transport radiation emergencies. RADSAFE has evolved from a number of previous such plans. It is based on the requirements of the emergency services, and draws on the principles of the national CHEMSAFE plan
Incidents at defence nuclear installations	Ministry of Defence
Industrial sites with large amounts of nuclear material	Health and Safety Executive
Advice to government, other agencies and the public on protection from radiological hazards	National Radiological Protection Board (NRPB, http://www.nrpb.org.uk/)

National Arrangements for Incidents Involving Radioactivity (NAIR). NAIR covers radiation incidents in public places such as damage to containers in transit, accidents to vehicles carrying radioactive material, discovery of actual or suspected radioactive substances in public places	NRPB co-ordinates NAIR, which is activated by the Police
	Annual memoranda are available from NRPB. Assistance is provided in two stages:
	    First-stage assistance comes from hospital radiation staff
	    Second-stage assistance comes from radiation staff from nuclear power stations or other similar establishments

Reception, treatment and decontamination of casualties at designated hospitals. Monitoring people and their personal belongings following exposure, by local medical physics departments. Plans for distributing potassium iodate tablets from local emergency departments. Information to the public and the media on health aspects of the accident. Collating advice from expert sources	Health authority

Continued

Table 4.13.1 *Continued*

Radiation incidents arising within the United Kingdom	
Telephone advice line	
Long-term follow-up of exposed persons for clinical or epidemiological purposes	
Advice on what food and drink can be consumed	Food Standards Agency
Advice on whether radioactive material can be flushed into the drains	Environment Agency/water utility

Radiation incidents arising outside the United Kingdom	
Overseas nuclear installations	Department of Environment, Transport and the Regions
	There is a national radiation monitoring network and emergency response system known as RIMNET, which enables any increases in radiation levels within the UK which arise from an overseas accident to be detected automatically
Nuclear-powered satellite accidents	Home Office

Box 4.13.1 Ionizing radiation

Ionizing radiation causes ionization when it passes through matter. It is either electromagnetic radiation (X-rays and gamma-rays) or fast-moving particles (alpha particles, beta particles, etc.).

These particles and rays release energy as they pass through biological tissues, resulting in damage. The effect of a dose of a particular form of radiation on a particular tissue is measured in sieverts (Sv).

The average annual exposure in the UK is 2.5 mSv. Of this 87% comes from natural background radiation (cosmic rays, granite, etc.), 12% comes from medical X-rays, 0.1% from nuclear discharges and 0.4% from fallout. The maximum permitted radiation from artificial sources is 1 mSv. Any dose of radiation increases the risk of developing cancer later in life over and above the existing background cancer rate. An average individual exposed to 5 mSv as a result of eating contaminated food in the first year after a radiation accident has a lifetime risk of about 1 in four thousand of developing fatal cancer. The lifetime risk of dying in a fire is about 1 per thousand, the lifetime risk of dying in a road traffic accident is 10 per thousand.

Early effects from radiation (physical illness within a month) require a very high dose, around 500 mSv. The average person in the UK received 0.1 mSv from the Chernobyl accident in 1986. In the event of a nuclear accident, sheltering or evacuation would be recommended to prevent a whole-body dose of 30 mSv (the ERL). This is well below the dose that could lead to physical symptoms.

Criteria are based on Emergency Reference Levels (ERL). ERLs are expressed in terms of the radiation dose to an individual that could be averted if the counter-measure is taken. For each counter-measure a lower and an upper ERL is recommended. The lower ERL is the smallest reduction in dose likely to offset the disadvantages of the countermeasure. If the estimated averted dose exceeds the lower ERL, then implementation of the countermeasure should be considered, but is not essential. The upper ERL is the reduction in dose for which the countermeasure would be justified in nearly all situations.

Action when a radiation incident occurs

- Enquire about:
  nature and scale of the incident;
  whether anyone has been, or is likely to be, exposed to radiation as a result of the accident and whether they can be traced;
  the likely clinical effect of exposure to the source of radiation;
  the extent and nature of any environmental contamination;
  the wider population that might have been exposed.
- Carry out an initial risk assessment.
- Consult with local, regional or national sources of expert advice (keep up-to-date contact details in written plan).
- Agree countermeasures, public information, follow-up.

4.14 Section 47 of the National Assistance Act 1948

Section 47 of the National Assistance Act 1948 allows an application to be made to a magistrate in the UK for an order to remove a person in need of care and attention to a hospital, nursing home or residential home. This power is invested in the local authority, which delegates it to a proper officer. Before the reorganization of local government in 1974, the proper officer was the Medical Officer of Health. In most areas the CCDC has rather inappropriately inherited this function.

The original provisions of the section required seven clear days' notice to be given to the person who was the subject of the application. However, it soon became clear that such a delay could cause further harm once a decision had been taken to use the Act. As a result, in 1951, the National Assistance (Amendment) Act was passed, which allowed removals to be effected without delay.

The criteria and procedures for the full order (1948) and the emergency order (1951) are compared in Table 4.14.1.

Definitions

Grave chronic disease	An illness which poses a threat to life.
Infirm	Unable to go to the toilet, wash, etc.
Insanitary conditions	There is no legal definition. Generally, insanitary is taken to mean poor, dirty conditions where there is a clear threat to health.
Proper care and attention	Person is unable to carry out essential basic daily living tasks either alone or with assistance—for example getting to the toilet, making a drink, getting in and out of bed, opening a window.

Table 4.14.1 Comparison of the criteria and procedures for the full order and the emergency order

Section 47 of the National Assistance Act 1948 (full order)	National Assistance (Amendment) Act 1951 (emergency order)
Seven days, clear notice must be given to the person who is the subject of the application	No notice or warning is required to be given to the person who is the subject of the order
The person must be:	*The person must be:*
Suffering from grave chronic disease *Or* Being aged, infirm or physically incapacitated, is living in insanitary conditions *And* Unable to devote to himself or herself, and not receiving from other persons, proper care and attention *And* Removal is necessary in the interests of the person or to prevent injury to the health of, or serious nuisance to, other persons	Suffering from grave chronic disease *Or* Being aged, infirm or physically incapacitated, is living in insanitary conditions *And* Unable to devote to himself or herself, and not receiving from other persons, proper care and attention
The order allows removal of person without delay to hospital, residential or nursing home	The order allows removal of person without delay to hospital, residential or nursing home
The order lasts for three months. The application is made in writing by the Environmental Services Department. The CCDC supplies a written statement and may attend court to give evidence. The assessing social worker may also provide a written report and attend court. The manager of the hospital or residential or nursing home into which the person is to be removed must signal their agreement to the court in writing. The person's GP may also be required to attend court. The person's GP should be asked to arrange ambulance transport	The order lasts for three weeks. The CCDC appears before a magistrate with a written certificate signed by the CCDC and another registered medical practitioner, usually the person's GP During office hours the CCDC will appear before a magistrate at the local magistrate's court. At other times a magistrate can be contacted through the local police station The manager of the hospital or residential or nursing home accommodation into which the person is to be removed should be in agreement. The person's GP should be asked to arrange ambulance transport
If it is expected that the person will resist being moved, then the police may be asked to be in attendance	If it is expected that the person will resist being moved, then the police may be asked to be in attendance
The court may extend the order for periods of up to three months	If an extension is required, an application for a full order must be made
An application may be made to revoke the order six weeks after it has been granted	There is no appeal
A review should be held by the end of the fourth week. This will allow time for an extension to be considered if necessary. Usually this is not necessary	A review should be held before the end of the second week. This will allow time for a full order to be considered if necessary. Usually this is not necessary

Requests for consideration of a compulsory removal order may come from various sources, including general practitioners and social services department staff.

These powers should be used only as a last resort, and alternatives for providing care and treatment at home or use of other legal powers (see Table 4.14.2) should be considered before opting for a compulsory removal.

Before an application is made, a case conference should be held if possible. There should be a comprehensive assessment of the person's circumstances. This should include liaison and consultation with anyone involved with their care such as their carer, close relatives, health services staff, home care staff, environmental health department staff, the person's GP and the local CCDC. A consultant geriatrician or psycho-geriatrician should be involved if it is likely that a hospital bed will be needed. If there is the possibility of mental health problems, the local mental health team should be involved.

The assessment should consider the health of the person, the level of risk to the person or others, the physical condition of the person's home and the health and nuisance risk this poses, whether there are problems with public utilities (gas, electric), whether there is a risk of fire, what attempts have already been made to resolve the situation and if there are grounds for guardianship or other action under the Mental Health Act 1983. All reasonable steps should be taken to maintain the person in their own home.

In some cases it may be difficult to gain entry to the person's home to carry out an assessment. Under Section 47 there is no right of entry, but often an existing care-worker or relative will be able assist the CCDC. Under the Police and Criminal Evidence Act 1984, a police officer may enter and search any premises for the purposes of saving life or limb or preventing serious damage to property. Section 129 of the Mental Health Act 1983 allows an approved social worker to interview a person in the course of his/her duties, and if conditions are believed to be insanitary, an environmental health officer can apply for a warrant to enter the premises under the Public Health Act 1936.

Even where the criteria appear to be met, it may not be appropriate to use a compulsory removal order. A person has the right to live as he/she wishes, and where a person is able to make an informed choice to remain at home and live in the way he/she desires, then this should be respected. Section 47 is not a compulsory treatment order, but most people accept treatment once they have been removed to hospital.

Possible impact of the Human Rights Act

The Human Rights Act 1998 comes into force in October 2000, and will make it unlawful for a public authority to act in a way which is incompatible with the European Convention on Human Rights (ECHR). Preliminary assessment suggests that detention under section 47 could be incompatible in one of three ways.

1 It may infringe the right to liberty (article 5 of ECHR), except in cases of 'the lawful detention of persons for the prevention of the spreading of infectious diseases, of persons of unsound mind, alcoholics or drug addicts or vagrants'.

Table 4.14.2 Possible outcomes of the assessment process

A package of services is put in place to meet the person's needs in their own home

Action under the National Assistance Act

Action under the Mental Health Act

Action by environmental health officers against filthy and verminous premises or articles under the Public Health Act 1936

The patient may be persuaded to attend hospital voluntarily. Home conditions may then be improved while the person is being treated in hospital

2 The lack of an appeal against detention under the 1951 Amendment and the six-week delay before an appeal against detention under the 1948 Act may contradict the entitlement 'to take proceedings by which the lawfulness of his detention shall be decided speedily by a court' (article 5(4)).

3 It may infringe the right to respect for private and family life (article 8), although article 8(2) allows interference with this right 'for the protection of health'.

Whilst definitive interpretation is awaited from the courts, the implications for the proper officer would seem to be:

• Be sure that a care plan to keep the person in their own home, or voluntary admission, is not possible.

• Check to make sure that patient is not suitable for compulsory admission under an Act less likely to infringe the ECHR, i.e. the Public Health (Control of Disease) Act 1984 or mental health legislation.

• Take legal advice on each individual case before using section 47.

4.15 Port health

The first port health controls were introduced in Venice in 1348. In modern times, reduction of the spread of international disease is co-ordinated by the World Health Organization, which administers the International Health Regulations. These regulations, which are particularly concerned with cholera, plague, smallpox and yellow fever, are usually incorporated into national law. The WHO regularly produces a list of 'infected areas' for use with these regulations.

In the UK there are separate regulations for ships, aircraft and international trains. These regulations give local authorities or port health authorities the powers to appoint medical officers and authorized port health officers (who could be non-medical, e.g. EHOs) to take action to prevent the entry of communicable diseases into the country. Neither the medical officers nor the port health officers are responsible for the medical care of individual passengers or crew. The medical officer is usually an employee of the corresponding health authority. Powers include inspection of vessels, examination of individuals and the provision of information.

Situations requiring the intervention of port health staff may include:

• Outbreak of food or water-borne disease due to (for example) in-flight catering or contaminated water on a passenger ship.

• Contamination of the interior of an aircraft with faeces or vomit.

• Rodents or insects on board which are capable of transmitting disease.

• Passengers or crew with viral haemorrhagic fever, yellow fever, plague, cholera, diphtheria or TB.

Contingency arrangements should be in place as, particularly with aircraft, little notice may be given of a situation which requires assessment and information gathering from a large number of individuals. Such contingency arrangements should cover personnel, space (including toilets), questionnaires, faecal sample kits/request forms and communications facilities.

A separate role, often undertaken by the same medical officer, is that of the Port Medical Inspector (PMI), who is responsible for medical advice to the immigration officer to protect public health. Provision of a PMI is a health authority responsibility.

Referrals to the PMI may include people coming to stay permanently in the UK, long-stay visitors (in excess of 6 months), people visiting for health reasons (to ensure they are self-supporting) and anyone who appears unwell. Such referrals may be medically examined, and in some ports may receive a chest X-ray. Unless entry is refused, details of the immigrant and the results of any examination are passed to the CCDC for the proposed area of residence. The effectiveness of such arrangements is currently under review.

4.16 Media relations

The media should be considered as an ally in protecting the health of the public. They are one of the most powerful influences upon the public. Relationships with the media should be developed proactively; good routine relationships with the media will make dealing with them during emergency situations very much easier.

Communicable disease issues arouse interest and anxiety in the public; this may seem irrational to a professional, however, the public have a right to be informed, and the press is usually the best route. In some circumstances the public and press may become hostile — avoiding the press, appearing evasive, misleading the public or lying are likely to make the situation worse.

Virtually all issues can be presented in a way that the public can understand. Professionals should not hide behind technical obfuscations.

Do not expect to have any control over material that you provide; press releases can be selectively quoted, and interviews can be edited. However, journalists are interested (usually) in accuracy.

Training

Anyone who is likely to deal with the media should undergo media training. This will help in understanding what the media need. Journalists often have a similar agenda to public health workers — they wish to inform and educate the public. If they encounter a group of professionals who understand their needs, and are trying to help, then the journalists are less likely to be antagonistic.

Identify people within the organization who are particularly good with the media — they may not be the most senior people.

Routine relationships

Develop regular contact with your local print and broadcast media. Be available to answer their questions; treat your local reporters as friends. If they trust you and rely on you as an authoritative source, it will make things much easier if a story is breaking.

Local papers may be willing to publish a regular column; this is a powerful way of getting health advice across. Use opportunities to publish in local papers, women's magazines, parents' magazines, etc. This will probably have a greater influence than publishing in the peer-reviewed medical press.

Have basic information packs available for journalists. These should describe the clinical features and importance of an infection and the salient epidemiological features and recent trends.

Outbreaks

During outbreak or emergency situations it is important to maintain good relations with the press. Journalists have a job to do; they can become intrusive, but they will understand that you have a job to do. Let the journalists know that they will be kept informed, that there will be regular briefings, daily or even twice daily. Ensure that the briefings do happen.

Appoint a media spokesperson and ensure that all media briefings are done through that person. The outbreak control team should coordinate the flow of information.

Messages

Decide beforehand what your key messages are — if possible discuss these with the journalist and discuss the questions that will be asked.

Decide if there are any areas that you do not wish to be drawn into.

Be honest and accurate; keep technical details to a minimum. Get the key message across first, then provide the reasoning behind it. Stress the facts and explain the context. Do not try to hide the truth or lie. If you are uncertain of the facts or some details, say so and offer to get the information.

Don't be drawn into areas you feel you cannot or should not discuss; be firm and polite and say that you cannot discuss that issue.

Try to avoid discussions of money and cost saving; stress public health action and your concern for safeguarding the public health. Avoid being drawn into speculation, or into criticisms of other groups. Behave as if you were always 'on the record'.

Press releases

Keep the press release short (8–10 paragraphs); make sure you have considered the message and the audience for the release. Consult a press officer. Get the most important message into the first paragraph and support it with a quote from a senior official. In the introduction describe Who, What, Where, When, Why/How. In the middle expand the story with supporting detail; conclude by summarizing and identifying the next steps.

Problems

The press might want access to cases or locations such as outbreak rooms for atmospheric pictures or interviews. These requests should be considered very carefully. Considerations of confidentiality and the smooth running of an investigation must come first. However, on occasion such photo opportunities might, by raising public awareness of an issue, be beneficial.

If things go wrong, remember that they can do so in the best of relations. Developing good relations with the media takes time and effort. If errors of fact appear in an article or you feel you have been misrepresented, contact the journalist and discuss them. If necessary talk to the editor.

4.17 Clinical governance and audit

Clinical governance provides a framework in which organizations involved in public health protection are accountable for continuously improving the quality of the services they provide and for safeguarding standards by creating an environment in which excellence will flourish.

The main components for clinical governance are the following:

• Clear lines of responsibility and accountability for the overall quality of the service provided.
• A comprehensive programme of quality improvement activities.
• Clear policies aimed at managing risks.
• Procedures for staff to identify and remedy poor performance.

The work of CDC departments does not fit neatly into these compartments, but a suitable breakdown could be as follows.

Responsibility

Clinical governance emphasizes that the organizational responsibility for quality lies at board level. In the case of communicable disease control in the UK, this responsibility lies with the District Health Authority (HA), perhaps via the Director of Public Health, who should be an executive member of the HA. The HA is responsible for adequately funding the district CDC service (see Box 4.17.1) and for encouraging an environment in which quality can flourish. The HA is also responsible for ensuring that other NHS services involved in communicable disease control—e.g. laboratories, chest clinics, STD clinics—have adequate clinical governance arrangements.

In practice, the executive responsibility for surveillance, prevention and control of communicable diseases (and other related functions) lies with the CCDC, who should therefore take the lead in assuring the quality of the district CDC function. The CCDC is also responsible for ensuring that support staff provide a quality service by encouraging training, openness, teamwork, the seeking of advice where appropriate, and performance review.

Box 4.17.1 Suggested staffing levels for district CDC departments	
Medical	Minimum of 1.0 whole time equivalent (wte) consultants per 400000 population. Extra consultant sessions in districts with more complex workload and for any non-CDC duties.
Nursing	Minimum of 1.0 per 400000 population. Extra nurse sessions in districts with large number of community settings (e.g. nursing homes).
Information scientist	0.2–0.5 per 400000 population. Minimum of 1 session per week.
Secretarial/ clerical/ data entry	Minimum of 1.5 wte per 400000 population. Must be telephone cover during working hours.

(Source: Report to NHS Executive, England, 1997.)

Quality improvement

CDC teams should complete a baseline self-assessment of their strengths and weaknesses. This could cover the following areas:

- Service structure, personnel and skills.
- Arrangements for on-call and for covering leave.
- Access to operational support and infrastructure within HA, e.g. administrative, IT, statistical expertise, communications, public relations.
- Access to specialist advice, library services and relevant Internet sites (e.g. Medline, Cochrane).
- Arrangements for multi-agency working, particularly Environmental Health Department and hospital control of infection teams. Should include relevant operational support from other health organizations (e.g. NHS Trusts and primary care groups in UK) for activities such as surveillance, contact tracing and incident control.
- Adequacy of surveillance: data access (timeliness, quality), analysis and dissemination.
- Completeness and updating of policies and plans.
- Use of evidence-based practice and mechanisms for disseminating good practice.
- Support to prevention and control in community settings.
- Mechanisms to maintain patient confidentiality.
- Multi-agency forum and committees (e.g. district control of infection, immunization) for agreeing policies and procedures.
- Audit and evaluation.

Departments may also wish to invite an external peer reviewer to comment on how their services compare with standard/best practice elsewhere.

The CCDC should formulate a prioritized action plan with clearly assigned responsibilities, in the light of the baseline assessment. This should then be discussed with the appropriate clinical governance lead.

One important element of quality improvement will be continuing professional development (CPD) for CDC staff. Each staff member should have a personal development plan, which should be discussed with their line manager. This could include training and updating in the following:

- Epidemiology and control of communicable diseases.
- Epidemiological methods and statistics for surveillance, outbreaks and research.
- Information technology.
- Infection control and environmental health.
- Management methods such as leadership, organization, supervisory skills, team working, time-management, presentation and media skills.
- New governmental, organizational or professional priorities.

Departmental CPD should include training and updating in on-call issues for all staff on the out-of-hours rota. Those whose routine work does not include a large component of CDC would benefit from attendance at a specialist course at least every three years.

Policies for managing risk

Such policies should include:
- Incident response plans for:
  - community outbreaks;
  - hospital outbreaks;
  - water-borne diseases;
  - instances requiring patient tracing, notification and helplines;
  - chemical incidents;
  - radiation incidents;
  - major emergencies.
- Incident plans need regular revision. If used in an incident, a written report should be produced. If not recently used, consideration should be given to a simulation exercise.
- Policies and procedures for dealing with common or serious diseases.
- A regularly updated on-call pack, which includes relevant policies and contact details for staff and other organizations.
- Good documentation of incidents and requests for advice.
- A system for reporting of complaints, problems encountered in delivering service, or poor outcomes.

Rectifying poor performance

In communicable disease control, this primarily revolves around clinical audit. In the UK, the role of the General Medical Council in revalidation will mean that doctors will need to be able to demonstrate that they are keeping themselves up to date and remain fit to practise in their chosen field.

- Clinical audit involves:
  - setting standards;
  - comparing actual performance to standards;
  - rectifying identified deficiencies.
- Audit should involve an element of peer review. One useful mechanism is to involve CCDC in neighbouring districts, perhaps as part of a Regional Audit Group. Where national standards do not exist, this group can devise regional ones on which to base audit.
- Suitable topics for audit might be:
  - adequacy of contingency plans;
  - adequacy of district surveillance systems for spotting outbreaks and analysing trends;
  - response of on-call staff (including partner organizations);
  - review of management of an actual outbreak;
  - review of response to (randomly selected) cases of meningococcal disease;
  - immunization uptake rates and methods used to improve them;
  - HIV prevention strategy.
- A report should be written on all significant outbreaks and incidents detailing the lessons learnt. More minor episodes (e.g. sporadic case of typhoid) can be discussed informally, e.g. at weekly departmental surveillance and information meetings.
- Discussion and monitoring of formal and informal complaints from the public or health professionals.

It is clear that the quality of CDC work and the ability to carry out clinical governance and audit are both dependent upon the level of resources available to the CDC department. None the less, the CCDC can use his/her leadership, management and professional skills to maximize the resources available and to prioritize their use; clinical governance is a tool that can be used to further those objectives.

Section 5
Communicable disease control in Europe

5.1 International collaboration in Europe

Infectious diseases do not respect national boundaries and outbreaks have the potential to involve more than one country. This has been increasingly recognized, as international travel and trade increases and as free trade areas within which goods and people circulate freely have developed. The World Health Organization has been responsible for collecting international data on infectious diseases, and administering the International Health Regulations, which have been the mainstay of the international response to communicable disease. However, new patterns of collaboration are required if countries are to be able to respond appropriately to international threats to health through sharing data and skills so that appropriate action can be taken at international level.

Within the European Union (EU), several collaborations have developed between national surveillance centres in response to this problem (Table 5.1.1). These have shown some remarkable successes in identifying outbreaks which would probably not have been identified otherwise, in assisting in the response to international outbreaks and in developing the framework for international collaborative action. These collaborations are based around experts in particular infections and around infrastructure developments.

The collaborations described are largely funded by the European Commission. However, WHO still has a leading role to play in the international control of communicable disease and is involved as a partner in many of the collaborations.

A number of international collaborations are described in Table 5.1.1 and the following sections describe the surveillance systems in each of the member states of the EU.

5.2 Austria

Contacts

Bundesministerium für Arbeit, Gesundheit und Soziales (Federal Ministry for Labour, Health, Social Affairs) http://www.bmags.gv.at.

Statutory notification systems

Legal framework
Ministry of Health is responsible for introducing changes in the statutory notification system.

Levels of responsibility
• Local responsibility for reporting: physicians and laboratories.
• Local responsibility for action: notifier is responsible for case management, contact tracing and contact management.
• National surveillance: Federal Ministry for Labour, Health, Social Affairs.

Notifiable diseases
39 diseases are notifiable. Financial incentives: none.

Case-definitions
In use for TB, AIDS, CJD and acute poliomyelitis.

Levels of reporting
Local level for reporting: 122 local health departments with an average population of 66 000. Regional level: 9 regions with an average population of 1 006 600.

Estimated time to inform national level
Up to 60 days.

Public health action
The responsibility for case management is held by the notifier. Control measures, including contact tracing and outbreak investigation, are generally the responsibility of the

Table 5.1.1 EU collaborations in communicable disease surveillance

Network	Description	Internet URL
EnterNet	EnterNet is an international network for the surveillance of human gastrointestinal infections, which monitors salmonellosis and *Escherichia coli* (VTEC) O157, including their antimicrobial resistance	http:www2.phls.co.uk/
EWGLI	EWGLI is a Legionnaires' disease surveillance network that includes all countries that are members of the EU and several countries outside the Union. The objectives of the network are to identify clusters of cases of Legionnaires' disease that may indicate the occurrence of a common source outbreak, to rapidly disseminate cluster alerts to collaborating centres, and to maintain and continually develop a European surveillance database	http://www.phls.co.uk/international/Ewgli/ewgli2.htm
EuroHIV	The surveillance of HIV/AIDS in Europe — EuroHIV: consists of the collection, analysis and dissemination of epidemiological data with the objectives of describing and better understanding the HIV epidemic and improving prevention and control	http://www.ceses.org/aidssurv/about.htm
EuroTB	The tuberculosis network was developed in response to epidemiological trends in Europe in the early 1990s. The network has led to clear benefits in descriptive epidemiology: in encouraging high quality standards, in involving laboratories and epidemiologists, in computerization of data	http://www.ceses.org/eurotb/eurotb.htm
ESEN	The aim of the European Sero-Epidemiology Network (ESEN) is to coordinate and harmonize the serological surveillance of immunity to vaccine preventable diseases in eight countries in Europe	
Eurosurveillance	The communication of information about European communicable disease prevention and control has been facilitated by the development of a monthly journal, *Eurosurveillance Monthly*, and a weekly e-mail newsletter. *Eurosurveillance Monthly* carries roundups of information and completed reports of field investigations and studies, whilst the weekly carries news of breaking events	http://www.eurosurv.org
Inventories	A number of inventories are being developed so that information about the available skills and capacity at European level is available. These inventories will include information about national reference laboratories, surveillance systems and vaccination programmes	
EPIET	The EPIET (European Programme of Intervention Epidemiology Training) is a 22-month programme whereby individuals from one EU member state country train in communicable disease epidemiology in another country, usually in one of the national centres. EPIET fellows meet regularly within a modular teaching programme, which other participants can also attend. The programme is backed by a coordination team that rigorously assures the quality of training	http://www.invs.sante.fr/epiet

public health service, primarily at local level with support from national level.

Data dissemination
A list of notifiable diseases is published by the Ministry monthly/yearly. In addition the national AIDS statistics (Östereichische AIDS-Statistik) are published monthly.

Flow chart of statutory notification
(Fig. 5.2.1)

Outbreak detection and investigation

Physicians' notifications and laboratory reports are collected at district and regional level. In the case of an outbreak the Ministry of Health has to be informed. Regional health administrations have the legal responsibility for detection, investigation and public health

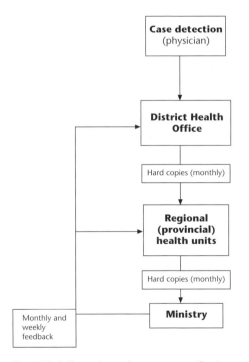

Fig. 5.2.1 Flow chart of statutory notification (Austria).

action in co-operation with the regional food and veterinary administration.

Prevention/prophylaxis

• Vaccine programme: DTPaP, MMR, Hib, HBV.
• Vaccination coverage: ~50% for MMR vaccinations, with strong regional variation.
• Antibiotics and malaria prophylaxis only available on prescription.

5.3 Belgium

Belgium is a federal state that is divided into three communities and three regions. The communities are based on language and culture (Flemish, French and German); they have responsibility for control of infectious diseases. Each has its own ministry (ministry of respective community, Administration of Public Health). In Brussels, where the Flemish community and the French community share responsibility, a community commission manages the control of infectious diseases. The three regions also have responsibilities in environmental and zoonotic disease control; again, each has its own ministry.

Contacts

Ministry of Social Affairs, Public Health and the Environment (http://www.health.fgov.be/).
Institut Scientifique de Santé Publique Louise Pasteur (Scientific Institute of Public Health (IPH) L. P.) — http://www.iph.fgov.be.

Statutory notification systems

Legal framework
Ministry of Health for each community is responsible for introducing changes in the statutory notification system.

Levels of responsibility

At Federal level the Ministry for Public Health responsibilities include:

- Inspection of drugs and food products.
- Control of imported diseases.

  Governments at community level responsibilities include:

- Prevention.
- Social and environmental-hygienic aspects of health.

  The administration of these community governments has a 'health inspector' per province in charge of surveillance and control of infectious diseases. The tasks are:

- Registration of notified cases of infectious diseases.
- Co-ordination and follow-up of control measures.
- Investigation and follow-up of outbreaks.
- Vaccination policy and its implementation.

  Governments at regional level are responsible for:

- Environmental and zoonotic disease control.
- Water quality and control of water-borne diseases.

  In Flanders, the community and regional authority are merged: the health inspector is responsible for the combined tasks. In Brussels, a separate authority (the Community Commission) carries the responsibility. As the German community is quite small, activities are undertaken by the French community.

Notifiable diseases

In the Flemish community 37 diseases are notifiable. In Brussels and the French community 42 diseases are notifiable. Financial incentives: none.

Case-definitions

In the Flemish community case-definitions are in use for most notifiable diseases and in the French community case-definitions are in use for all notifiable diseases.

Levels of reporting

Local level for reporting: usually at the level of the province, with an average population size of 900 000 (250 000–1 600 000).

Estimated time to inform national level

Two days in the Flemish community and up to 45 days in the French community.

Public health action

The responsibility for case management is held by the notifier. Control measures including contact tracing and outbreak investigation are generally the responsibility of the public health service, primarily on local level with support from the administration at the central (community) level. Support can also be provided by the IPH.

Data dissemination

In Flanders an epidemiological bulletin, the *Epidemiologisch Bulletin van de Vlaamse Gemenschap* is published (http://www.wvc.vlaanderen.be/epidemiologisch_bulletin/). It contains tables with notification data. An annual report is also produced. In the French community, the Direction Général de la Santé publishes data on a monthly basis in the *Relevé mensuel de maladies transmissibles*. At the IPH, the monthly data from sentinel laboratories are accessible via Internet (http://www.iph.fgov.be/epidemio/epinl/plabnl/index.htm).

Flow chart of statutory notification
(Fig. 5.3.1)

Outbreak detection and investigation

A variety of sources of information are used to detect possible outbreaks (physicians' notifications, laboratory reporting, telephone calls from the public, absence notification systems). The Health Inspectors of the communities have the legal responsibility for detection, investigation and public health action within their community in co-operation with other local/regional authorities (environmental health, veterinarians, etc.). Other national authorities may also then be involved.

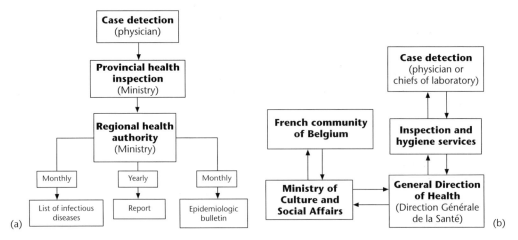

Fig. 5.3.1 Flow chart of statutory notification (Belgium). (a) Flanders; (b) French community (including data from the German community).

Prevention/prophylaxis

• Vaccine programme: DTP, Hib, HBV, MMR.
• Vaccination coverage: >95% for DTP, ~80% for other vaccinations (Flemish community).
• Antibiotics and malaria prophylaxis only available on prescription.

5.4 Denmark

Contacts

Sundhedsstyrelsen (SST)—National Board of Health—http://www.sst.dk.
Department of Epidemiology, Statens Serum Institute (SSI)—http://www.ssi.dk.

Statutory notification systems

Legal framework
The National Board of Health and the Ministry of Health have the responsibility for modifications.

Levels of responsibility
• Local responsibility for reporting: all physicians are obliged by law to notify all cases that fulfil the criteria for notifiable diseases.
• Local responsibility for action: Medical Officers of Health (MOHs) at departmental level.
• National surveillance: Statens Serum Institut.

Notifiable diseases
Thirty-three diseases are notifiable on person identifiable basis, 4 diseases are notifiable on an anonymous basis. No financial incentives are given to physicians to notify. Laboratories report 5 diseases to Statens Serum Institut as well as the number of positive and negative HIV-test results. All blood banks report screening results of blood donors for virological markers.

Case-definitions
Are in use for all notifiable diseases.

Levels of reporting
Local level for reporting: 15 Departments with MOHs—with an average population size of 350 000 (45 000–625 000). National population: 5.3 million inhabitants.

Estimated time to inform national level

Varies for different diseases. Considerable time-delays occur; range from 2 days to several weeks for national level between diagnosis and receipt at national level.

Public health action

The responsibility for case management is held by the notifier. Control measures, including contact tracing and outbreak investigation, are the responsibility of the local MOH, with support from national level (SSI).

Data dissemination

An epidemiological bulletin, the *Epi-Nyt (Epi-News)* is published weekly at national level (http://www.ssi.dk/en/index.htlm). The data for notifiable diseases are published quarterly/yearly. On local level feedback is given in yearly reports from the MOHs.

Flow chart of statutory notification
(Fig. 5.4.1)

Outbreak detection and investigation

Physicians are required by law to report any abnormal event or outbreak of any disease immediately by phone to the local Department of MOHs. They also have to notify to both the MOHs and to the national level (Statens Serum Institut) by mail using a written form. Local and national reference laboratories also detect and report outbreaks. The MOHs have the responsibility for outbreak control at regional/local level. The Statens Serum Institut has the national responsibility as a reference centre for surveillance and will be involved in outbreak investigation/control on request. Statens Serum Institut has a microbiologist on duty 24 h/day.

Prevention/prophylaxis

• Vaccination programme: DTPaP, Hib, MMR, OPV.
• Vaccination coverage: ~85% for MMR vaccinations.
• Antibiotics and malaria prophylaxis only available on prescription.

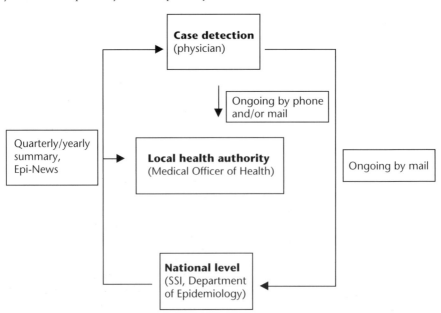

Fig. 5.4.1 Flow chart of statutory notification (Denmark).

5.5 Finland

Contacts

Elintarvikevirasto (National Food Administration) http://www.elintarvikeviras.fi.

Kansanterveyslaitas (KTL) (National Public Health Institute) http://www.ktl.fi.

Eläinlääkintä-ja elintarvikelaitos (EELA, National Veterinary and Food Research Institute) http://www.mmm.fi/hallinnon-ala/eela.

Statutory notification systems

Legal framework
The law and act on communicable diseases (1986, last amendment 1997) regulates surveillance and control of infectious diseases. The Ministry of Health is responsible for introducing changes in the statutory notification system.

Levels of responsibility
• Local responsibilities for reporting and action: physicians in local health centres are responsible for detection of cases and necessary action for control. They are assisted by infectious disease specialists and microbiologists. Veterinary and food control authorities are involved in food-borne outbreak surveillance and are responsible for control measures.
• National surveillance: KTL.

Notifiable diseases
Seventy-nine diseases classified into three categories are notifiable. Two systems coexist within the surveillance system. For some diseases both the physician and the laboratory must report the case, for the others only laboratory reports are collected (more than half of all infections). The laboratories use routine reporting to remind the treating physician to notify whenever appropriate. Financial incentives: none.

Case-definitions
Are in use for all notifiable diseases.

Levels of reporting
452 local health units with an average population size of 11 000 and 22 regions with an average population size of 230 000.

Estimated time to inform national level
Laboratory notifications are sent directly to the national level at KTL, reaching it in an average of 5 working days. Physician notifications are sent through the regional level to the national level, which takes approximately two weeks.

Public health action
The responsibility for case management is held by the notifier. Control measures including contact tracing and outbreak investigation are generally the responsibility of the public health service, primarily at local level with support from national level.

Data dissemination
All registry data are compiled and arranged at KTL and displayed on the website (www.ktl.fi) of the Institute and are accessible to all involved health authorities. A weekly updated www-version including comments is publicly accessible. The format allows further analysis by the user. Figures and summary comments are routinely reported in the monthly bulletin, the *Kansanterveys-lehti*. Data on laboratory findings are published monthly via the Internet (http://www.ktl.fi). In addition annual reports are published.

Flow chart of statutory notification
(Fig. 5.5.1)

Outbreak detection and investigation

In outbreak situations local health authorities are primarily responsible for assessment and action. In cases where several municipalities are involved, the hospital district specialist acts as co-ordinator and consultant. KTL is in-

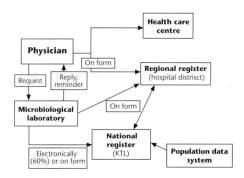

Fig. 5.5.1 Flow chart of statutory notification (Finland).

volved in wider outbreaks and provides co-ordination and expert help.

Prevention/prophylaxis

• Vaccination coverage: >98% for all vaccinations.
• Antibiotics and malaria prophylaxis only available on prescription.

5.6 France

Contacts

Direction Générale de la Santé (DGS) ministry in charge of public health — http://www. sante.gouv.fr.

Institut de Veille Sanitaire (National Public Health Surveillance Institute) (InVS). http://www.invs.sante.fr.

Statutory notification systems

Legal framework
DGS is responsible for introducing changes in the statutory notification system.

Levels of responsibility
• Local responsibility for reporting: physi-cians are obliged by law to notify cases that ful-fil the criteria for notification.
• Local responsibility for action: the local health departments (DDASS) are responsible for public health action.
• National surveillance: DGS is responsible for introducing modifications in the notification system. The InVS (Infectious Disease Unit) and DGS are involved in managing surveillance at national level.

Notifiable diseases
Twenty-three diseases are notifiable. Physi-cians notify individual cases anonymously to the DDASS using standardized forms. Intro-duction of two classes for notification diseases is planned. They will differentiate between diseases that require immediate action (e.g. meningococcal meningitis) and those used for epidemiological monitoring only (e.g. HIV). Financial incentive: none.

Case-definitions
Are in use for all notifiable diseases.

Levels of reporting
Local level for reporting: 100 DDASSs — with an average population size of 570 000 (75 000–2 500 000). National population: 57 million inhabitants.

Estimated time to inform national level
In general 7 days for local level and 11 days for national level, varying for different diseases.

Public health action
The responsibility for case management is held by the notifier. Control measures in-cluding outbreak investigation are generally the responsibility of the public health service, primarily at local level with support from regional and national level. InVS performs trend analysis and outbreak detection based on surveillance data. A computerized alert system is used (http://www.invs.sante.fr/do_fr).

Data dissemination
An epidemiological bulletin, the *Bulletin*

Épidemiologique Hebdomadaire, is published weekly at national level (http://www.invs.sante.fr/beh) by DGS. In addition annual reports (6-monthly for AIDS) are provided (http://www. invs.sante.fr/.

Flow chart of statutory notification
(Fig. 5.6.1)

Outbreak detection and investigation

Any health professional should inform the local health authority (DDASS) of any abnormal event or outbreak of any disease. The local health authority is responsible for investigation and control. The DDASS can respond by asking for the help of regional (cellules interegionales d'épidemiologie) or national level (InVS) for the investigation. Control of the outbreak is the task of the DDASS or DGS. Depending on the type of outbreak (e.g. food borne outbreaks) the Ministries of Agriculture, Finance or Consumers can be involved.

Regional or national outbreaks are investigated by InVS.

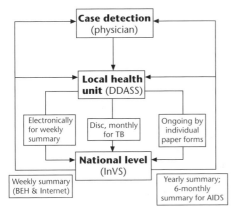

Fig. 5.6.1 Flow chart of statutory notification (France). DDASS, Direction Départementale des Affaires Sanitaires et Sociales; InVS, Institut de Veille Sanitaire; BEH, *Bulletin Epidémiologique Hebdomadaire*.

Prevention/prophylaxis

• Vaccine programme: DTPP, MMR, Hib, BCG, HBV.
• Vaccination coverage: 80–90% for MMR vaccinations.
• Antibiotics and malaria prophylaxis only available on prescription.

5.7 Germany

Contacts

Bundesministerium für Gesundheit (BMG) (Federal Ministry for Health) http://www.bmgesundheit.de.
Robert Koch Institute (RKI) (Federal Institute of Communicable and Non-Communicable Diseases) http://www.rki.de.
Statistisches Bundesamt (Federal Statistical Office) http://www.statistik-bund.de.

Statutory notification systems

Legal framework
The Ministry of Health is responsible for introducing changes in the statutory notification system; new legislation from 2001.

Levels of responsibility
• Local responsibility for reporting: physicians and laboratories.
• Local responsibility for action: local health departments (Gesundheitsämter) in co-operation with physicians and hospitals.
• National surveillance: Robert Koch Institute in co-operation with the 16 states, as in the federal system in Germany the responsibility for health is at state level.

Notifiable diseases
The law distinguishes 4 groups, which differ by disease-related events and have a differing amount of data to be notified within different time intervals. Financial incentives: none.

Case-definitions

Case-definitions are developed and in use for all diseases.

Levels of reporting

The country is divided into 439 districts, each with a district health authority (*Gesundheits-amt*). The average population size is 186 000 (20 000–3 500 000). These districts belong to regions which form 16 states with an average population size of 5 100 000 inhabitants (700 000–18 000 000).

Estimated time to inform national level

Up to 7 days for regional level and 14 days for national level.

Public health action

The responsibility for case management is held by the notifier. Control measures including contact tracing and outbreak investigation are generally the responsibility of the public health service, primarily on local level with support from state and national level.

Data dissemination

An epidemiological bulletin, the *Epidemiologisches Bulletin*, is published by the Robert-Koch Institute at national level every week. It includes tables of notified diseases and can be accessed via Internet (http://www.rki.de/INFEKT/EPIBULL/EPI.HTM). A statistical annual report is published by the Federal Statistical Office (http://www.statistik-bund.de). In addition, regular feedback is given by institutions on regional and state level.

Flow chart of statutory notification

(Fig. 5.7.1)

Outbreak detection and investigation

A variety of information sources are used to detect possible outbreaks. The information is forwarded to district health authorities (*Gesundheitsämter*), which are responsible for investigation and for public health action at the local level. The Gesundheitsämter report

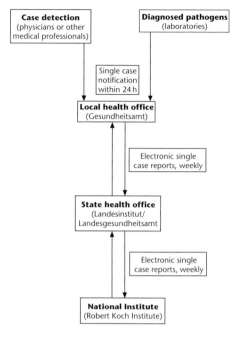

Fig. 5.7.1 Flow chart of statutory notification (Germany).

to the State Health Department, which is responsible for outbreak detection and management at the regional level. The State Health Department reports to the Robert Koch Institute, which has the national responsibility for outbreak control.

Prevention/prophylaxis

• Recommended vaccinations: DTaP, MMR, Hib, IPV, HBV.
• Antibiotics and malaria prophylaxis only available on prescription.

5.8 Greece

Contacts

Ministry of Health and Welfare, 17 Aris-

totelous Str., GR-10553 Athens (http://www.
minagric.gr/greek/index.shtml).

Hellenic Centre for the control of AIDS and
STDs (http://www.ncsi.gr).

National Centre for Surveillance and Intervention (http://www.ncsi.gr) (Tel.0030–
18840770).

Statutory notification systems

Legal framework

The Ministry of Health is responsible for introducing changes in the statutory notification
system.

Notifiable diseases

Twenty-nine diseases are notifiable. Financial
incentive: none.

Case-definitions

Are in use for acute polio and AIDS.

Levels of reporting

Fifty-four local health units with an average
population size of 200 000 and 13 regions with
an average population size of 800 000.

Estimated time to inform national level

One week.

Public health action

The responsibility for case management is
held by the notifier. Control measures including contact tracing and outbreak investigation
are generally the responsibility of the public
health service, primarily on local level with
support from national level.

Data dissemination

A monthly report is published (http://www.
ncsi.gr).

Flow chart of statutory notification

(Fig. 5.8.1)

Outbreak detection and investigation

Physicians notify cases to the prefecture public
health division, which is responsible for case

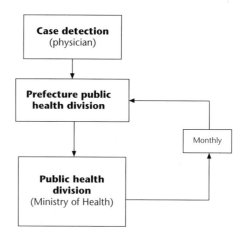

Fig. 5.8.1 Flow chart of statutory notification
(Greece).

investigation. Monthly aggregate data are sent
to the Ministry of Health, where a monthly
report is generated and disseminated as feedback. The national Centre for Surveillance and
Intervention was established in 1997. It aims
to computerize the notification system and
transmission of data. Data are analysed at
the national centre to detect and investigate
outbreaks.

Prevention/prophylaxis

• Vaccine programme: MMR, DTP, HBV,
meningitis in case of outbreak.
• Antibiotics and malaria prophylaxis only
available on prescription.

5.9 Republic of Ireland

Contacts

An Roinn Sláinte agus Leanaí (Department of
Health and Children) (http://www.doh.ie).

National Disease Surveillance Centre
(http://www.ndsc.ie).

Virus Reference Laboratory: http://www.ucd.i.e./~virusref/vrlhome.html.

Statutory notification systems

Legal framework
Notification is required under the Infectious Diseases Regulations of 1981. The Ministry of Health is responsible for introducing changes in the statutory notification system.

Levels of responsibility
• Local responsibility for reporting: physician caring for the case.
• Local responsibility for action: coordinated through the regional health boards.
• National surveillance: National Disease Surveillance Centre recently established to undertake analyses and co-ordination at national level.

Notifiable diseases
Fifty diseases are notifiable. Financial incentive: 2 Euro.

Case-definitions
Are not in use for notifiable diseases.

Levels of reporting
Eight regional health boards with an average population size of 250 000.

Estimated time to inform national level
Ten days for regional level and 17 days for national level.

Public health action
Responsibility for case management is held by the notifier. Control measures including contact tracing and outbreak investigation are generally the responsibility of the public health service, primarily at local level with support from national level.

Data dissemination
The NDSC publishes monthly summary data in *EPI-Insight* (www.ndsc.ie). The Virus Reference Laboratory issues a bulletin, the *Virus*

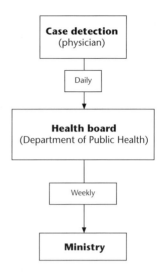

Fig. 5.9.1 Flow chart of statutory notification (Republic of Ireland).

Alert (http://www.ucd.ie/~virusref/vrlhome.html).

Flow chart of statutory notification
(Fig. 5.9.1)

Outbreak detection and investigation

A new National Disease Surveillance Centre has been established and has responsibilities in national outbreak control, liaising with laboratories and the Food Safety Authority.

Prevention/prophylaxis

• Vaccine programme: DTP, MMR, Hib.
• Antibiotics and malaria prophylaxis only available on prescription.

5.10 Italy

Contacts

Ministry of Health—http://www.sanita.it/malinf.

Instituto Superiore di Sanità (ISS) (National Institute of Health) http://www.iss.it.

Statutory notification systems

Legal framework
The Ministry of Health is responsible for introducing changes in the statutory notification system. This is defined by law. The list of specific communicable diseases was last revised in 1990.

Levels of responsibility
• Local responsibility for reporting: physicians are obliged by law to notify cases that fulfil the criteria for notification.
• Local responsibility for action: the local health units (USL) are responsible for public health action.
• National surveillance: the Ministry of Health is responsible for introducing modifications in the notification system.

Notifiable diseases
Forty-eight diseases, divided into 5 classes, are notifiable. These differ in the flow of information and by the degree of ascertainment requested. For each class a specific form exists. Financial incentive: none.

Case-definitions
In use for most notifiable diseases.

Levels of reporting
Two hundred and twenty-eight local health units with an average population size of 250 000 and 20 regions with an average population size of 2 850 000.

Estimated time to inform national level
Seven days for local level, 40 days for regional level and 90 days for national level.

Public health action
Responsibility for case management is held by the notifier. Control measures including contact tracing and outbreak investigation are generally the responsibility of the public

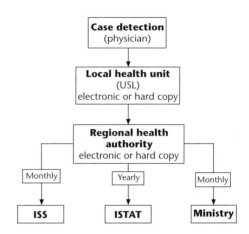

Fig. 5.10.1 Flow chart of statutory notification (Italy). ISS, Instituto Superiore di Sanità; ISTAT, Instituto Nazionale di Statistica; USL, Unità Sanitaria Locale.

health service, primarily on local level, with support from national level.

Data dissemination
An epidemiological bulletin, the *Bollettino epidemiologico*, is published by the Ministry of Health at national level every 6 months on paper. Data are published on the Internet (http://www.sanita.it/malinf/bollepid/indice.htm).

Flow chart of statutory notification
(Fig. 5.10.1)

Outbreak detection and investigation

Unusual events are reported informally to the infectious disease unit at regional and national level by telephone. Outbreak investigations are mainly performed by local health departments. The National Institute of Health performs field investigations only by request of the Ministry of Health or the regional authority.

Prevention/prophylaxis

• Vaccine programme: DTP, IPV/OPV, MMR.

(http://www.sanita.it/malinf/normativ/doc/d
m7–4_99.doc).
• Vaccination coverage: ~60% for MMR and
>95% for DTP vaccinations.
• Antibiotics and malaria prophylaxis only
available on prescription.

5.11 Luxemburg

Contact

Direction de la Santé—(http://www.santel.
lu/MIN/).

Statutory notification systems

Legal framework
Notification of communicable diseases is
defined by law. Last changed in 1997. The
Ministry of Health is responsible for introducing changes in the statutory notification
system.

Notifiable diseases
Thirty seven diseases grouped in 4 classes are
notifiable. Financial incentive: 2 Euro.

Case-definitions
Are in use for respiratory TB and AIDS.

Levels of reporting
One level of reporting with 418 000
inhabitants.

Estimated time to inform national level
2 days.

Public health action
Responsibility for case management is held
by the notifier. Control measures including
contact tracing and outbreak investigation
are generally the responsibility of the public
health service a technical division of the Ministry of Health.

Data dissemination
The *Memorial* is published by the Ministry of

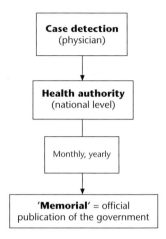

Fig. 5.11.1 Flow chart of statutory notification
(Luxemburg).

Health at national level every month and a
yearly summary report is published.

Flow chart of statutory notification
(Fig. 5.11.1)

Prevention/prophylaxis

• Vaccine programme: MMR, HBV, DTP,
IPV.
• Vaccination coverage: 98% for all
vaccinations.
• Antibiotics and malaria prophylaxis only
available on prescription.

5.12 The Netherlands

Contacts

Ministry of Health, Welfare and Sports
(VWS)—http://www.minvws.nl.
National Institute of Public Health and the
Environment (RIVM)—http://www.rivm.nl.
National Coordinating Centre for Com-
municable Disease Outbreak Management
(LCI)—http://www.lci.lcr.nl/.

Statutory notification systems

Legal framework
The Ministry of Health is responsible for introducing changes in the statutory notification system; new legislation was implemented in 1999.

Levels of responsibility
• Local responsibility for reporting: physicians, municipal health services (GGD).
• Local responsibility for action: municipal health services (GGD).
• National surveillance: RIVM.

Notifiable diseases
30 diseases are notifiable in 3 groups; Group A (only polio): cases have to be notified immediately if there is a suspected case; Group B (19 diseases): cases have to be notified by the physician after diagnosis within 24 h; Group C (10 diseases): positive laboratory test results have to be notified. Financial incentive: none.

Case-definitions
In use for all notifiable diseases.

Levels of reporting
Local level for reporting—municipal health services (GGD), with an average population size of 285000 (120000–750000). National population: 15 million inhabitants.

Estimated time to inform national level
In general less than a week.

Public health action
Responsibility for case management is held by the notifier. Control measures, including contact tracing and outbreak investigation, are generally the responsibility of the public health service, primarily at local level with support from national level.

Data dissemination
An epidemiological bulletin, the *Infectieziekten Bulletin* is published at national level every 4 weeks (http://www.isis.rivm.nl/inf_bul/

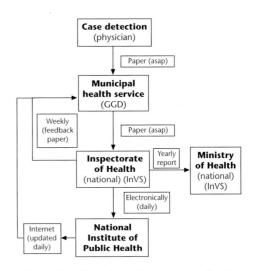

Fig. 5.12.1 Flow chart of statutory notification (The Netherlands).

home_bul.html). Feedback of data, updated daily, is available via the Internet (http://www.isis. rivm.nl).

Flow chart of statutory notification
(Fig. 5.12.1)

Outbreak detection and investigation

Various sources are used to detect possible outbreaks (physicians' notifications, laboratory reporting, telephone calls from the public). Notifications from physicians and laboratory reports are sent to the municipal health departments (GGD). When appropriate, the GGD sends a notification form to the Health Inspectorate (administrative action). When necessary, the National Co-ordinating Centre for Communicable Disease Outbreak Management (LCI) is informed (consultation and assistance). Directors of all health-care facilities are required by law to notify unusually high occurrence or severity. The LCI co-ordinates investigations, summons the outbreak management team, and informs those individuals responsible for decision-making (under the responsibility of the Ministry of Health). The national outbreak management team recommends the most appropriate interventions.

Prevention/prophylaxis

- Vaccine programme: DTPP, MMR, Hib.
- Vaccination coverage: >90% for all vaccinations.
- Antibiotics and malaria prophylaxis only available on prescription.

5.13 Norway

Contacts

Ministry of Health—http://www.odin.dep.no/.

Statens Institutt for Folkehelse (Folkehelsa) (National Institute of Public Health, NIPH)—http://www.folkehelsa.no/.

Statutory notification systems

Legal framework
Notification is based on the Communicable Diseases Control Act of 1995. The Norwegian Board of Health is responsible for introducing changes in the statutory notification system.

Levels of responsibility
- Local responsibility for reporting: physicians and medical microbiological laboratories which detect a notifiable disease are obliged to notify.
- Local responsibility for action: the Public Health Officer (head physician in the municipality) is responsible for infectious disease control.
- National surveillance: National Institute of Public Health is responsible for the running of the surveillance system. The Norwegian Board of Health is responsible for introducing changes in the statutory notification system.

Notifiable diseases
Sixty-seven diseases divided into 4 groups are notifiable. Financial incentives: none.

Case-definitions
In use for all notifiable diseases.

Levels of reporting
Four hundred and thirty-five Local Health Units with an average population size of 10 000.

Estimated time to inform national level
3 days.

Public health action
Responsibility for case management is held by the notifier. Control measures including contact tracing and outbreak investigation are generally the responsibility of the public health service, primarily on local level with support from national level.

Data dissemination
An epidemiological bulletin, the *MSIS Report*, is published by the National Institute of Public Health at national level every week. Infectious disease statutory notification data are accessible on the Internet (http://www.folkehelsa.no).

Flow chart of statutory notification
(Fig. 5.13.1)

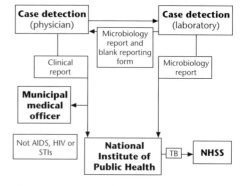

Fig. 5.13.1 Flow chart of statutory notification (Norway).

Outbreak detection and investigation

The main sources for information on outbreaks are the national notification system for infectious diseases (combined clinical and laboratory) and telephone calls from doctors, the media and the public. The municipal medical officers have the legal responsibility for detection, investigation and public health actions within their municipality, in co-operation with other local authorities. If more than one municipality is involved or if the outbreak is unusually severe, outbreak investigations and public health actions are undertaken in close co-operation with the NIPH. The NIPH is the national expert centre for surveillance and can be involved in outbreak investigations on request.

Prevention/prophylaxis

• Vaccine programme: DTPa, IPV, Hib, MMR, BCG.
• Vaccination coverage: 90–95% for all vaccinations.
• Antibiotics and malaria prophylaxis available only on prescription.

5.14 Portugal

Contacts

Direccao General de Saùde (Directorate General for Health, Ministry of Health) — http:// www.dgsaude.pt.
Instituto Nacional de Saúde Dr Ricardo Jorge (National Institute of Health) — http:// www. insarj.pt.

Statutory notification systems

Legal framework
Ministry of Health is responsible for introducing changes to the statutory notification system.

Levels of responsibility
• Local responsibility for reporting: every physician identifying a case (within 48 h).
• Local responsibility for action: treatment of individual cases by identifying physician; public health action and epidemiological control is by the local public health department.
• National surveillance: National Director of Health from the Directorate General of Health. The National Institute of Health is legally responsible for communicable disease surveillance, although it is not directly involved in the management of notifications.

Notifiable diseases
Forty-six diseases are notifiable. Financial incentives: none.

Case definitions
Are available for all notifiable diseases from 1999.

Levels of reporting
Six hundred and thirty local health units with an average population size of 16 000 and 20 regions (18 districts and 2 autonomous regions) with an average population size of 500 000 (128 000–2 050 000).

Estimated time to inform national level
9 days for local level and 17 days for national level.

Public health action
The responsibility for case management is held by the notifier. Control measures, including contact tracing and outbreak investigation, are generally the responsibility of the public health service, primarily on local level with support from national level.

Data dissemination
The *Saúde em números* (Epidemiological Bulletin) is published by the Directorate General for Health at national level 4 times a year. Yearly statistics on mandatory notifiable

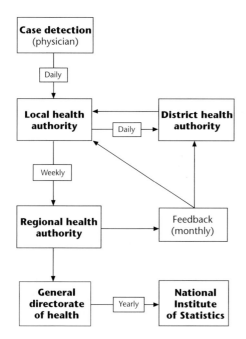

Fig. 5.14.1 Flow chart of statutory notification (Portugal).

diseases are published on the internet (http://www. dgsaude.pt). Special bulletins are released when needed.

Flow chart of statutory notification
(Fig. 5.14.1)

Outbreak detection and investigation

The Division of Epidemiology of the Ministry of Health checks notifications daily. If necessary the information is checked by contact with the notifier or the relevant local health department. An epidemiological investigation can be initiated through the decision of the agency responsible for communicable disease surveillance. This should then be carried out by the local health department.

Prevention/prophylaxis

• Vaccine programme: BCG, HBV, OPV, Hib,

DTP, Td, MMR (see http://www.dgsaude.pt/ profissionais/ pnv_ot.html).
• Vaccination coverage: near 95% for all vaccinations.
• Antibiotics and malaria prophylaxis are generally only available on prescription.

5.15 Spain

Contacts

Ministerio de Sanidad y Consumo Dirección General de Salud Publica (Ministry of Health and Consumers' Affairs) http://www.msc.es.

Instituto de Salud 'Carlos III' (National Institute of Health) http://www.isciii.es.

Statutory notification systems

Legal framework
Ministry of Health is responsible for introducing changes in the statutory notification system. The autonomous regions have an important role in determining policy.

Levels of responsibility
All physicians are obliged by law to notify all cases that fulfil the criteria for notification.
• Local responsibility for reporting: the regional health departments in each autonomous region.
• Local responsibility for action: the regional health departments in each autonomous region.
• National surveillance: the Centro Nacional de Epidemiología is involved in managing surveillance at national level.

Notifiable diseases
Thirty-one diseases are notifiable. Financial incentives: none.

Case-definitions
Are in use for all notifiable diseases.

Levels of reporting

Fifty-two provincial health units with an average population size of 756000 and 19 regions with an average population size of 2100000.

Estimated time to inform national level

Maximum: 21 days for national level—depends on the protocol for each disease.

Public health action

The responsibility for case management is held by the notifier. Control measures, including contact tracing and outbreak investigation, are generally the responsibility of the public health service, primarily on local level with support from national level.

Data dissemination

An epidemiological bulletin, the *Boletín Epidemiológico Semanal*, is published by the National Institute Health at national level (http://www.isciii.es/cne). Other regional and local bulletins are published.

Flow chart of statutory notification

(Fig. 5.15.1)

Non-statutory surveillance systems

A laboratory reporting system, based on the notification of microbiological identifications at hospital laboratories, will become statutory from January 2001.

Outbreak detection and investigation

The notification of outbreaks is mandatory and standardized. All outbreaks must be reported immediately at regional level. At national level it is obligatory to report immediately only those outbreaks which, by law, are defined as being 'supracomunitario' (considered to be of national interest), in order to facilitate their rapid control, whereas other outbreaks are reported quarterly. Outbreak investigations as well as necessary control measures are carried out by the health authorities of the autonomous regions.

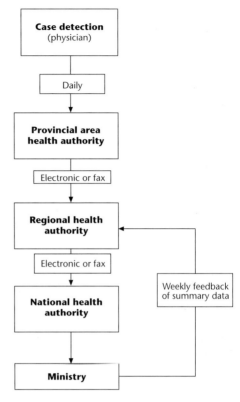

Fig. 5.15.1 Flow chart of statutory notification (Spain). The primary notifications are forwarded using a variety of systems: mail, fax, telephone, e-mail, etc. Presently all the regions transmit data via e-mail. A network is being developed for the National Epidemiological Surveillance Network which will permit the flow of data from the local level.

Prevention/prophylaxis

• Vaccine programme: DTP, polio, MMR, Hib, HBV.
• Vaccination coverage: >95% for DTP, polio, MMR.

5.16 Sweden

Contacts

Ministry of Social Affairs—http://www. doh. gov.uk/links/sweden.htm.
National Board of Health and Welfare—http://www.sos.se.
Swedish Institute for Infectious Disease Control (SMI)—http://www.smittskyddsin-stitutet.se.

Statutory notification systems

Legal framework
Ministry of Health is responsible for changes in the law concerning infectious disease surveillance and control.

Levels of responsibility
• Local responsibility for reporting: physicians and laboratories are obliged by law to notify cases that fulfil the criteria for notification.
• Local responsibility for action: the County Medical Officers for Communicable Disease Control are responsible for public health action.
• National surveillance: The National Board of Health and Welfare is responsible for introducing modifications in the notification system. The SMI is responsible for managing surveillance at national level.

Notifiable diseases
Fifty-three diseases are notifiable. Physicians notify individual cases with a unique identification number. A code is used for STIs. Notification is done in parallel to the County Medical Officer and to the SMI. A computerized notification system (SmiNet), both on county and national level, has been in use since 1997. Financial incentives: none.

Case-definitions
In use for all notifiable diseases.

Levels of reporting
21 counties with an average population size of

422 000 (57 000–1 803 000). National population 8 861 426.

Estimated time to inform national level
Notification should in general be done within 24 h.

Public health action
The notifier holds the responsibility for case management. Control measures, including contact tracing and outbreak investigation, are generally the responsibility of the County Medical Officer, with support from the national level.

Data dissemination
An epidemiological bulletin, *Smittskydd*, is published by the SMI every month. Local data and aggregated national data are accessible to the County Medical Officer through the SmiNet. Compiled national statistics are published in the yearly report of the SMI. Monthly and yearly national data are accessible to the public on http://www.smittskyddsinsti-tutet.se.

Flow chart of statutory notification
(Fig. 5.16.1)

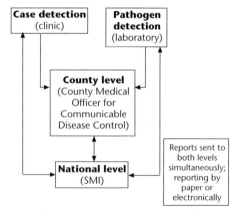

Fig. 5.16.1 Flow chart of statutory notification (Sweden). SMI, Smittskyddsinstitutet (Swedish Institute for Infectious Disease Control).

Non-statutory surveillance systems

STIs are notified numerically by all regional labs on voluntary basis.

Outbreak detection and investigation

Physicians' notifications, laboratory reporting and telephone calls from the public are used for outbreak detection at local and national level. The County Medical Officers are responsible for investigation and control. They can ask the help of regional epidemiological units or the national unit (SMI). Depending on the kind of the outbreak, the National Veterinary Institute (http://www.sva.se), Swedish Board of Agriculture (http://www.sjv.se) and the National Food Administration (http://www.slv.se) may also be involved.

Prevention/prophylaxis

• Vaccine programme: See http://www.euvax. org/main.html.
• Vaccination coverage: >95% for MMR vaccinations.
• Antibiotics and malaria prophylaxis available on prescription only.

5.17 Switzerland

Contacts

Bundesamt für Gesundheit (BAG)—Swiss Federal Office of Public Health. http://www. admin.ch/bag.

Statutory notification systems

Legal framework
Epidemics Act and Federal Regulations. The Ministry of Health is responsible for amendments of the statutory notification regulations.

Levels of responsibility
• Local responsibility for reporting: primarily by microbiology laboratories to both the cantonal physician and the BAG. Statutory notification by physicians is restricted to diseases which may require prompt public health action on suspicion (e.g. meningococcal disease) and to those with a clinical diagnosis (e.g. tetanus).
• Local responsibility for action: physicians treating patients and cantonal physicians.
• National surveillance: the responsibility for control lies with the 26 cantons. The BAG has a co-ordinating and supervisory function, and issues national recommendations for surveillance and control.

Notifiable diseases
Thirty-five conditions are notifiable, including adverse reactions to vaccines and clusters of cases. Financial incentives: none.

Case-definitions
The system includes notification criteria and case-definitions. The former apply to notifying laboratories and physicians and are detailed on notification forms. The latter refer to statistical analyses at the BAG, where only a few case-definitions are in use (e.g. invasive meningococcal disease).

Levels of reporting
Twenty-six cantons with a population size varying from 14 000 to 1 200 000.

Estimated time to inform national levels
7 days.

Public health action
The responsibility for case management is held by the notifying physician. Control measures, which include contact tracing and outbreak investigation, are the responsibility of the public health service, primarily the cantonal physicians, supported by the BAG. International infectious disease affairs are the responsibility of the BAG.

Data dissemination
An epidemiological bulletin, the *Bulletin de*

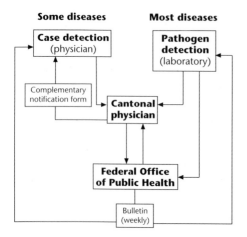

Fig. 5.17.1 Flow chart of statutory notification (Switzerland).

l'Office fédéral de la santé publique/Bulletin des Bundesamtes für Gesundheit is published weekly by the BAG. Weekly data, maps and graphs and comparisons with previous reporting periods are made available to the public on: http://www.admin.ch/bag/infreporting.

Flow chart of statutory notification
(Fig. 5.17.1)

Outbreak detection and investigation

There is no national system for outbreak control in Switzerland. Outbreak management is in the responsibility of the 26 cantons. The role of the Swiss Federal Office of Public Health is mainly to co-ordinate control activities. The Federal Office can only take actions in exceptional situations. Physicians and laboratories are required by law to report unusually high frequencies of infectious diseases to the cantonal physician, who then has to inform the Swiss Federal Office of Public Health. The Federal Office issues guidelines for outbreak investigations and supports local actions on demand.

Prevention/prophylaxis

• Vaccine programme: the BAG is responsible for the national vaccination plan.
• Vaccination coverage: no national instrument exists for continuous monitoring of coverage of target age groups by vaccines included in the national vaccination plan. However, the BAG mandates ad hoc studies.
• Antibiotics and drugs for malaria prophylaxis are only available on prescription.

5.18   United Kingdom

Contacts

Vary for England, Wales, Scotland and Northern Ireland (see Appendix 1).

Statutory notification systems

Legal framework
The relevant Department of Health is responsible for introducing changes in the statutory notification system.

Notifiable diseases
In England and Wales 30 diseases are notifiable (Table 4.2.1). The lists of notifiable diseases are slightly different for Scotland and Northern Ireland; *c.* 3.5 Euro are given to physicians as financial incentive to notify.

Case-definitions
In England and Wales and Northern Ireland case-definitions are in use only for food poisoning. In Scotland case-definitions for acute polio, rabies, diphtheria, smallpox, unspecific viral haemorrhagic fever and food poisoning are used.

Levels of reporting
England and Wales: 376 local authorities with an average population size of 130 000 and 9

regions with an average population size of 5 800 000. *Northern Ireland*: 4 local health and social services boards with an average population size of 410 000. *Scotland*: 15 local health boards with an average population size of 341 000.

Estimated time to inform national level
England and Wales: 7 days for local level and 19 days for national level.
Northern Ireland and Scotland: 7 days for local level and 14 days for national level.

Public health action
The notifier has responsibility for case management. Control measures, including contact tracing and outbreak investigation, are generally the responsibility of the consultant for communicable disease control of the health authority in which the case is resident. Regional and national support are available from the PHLS Communicable Disease Surveillance Centre (or SCIEH in Scotland).

Data dissemination
England and Wales: An epidemiological bulletin, the *CDR Weekly* is published by the Public Health Laboratory Service every week (http://www.phls.co.uk/publications/cdr.htm) Annual reports are also published. Information is available to the public via the PHLS web-site.

Scotland: An epidemiological bulletin, the *SCIEH Weekly report* is published by the Scottish Centre for Infection and Environmental Health every week. A report with corrected data is published quarterly, and annually. *Epi-Net*, an internet network, and e-mail is used for urgent messages. It is accessible via CDSC home page (http://www.open.gov.uk/cdsc/cdschome.htm).

Northern Ireland: A *Communicable Disease Monthly Report* is published by CDSC (Northern Ireland).

A national (UK) quarterly journal (*Communicable Diseases and Public Health*), giving detailed reports and articles, is also published (http://www.phls.co.uk/publications/cdph.htm).

Flow chart of statutory notification
(Fig. 5.18.1)

Non-statutory surveillance systems (NSSS)
Laboratory reporting is non-statutory (although the Department of Health recommends that all NHS and PHLS laboratories should take part in the system). Laboratories report to regional units of CDSC, increasingly via an electronic reporting system (CoSurv), which then reports to the national centre. Feedback is provided via regional newsletters and the national *CDR Weekly*.

Outbreak detection and investigation

Northern Ireland
A variety of sources of information (physicians' notifications, laboratory reporting, telephone calls from the public, etc.) are used to detect possible outbreaks. Notifications from physicians are made to the CCDC at Health Board, with outbreaks reported by telephone or e-mail to CDSC (NI). Laboratory reports are made to CCDC and copies to CDSC (NI). The Directors of Public Health have the legal responsibility for detection, investigation and public health actions within their area. If more than one board area is involved or if the outbreak is unusually severe, outbreak investigations and public health actions are done in co-operation with CDSC (NI). CDSC (NI) has responsibility for surveillance at regional level and will be involved in outbreak investigation and control at the request of either the Director of Public Health or the Chief Medical Officer (NI).

Scotland
A variety of sources of information (physicians' notifications, laboratory reporting, telephone calls from the public, etc.) are used to detect possible outbreaks. Notifications are made to the designated medical officer at the relevant health authority, who is usually a public health physician from the correspond-

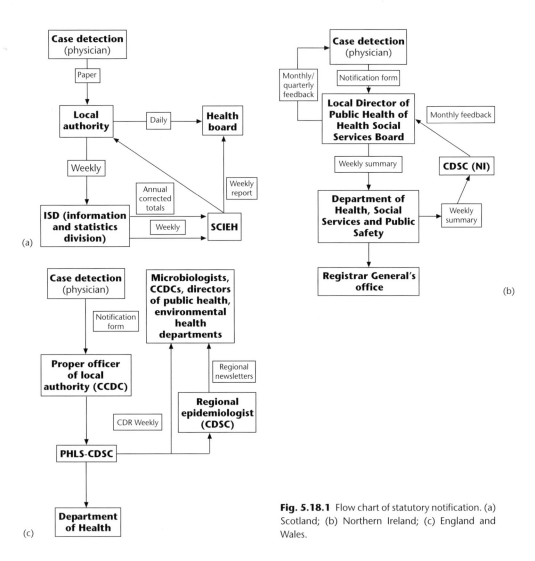

Fig. 5.18.1 Flow chart of statutory notification. (a) Scotland; (b) Northern Ireland; (c) England and Wales.

ing health board. There is also a list of infections reportable to the Scottish Office. Outbreaks are usually investigated by the Consultant in Public Health (Environmental Health) of the local health board, with assistance from SCIEH as appropriate.

England and Wales

A variety of sources of information (physicians' notifications, laboratory reporting, telephone calls from the public, etc.) are used to detect possible outbreaks. Notifications from physicians are made to the proper officer of the local authority (usually the CCDC at the corresponding health authority). Outbreaks are reported by telephone. Laboratory reports are made to the CCDC (by local arrangement) and CDSC (as 'CDR' reports), often by 'CoSurv' electronic reporting. The CCDC has executive responsibility for detection, investigation and public health actions within their area. If more than one district is involved or if the outbreak is unusually severe or complex, outbreak investigations and public health actions are carried out in co-operation with the regional or national tier of CDSC.

Prevention/prophylaxis

- Vaccine programme: see Box 4.7.1.
- Vaccination coverage: ~90% for MMR and >95% for DTP vaccinations.
- Antibiotics only available on prescription. Chloroquine and proguanil can be purchased without a prescription.

Appendices

Appendix 1: Useful addresses and telephone numbers (UK)

The World Health Organization
Regional Office for Europe (EURO)
8, Scherfigsvej, DK-2100 Copenhagen 0, Denmark
Tel: 0045 39171717

European Union
Public Health Directorate, DG Health and Consumer Protection, European Commission, L-2920 Luxembourg
Tel: 00 352 43011

Public Health Laboratory Service (PHLS)
61 Colindale Avenue, London NW9 5EQ.

Communicable Disease Surveillance Centre (CDSC)
Tel: 0208-200-6868

PHLS Headquarters
Tel: 0208-200-1295

Central Public Health Laboratory
Tel: 0208-200-4400

CDSC Wales
Tel: 02920-521997

CDSC Northern Ireland
Tel: 02890-263765

Scottish Centre for Infection and Environmental Health (SCIEH)
Clifton House, Clifton Place, Glasgow, G3 7LN
Tel: 0141-300-1100

Departments of Health
• Richmond House, 79 Whitehall, London SW1A 2NS
Switchboard: 0207-210-3000
Duty Medical Officer (out of hours): 0207-210-5371
Press Office: 0207-210-5228

• Health aspects of Environment and Food
Skipton House, 80 London Road, London SE1 6XZ

Food safety/food hazards
Tel: 0207-972-5055

• Health Promotion Division, Wellington House, 135 Waterloo Road, London SE1 8UG

Immunization
Tel: 0207-972-4488
TB, influenza, travel
Tel: 0207-972-4480
HIV
Tel: 0207-972-4382
Hepatitis, VHFs
Tel: 0207-972-4479

• Welsh Office Health Strategy Division
Cathays Park, Cardiff CF1 3NQ

Food safety/food hazards
Tel: 02920-823468
Out of hours: 02920-825111

• Scottish Office Department of Health
St Andrews House, Edinburgh EH1 3DG

Food safety/food hazards (via Agriculture Dept)
Tel: 0131-244-2178
Health Policy Unit (and out of hours for food)
Tel: 0131-556-8400

• Northern Ireland Department of Health and Social Services,
Castle Buildings, Stormont, Belfast BT4 3PP
Tel: 02890-520000

Food Standards Agency
Ergon House, 17 Smith Square, London SW1P 3JR
Switchboard: 0845-757-3012
(MAFF) Duty Officer: 0207-270-8960

Centre for Applied Microbiology and Research (CAMR)
Porton Down, Salisbury SP4 0JG
Tel: 01980-612100

PHLS Malaria Reference Laboratory
London School of Hygiene and Tropical Medicine, Keppel St, London WC1E 7HT (Advisory service for health professionals only)
Tel: 0207-636-3924
Laboratory Tel: 0207-927-2427

Clinical infectious disease units
Hospital for Tropical Diseases, London
Tel: 0207-387-4411
Coppetts Wood Hospital, London*
Tel: 0208-883-9792
Newcastle General Hospital, Newcastle-upon-Tyne*
Tel: 0191-273-8811
Heartlands Hospital, Birmingham
Tel: 0121-424-2000
Churchill Hospital, Oxford
Tel: 01865-225214
University Hospital (Fazakerley), Liverpool
Tel: 0151-525-5980
North Manchester General Hospital
Tel: 0161-795-4567
Southmead Hospital, Bristol
Tel: 0117-950-5050

* High Security Unit suitable for viral haemor-rhagic fevers.

Poison information services
Belfast
Tel: 02890-240503
Birmingham
Tel: 0121-507-5588
Cardiff
Tel: 029-2070-9901
Edinburgh
Tel: 0131-536-2300
Leeds
Tel: 0113-243-0715
London
Tel: 0207-635-9191
Newcastle
Tel: 0191-282-0300

Advice lines available to general public
National AIDS Helpline
Tel: 0800-567123
Hospital for Tropical Diseases Travel Clinic
Tel: 0839-337733*

Malaria Reference Laboratory Helpline
Tel: 0891-600350*
Medical Advisory Service for Travellers Abroad
Tel: 0891-224100*
Liverpool School of Tropical Medicine Travel Advice Line
Tel: 0891-172111*
National Meningitis Trust
Tel: 0845-6000-800
Meningitis Research Foundation
Tel: 0808-800-3344

* Subject to premium rate call charges.

You will also need to know how to contact the following out of hours:
Senior officers of your health authority:
    Chairman;
    Chief Executive;
    DPH;
    CCDC;
    Press Officer;
    Legal adviser
Environmental health Staff:
    Senior officers;
    EHO on-call
Local microbiologists
Nearest public health laboratory
Local ID physician
Local water company
Local magistrates
Local hospital managers
CCDC from adjacent districts

Appendix 2: Guidance documents and books

Blood-borne viruses

UK Health Departments. *AIDS/HIV Infected Health Care Workers: Guidance on the Management of Infected Health Care Workers and Patient Notification.* London: Department of Health, 1998. (Available from http://www.open.gov.uk/doh/aids.htm, or PO Box 410, Wetherby, LS23 7LN, UK).

UK Health Departments. *HIV Post-Exposure Prophylaxis: Guidance from the UK Chief Medical Officers' Expert Advisory Group on AIDS.* London: Department of Health, 2000. (Available from http://www.doh.gov.uk/eaga/index.htm).

Department of Health. *Protecting Health Care Workers and Patients from Hepatitis B*: HSG (93) 40. London: Department of Health, 1993.

Department of Health. Addendum to HSG(93)40: *Protecting Healthcare Workers and Patients from Hepatitis B*. London: Department of Health, 1996.

NHS Executive (England). *Hepatitis B Infected Health Care workers. Guidance on Implementation of Health Service Circular 2000/020*. Leeds: NHS Executive, 2000. (Available on http://www.doh.gov.uk/nhsexec/hepatitisb. htm).

UK Health Departments. *Guidance for Clinical Health Care Workers: Protection against Infection with Blood-borne Viruses. Recommendations of the Expert Advisory Group on AIDS and the Advisory Group on Hepatitis*. London: UK Health Departments, 1998.

Ramsay R. Guidance on the investigation and management of occupational exposure to hepatitis C. *Commun Dis Public Health* 1999; **2**: 258–262.

Gastrointestinal disease

PHLS Salmonella Subcommittee. The prevention of human transmission of gastrointestinal infections, infestations and bacterial infections. *Commun Dis Rep CDR Rev* 1995; **5**: R158–172.

Department of Health. *Management of Outbreaks of Foodborne Illness*. London: Department of Health, 1994. (Copies from BAPS, Health Publication Centre, Heywood Stores, Manchester Road, Heywood, OL10 2PZ).

Subcommittee of the PHLS Advisory Committee on Gastrointestinal Infections. Guidelines for the control of infections with Vero cytotoxin producing *Escherichia coli* (VTEC). *Commun Dis Public Health* 2000; **3**: 14–23.

Viral gastroenteritis subcommittee of the PHLS Virology Committee. (1993) Outbreaks of gastroenteritis associated with SRSVs. *PHLS Microbiol Digest* **10 (1)**, 2–8. (NB: Revision due 2001).

Bouchier IT (Chairman). *Cryptosporidium in Water Supplies*. Third report of the group of experts to: Department of Environment, Transport, and the Region and the Department of Health. London: DETR, 1998.

Strength of association between human illness and water: revised definitions for use in outbreak investigations. *Commun Dis Rep CDR Wkly* 1996; **6**: 65–68.

Hunter PR. Advice on the response from public and environmental health to the detection of cryptosporidial oocysts in treated drinking water. *Commun Dis Public Health* 2000; **3**: 24–27.

Department of Health Expert Working Party. *Food Handlers', Fitness to Work: Guidance for Food Businesses, Enforcement Officers and Health Professionals*. London: Department of Health, 1995.

Immunization

Department of Health. *Immunisation against Infectious Diseases*. London: HMSO, 1996. (ISBN 0-11-321-815-X).

Imported infection and travel advice

World Health Organization. *International Travel and Health. Vaccination Requirements and Travel Advice*. Geneva: WHO, 2000. (ISBN: 92 4 158025 9).

Department of Health. *Health Information for Overseas Travel*. London: HMSO, 1995. (ISBN 0-11-321-833-8).

Bradley DJ, Warhurst DC. Guidelines for the prevention of malaria in travellers from the United Kingdom. *Commun Dis Rep CDR Rev* 1997; **7**: R138–R151.

Advisory Committee on Dangerous Pathogens. *Management and Control of Viral Haemorrhagic Fevers*. London: The Stationary Office, 1996. (ISBN: 0-11-321860-5). http://www.doh.gov.uk/acdp.htm

Begg N. *Manual for the Management and Control of Diphtheria in the European Region and Control of Diphtheria in the European Region.* Copenhagen: WHO Regional Office for Europe, 1994.

Bonnet JM, Begg NT. Control of diphtheria: guidance for consultants in communicable disease control. *Commun Dis Public Health* 1999; **2**: 242–249.

Department of Health. *Memorandum on Rabies. Prevention and Control.* London: Department of Health, 2000. (Available from http://www.doh.gov.uk/memorandumrabies).

Infection control

Public Health Medicine Environmental Group. *Guidelines for the Control of Infection in Residential Homes and Nursing Homes.* London: Department of Health, 1996.

Healing TD, Hoffman PN, Young SEJ. The infection hazards of human cadavers. *Commun Dis Rep CDR Rev* 1995; **5**: R61–68.

Combined Working Party of the British Society of Antimicrobial Chemotherapy, the Hospital Infection Society and the Infection Control Nurses Association. Revised guidelines for the control of methicillin-resistant *Staphylococcus aureus* in hospital. *J Hosp Inf* 1998; **39**: 253–290.

Meningococcal infection and meningitis

PHLS Meningococcal Infections Working Group. Control of meningococcal disease: guidance for consultants for communicable disease control. *Commun Dis Rep CDR Rev* 1995; **5**: R189–195.

Stuart JM, Monk PN, Lewis DA, *et al.* (for PHLS Meningococcal Infections Working Group and PHMEG). Management of clusters of meningococcal disease. *Commun Dis Rep CDR Rev* 1997; **7**: R3–R5.

Kaczmarski PB, Cartwright KAV. Control of meningococcal disease: Guidance for microbiologists. *Commun Dis Rep CDR Rev* 1995; **5**: R196–R198.

Committee of Vice-Chancellors and Principals of the Universities of the United Kingdom. *Managing Meningitis in Higher Education Institutions.* London: Committee of Vice-Chancellors and Principals of the Universities of the United Kingdom, 1998.

Cartwright KAV, Begg NT, Rudd P. Use of vaccines and antibiotic prophylaxis in contacts and cases of *Haemophilus influenzae* type b (Hib) disease. *Commun Dis Rep CDR Rev* 1984; **4**: R16–17.

Tuberculosis

Subcommittee of the Joint Tuberculosis Committee of the British Thoracic Society. Control and prevention of tuberculosis in the United Kingdom: Code of Practice 2000. *Thorax* 2000; **55**: 887–901.

Interdepartmental Working Group on Tuberculosis. *Recommendations for the Prevention and Control of Tuberculosis at Local Level.* London: Department of Health and Welsh Office, 1996.

Interdepartmental Working Group on Tuberculosis. *The Prevention and Control of Tuberculosis in the United Kingdom. UK Guidance on the Prevention and Control of Transmission of: 1. HIV Related Tuberculosis, 2. Drug Resistant, Including Multiple Drug-Resistant Tuberculosis.* London: Department of Health and Welsh Office, 1998.

Joint Tuberculosis Committee of the British Thoracic Society (1998). Chemotherapy and management of tuberculosis in the United Kingdom: recommendations 1998. *Thorax* 1998; **49**: 1193–1200.

Other

Saunders CGP, Joseph CA, Watson JM. Investigating a single case of Legionnaires' disease: Guidance for consultants in communicable disease control. *Commun Dis Rep CDR Rev* 1994; **10**: R112–R114. (Revision due 2001).

Murray V (ed). *Major Chemical Disasters— Medical Aspects of Management.* Oxford: Royal Society of Medicine Services, 1990.

Guidance for the control of parvovirus B19 infection in healthcare settings and the community. *J Public Health Med* 1999; **21**: 439–446.

General

Guidance on Infection Control in Schools and Nurseries (poster). London: Department of Health, 1999. (Summary database of the evidence for the exclusion periods and comments on poster available via PHLS web-site).

Joint Formulary Committee. *British National Formulary*. London: British Medical Association, 2000.

Directory of CsCDC and MOsEH in England and Wales and Northern Ireland. PHLS Communicable Disease Surveillance Centre, 8th Edition (or "ComDisc" from CDSC).

Department of Health and Welsh Office Public Health Legal Information Unit. *Communicable Disease Control: a Practical Guide to the Law for Health and Local Authorities in England and Wales*. London: Department of Health, 1994.

Acheson ED. *Public Health in England: the Report of the Committee of Inquiry into the Future Development of the Public Health Function*. London: Department of Health, 1988.

Index

Note: page numbers in *italics* refer to figures and boxes, those in **bold** refer to tables

337